ANALYSIS OF BIOMARKER DATA

ANALYSIS OF BIOMARKER DATA

A Practical Guide

STEPHEN W. LOONEY
Department of Biostatistics and Epidemiology
Georgia Regents University
Augusta, Georgia

JOSEPH L. HAGAN
Texas Children's Hospital
Houston, Texas

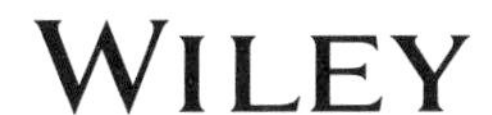

Published by John Wiley & Sons, Inc., Hoboken, New Jersey.
Published simultaneously in Canada.

Library of Congress Cataloging-in-Publication Data

Looney, Stephen W., author.
Analysis of biomarker data : a practical guide / Stephen W. Looney, Joseph L. Hagan.
p. ; cm.
Includes bibliographical references and index.
ISBN 978-1-118-02755-4 (cloth)
I. Hagan, Joseph L., author. II. Title.
[DNLM: 1. Biological Markers–analysis. 2. Data Interpretation, Statistical. 3. Models, Statistical. QW 541]
R857.B54
610.28′4–dc23

2014024697

Printed in the United States of America

10 9 8 7 6 5 4 3 2 1

To my students
–Stephen W. Looney

To S.L., my mentor and friend
–Joseph L. Hagan

CONTENTS

PREFACE

As the title indicates, this book is intended to be a practical guide for the statistical analysis of biomarker data. To us, such a guide should include information on the proper application of statistical methods that are most commonly used to analyze biomarker data, with special emphasis placed on the underlying assumptions. This includes recommendations concerning: (1) preferred methods for determining whether or not the underlying assumptions are valid for a particular set of biomarker data and (2) how to proceed if the underlying assumptions appear to be violated. In addition to emphasizing the underlying assumptions, we have also placed considerable emphasis on computational issues related to the methods most commonly used to analyze biomarker data. To the greatest extent possible, we have provided software (primarily SAS® code) for performing the statistical methods that we recommend. All of this software, along with the complete data sets for all of the examples, is included in the Software Appendix that is available on the companion website for this textbook. For many of the examples, the complete data set, along with the computer code for analyzing the data, are also provided in the text.

Our intention has been to present our descriptions of the statistical methods that are included in this textbook at a fairly low technical level; however, we have provided all of the necessary formulas for those who are interested in the more theoretical aspects of these methods. By including these formulas, we hoped to achieve two goals: (1) to provide sufficient information for those who wish to program these methods themselves, using Excel, R or C++, for example and (2) to provide the mathematical details for those who are interested in the theoretical foundations of these methods. Sections that we feel are unusually technical (in terms of extensive use of formulas and/or theoretical development) are marked with an asterisk (*) and can be safely skipped without loss of continuity. Overall, the presentation in this textbook does not require familiarity with calculus or matrix algebra. Generally speaking, a sufficient background for the material in this book would be the equivalent of a two-semester statistical methods sequence at the advanced undergraduate or introductory graduate level. Minimal requirements include a good working knowledge of basic statistical inference (point and interval estimation and hypothesis testing), as well as some familiarity with correlation analysis, chi-square analysis, and nonparametric statistics. Chapter 3 contains a review of the basic statistical concepts and methods that we consider to be sufficient prerequisites for the material in Chapters 4 and 5.

One may question our choice of statistical methods included in this book. For example, there is very little discussion of multivariable models, although we do provide a very elementary description of multiple linear regression in Chapter 3. We also briefly mention multiple logistic regression in several places. We realize the importance of the application of these and other multivariable methods in biomarker research (e.g., in the analysis of survival data or longitudinal data), but feel that we cannot fully address the numerous complex considerations involved in the appropriate use of these methods within the limited scope of this book. There is very heavy emphasis (some may say too heavy) in this book on testing distributional assumptions, and on nonparametric and exact methods. As illustrated in Section 4.2, investigators often state that they used a data transformation or nonparametric method to analyze their biomarker data due to "extreme skewness" (or similar language); however, very rarely do they provide any statistical justification for following this course of action. Many of the studies involving biomarker data that we have worked on as collaborating statisticians have had very small sample sizes (some as small as 5 or 6), hence the strong emphasis on exact methods. Another area that some may say has received too much emphasis in this book is the assessment of the reliability and validity of a biomarker. We feel that this aspect of biomarker development is too often ignored (or given only minimal attention) in the biomarker literature. Thus, one of our goals in writing this textbook has been to provide sufficient background knowledge and software tools so that it will be easier for investigators to undertake a more thorough assessment of these important characteristics of a newly proposed biomarker.

Wherever possible, we have illustrated the statistical methods included in this textbook with examples that make use of "real" data. Most of these data sets were taken (or adapted) from the biomarker literature, or from unpublished studies we participated in as collaborators. In some instances, we have used hypothetical data (which we hope are also realistic) when the "real data," we needed to illustrate a particular point were not readily available. Most of these hypothetical data sets were constructed so that they retained certain key features of the published study on which they were based.

We have not written this book with the anticipation that it would be used as the primary textbook for a course on the statistical analysis of biomarker data; however, it could be used for that purpose for a summer course, an independent study, or a graduate seminar. With this in mind, we have included a small number of problems (and solutions) at the end of each chapter. We consider our primary audience for this textbook to consist of investigators who wish to perform their own analyses of biomarker data; this includes toxicologists, pharmacologists, epidemiologists, environmental and clinical laboratory scientists, and other professionals in the health and environmental sciences. Statisticians who routinely analyze and interpret biomarker data could also find it to be of interest. Since most of the statistical techniques that we discuss in this book also apply to surrogate markers (or, more accurately, surrogate endpoints), professionals who work in the areas of pharmaceutical and chemical product development could also find this book to be useful. Our goal has been to provide enough practical information (including software code and software recommendations) to facilitate the statistical analysis of biomarker data for all of these individuals.

ACKNOWLEDGEMENTS

We gratefully acknowledge the contributions of Courtney McCracken, who graciously allowed us to use excerpts from her doctoral dissertation as the basis for Section 4.8 of this text, which deals with estimating correlation coefficients when both variables are subject to limits of detection. Jennifer Waller graciously provided basic SAS® code for calculating improved confidence intervals for correlation coefficients, which we expanded into the SAS code we provide in Section 4.5. We are grateful to our collaborators, Ganesan Ramesh, Allison Hunter Buchanan, Mary Stuart, Michelle Reid, Joe Miller, Jack Price, Luis Espinoza, and Jason Goldberg for their kind permission to reproduce their research data here. We also wish to acknowledge the generosity of our colleagues Ioannis Dimakos, Paul Juneau, Nancy Cheng, Stuart Gansky, Allison Deal, Chuck Coleman, and Mark Solak for their permission to reproduce their SAS code. We gratefully acknowledge Cindy Oxford and Teresa McVeigh for their editorial assistance in the final stages of the development of this manuscript.

We wish to express our sincere appreciation to Susanne Steitz-Filler, Senior Editor for Mathematics and Statistics at John Wiley and Sons, for her encouragement, assistance, and most of all, patience, throughout the development of this manuscript. Sari Friedman, Senior Editorial Assistant for Mathematics and Statistics at Wiley, also provided very helpful advice and assistance.

1

INTRODUCTION

1.1 WHAT IS A BIOMARKER?

According to the *Dictionary of Epidemiology*, a *biomarker* (or *biological marker*) is "a cellular, biochemical, or molecular indicator of exposure; of biological, subclinical, or clinical effects; or of possible susceptibility" (Porta 2008, p. 21). As Porta points out, the term "biomarker" is often ambiguous; this is perhaps an indication that there is insufficient understanding of the pathophysiological or mechanistic role of the "marker."

The ambiguity may also be due to the fact that biomarkers are involved in one way or another with so many different disciplines (clinical trialists, statisticians, regulators, etc.) and clinical research applications. In fact, there is so much potential ambiguity associated with the term "biomarker" that several efforts have been made to provide a formal definition of exactly what a biomarker is.

For example, in a 1987 US National Research Council report, biomarkers were defined to be "indicators signaling events in biological systems or samples." In 2001, a Biomarkers Definitions Working Group (BDWG), convened by the US National Institutes of Health, proposed the following definition of biological marker (biomarker): "A characteristic that is objectively measured and evaluated as an indicator of normal biological processes, pathogenic processes, or pharmacologic responses to a therapeutic intervention."

As interest in the development, validation, and application of new biomarkers has increased, numerous classification systems for biomarkers have been proposed. These include Type 0–Type 6 biomarkers; Type I and II biomarkers (Mildvan et al.

Analysis of Biomarker Data: A Practical Guide, First Edition. Stephen W. Looney and Joseph L. Hagan.

1997); prognostic and predictive biomarkers; genomic, proteomic, and combinatorial biomarkers; screening and stratification biomarkers, and so on. (See Table 1 of DeCaprio (2006) for details.) Most of these classification systems reflect the intended use of the biomarker data in a particular discipline; however, all biomarkers are related in the sense that each of them is designed to be an "indicator" of something, as noted in the *Dictionary of Epidemiology* definition cited above. Our primary focus in this book is on markers of exposure, although the statistical techniques we describe can be applied to almost any type of biomarker. By using "real" data taken from published biomarker studies to exemplify the proper application of these techniques, we have tried to illustrate the broad applicability of statistical methods in the analysis of biomarker data, regardless of the particular type of biomarker that is being considered.

1.2 BIOMARKERS VERSUS SURROGATE ENDPOINTS

In their report describing preferred definitions for biomarkers and surrogate endpoints, the BDWG defined a *clinical endpoint* as: "A characteristic or variable that reflects how a patient feels, functions, or survives." They then defined a *surrogate endpoint* as: "A biomarker that is intended to substitute for a clinical endpoint." A surrogate endpoint is thus expected to "predict clinical benefit (or harm or lack of benefit or harm) based on epidemiologic, therapeutic, pathophysiologic, or other scientific evidence." As they pointed out, all surrogate endpoints are biomarkers, but not all biomarkers are surrogate endpoints. In fact, "it is likely that only a few biomarkers will achieve surrogate endpoint status." (Note that they discouraged the use of the term *surrogate marker*, and advocated the exclusive use of *surrogate endpoint* instead (BDWG 2001, p. 91).)

Because of the requirement that one must be able to substitute a surrogate endpoint in place of the corresponding clinical endpoint, the process of validating a surrogate endpoint goes far beyond what is usually required when validating a biomarker (see Chapter 5). In fact, the BDWG claimed that the term *validation* is unsuitable for describing the process of linking biomarkers to clinical endpoints; they proposed that the process of determining surrogate endpoint status be referred to as *evaluation*. They reserved use of *validation* to describe the process of addressing what they referred to as the "performance characteristics" (e.g., sensitivity, specificity, and reproducibility) of a measurement process or assay technique. This is consistent with our use of the term *biomarker validation* in Chapter 5.

Because of the complexity involved in evaluating a surrogate endpoint, various approaches have been proposed, almost all of which involve examining the effect of a treatment for the clinical endpoint (typically referred to as the "disease") on the surrogate for the endpoint. In a landmark paper, Prentice (1989) formulated a definition of surrogate endpoints and defined a set of operational criteria for their evaluation. In their subsequent work, Freedman et al. (1992) proposed that one should focus attention on the proportion of the treatment effect explained by the surrogate for the disease endpoint, whereas Buyse and Molenberghs (1998) proposed that the primary focus should be on the *relative effect* of the treatment on the surrogate. Various authors also advocated the use of meta-analytic data in the evaluation of a surrogate endpoint (Freedman et al. 1992; Lin et al. 1997; Daniels and Hughes 1997). The application of meta-analytic techniques to surrogate endpoint evaluation was further developed by Buyse et al. (2000); Gail et al. (2000); Molenberghs et al. (2002); and others. The very comprehensive textbook edited by Burzykowski et al. (2005) thoroughly discuss all of these statistical approaches and subsequent developments. The Institute of Medicine report (Micheel and Ball 2010) approaches the evaluation of surrogate endpoints from a more clinical perspective.

Although surrogate endpoints are certainly a very important special case of biomarkers, we feel that the specialized techniques developed for evaluating them, especially as these techniques relate to treatment of the clinical endpoint, are beyond the scope of this text. Hence, we do not discuss surrogate endpoints as a separate topic elsewhere in this book. However, the methods that we describe for analyzing biomarker data and validating a biomarker (as defined by BDWG), certainly apply to surrogate endpoints as well.

1.3 ORGANIZATION OF THIS BOOK

In Chapter 1, we define what we mean by a biomarker and then describe our understanding of the differences and similarities between biomarkers and surrogate endpoints.

In Chapter 2, we cover basic principles of effective design of a study that will make use of biomarker data, including selecting the most appropriate type of study design (cross-sectional, case–control, etc.), choosing the appropriate measure of association once the type of design has been selected, designing the statistical analysis that will be applied to the study data once they have been obtained, and choosing the appropriate sample size for the study that is being planned. We also describe several features of what we consider to be the effective presentation of statistical results once the study data have been analyzed.

In Chapter 3, we provide a survey of elementary statistical methods that are widely used when analyzing biomarker data. To be specific, the methods that we cover include: graphical and tabular summaries; descriptive statistics; basic concepts of statistical inference, including point estimation, confidence interval estimation, and hypothesis testing; comparisons of means between two groups and among more than two groups; statistical inference for correlation coefficients; simple and multiple linear regression; and analysis of cross-classified data, including the chi-square test of independence and methods for comparing proportions across two or more groups. Our intention in this chapter is not to provide comprehensive coverage of all of elementary statistical methods, but rather to describe selected methods in sufficient detail so that someone who is relatively inexperienced in the application of statistics will be able to carry out these analyses appropriately and with a minimum of effort.

In Chapter 4, we describe various “challenges” that one is likely to encounter in the analysis of biomarker data and offer our recommendations on preferred methods for dealing with them. These challenges include: (1) violations of underlying assumptions (normality, homogeneity of variance), (2) lack of independence between the groups being compared, (3) proper analysis of correlated data, (4) clustered data, (5) contaminated data, (6) non-detectable observations, (7) choosing the appropriate measure of association between predictor and outcome, and (8) choosing the appropriate method of analysis for cross-classified data (i.e., contingency tables). Each of these challenges is illustrated using data from a "real" biomarker study, most of which were taken from the scientific literature.

In Chapter 5, we provide a detailed discussion of the methods we recommend for evaluating the quality of a newly proposed (or existing) biomarker (also called *biomarker validation*). Our focus is on establishing that the biomarker has adequate reliability and validity.

Throughout Chapters 3–5, we provide what we hope is sufficient mathematical detail for those who are interested, but our primary emphasis is on the proper application of the statistical methods. Sections marked with an asterisk (*) contain a more theoretical treatment of the topic at hand and can safely be omitted without loss of continuity with the remainder of the text.

To the greatest extent possible, we provide software code for performing the statistical methods that we describe. Our software of choice is SAS because of its flexibility and widespread use in industry, government, and academia; but, in some instances, we also indicate how to perform an analysis using R (R Core Development Team 2014) or other statistical software (SPSS, STATA, etc.). The data sets for the fully worked examples in the book are provided along with the code used to analyze them. Shorter segments of code are included in the body of the text and are available on the companion website; longer segments are not provided in the text, but are available on the website.

We do not anticipate that the primary audience for this textbook will be students, so we have not provided extensive problem sets. However, we do recognize that exercises (with solutions) are an effective tool for anyone who is trying to learn how to perform a particular type of statistical analysis for the first time, or for someone who is trying to refresh their memory of statistical methods that they may have studied years ago. From personal experience, we know that exercises with solutions can be extremely helpful for experienced statisticians who are trying to learn about a statistical method they have never used before, or about applications of certain statistical methods in a scientific field that is new to them. Exercises with solutions are also useful as "test cases," when someone is trying to write their own software to carry out a statistical method for which easily accessible software is not available. With this in mind, we have provided small problem sets at the end of Chapters 3, 4, and 5. These contain exercises that are similar to the worked examples included in the text. To the greatest extent possible, these exercises are based on "real" data taken from published biomarker studies. Solutions to these exercises, including the SAS or R code needed to carry out the analyses, are provided at the end of the text.

2

DESIGNING BIOMARKER STUDIES

2.1 INTRODUCTION

In Chapters 3–5 of this book, we focus our discussion on what is to be done once the study data are ready to be analyzed. However, in this chapter, our primary concern is with planning the study so that the methods described in those chapters can be properly applied to yield valid study results.

The same issues that one must deal with in any type of research that involves the quantitative examination of data are also relevant when designing studies that involve biomarkers. Generally, the first step is to formulate a research question that involves one or more measurable phenomena (e.g., "Is exposure to second-hand smoke related to lung cancer?"). Next, one must determine the best way to detect or measure these entities (cotinine levels in urine, lung biopsy, etc.). For the discussion in this chapter and throughout this text, at least one of the measurable entities will be a biomarker. Once the measurement processes to be used in the study have been completely specified and carefully described in the study protocol, one must then specify exactly how the study will be conducted. This typically requires (1) the selection of a study design (cross-sectional, case–control, cohort, randomized trial, etc.); (2) the identification of a target population, accessible population, intended sample, and actual sample; (3) a detailed description of exactly how the study data will be collected from the actual sample; (4) a description of the statistical methods to be applied once the study data have been collected and entered into the study database; and (5) a determination of the sample size required for the intended study. (See Hulley et al. (2013) for an excellent description of the process of designing

Analysis of Biomarker Data: A Practical Guide, First Edition. Stephen W. Looney and Joseph L. Hagan.

clinical research studies.) *Each of the above steps (1)–(5) should be carried out prior to performing the study and collecting the study data.*

Once steps (1)–(5) above have been performed and sufficient resources have been acquired for conducting the study, the study can begin. Eventually, the study will be completed and the research data will be entered into the study database and prepared for analysis. This process typically requires "cleaning" the data to remove mis-entered or otherwise faulty data points. Note that *all* data cleaning, editing, etc., must be accomplished *prior* to beginning any statistical analyses. If data errors are found after the statistical analyses have been completed, this usually means that all of the analyses will have to be repeated. This is why double entry and other methods should be used to ensure that the computerized research data are of the highest possible quality before any analyses are begun.

Of course, it is extremely important that the sample size for the study was appropriately determined prior to data collection: an n that is too small typically yields insufficient statistical power and imprecise estimation (resulting in a lack of statistical significance); an n that is too large leads to waste of resources and statistically significant results that lack practical significance. This text is primarily devoted to describing and illustrating appropriate methods for analyzing biomarker data; however, as the need arises, we will also discuss methods for determining the appropriate sample size since even the most carefully selected statistical procedures will not perform well if the sample size is too small.

2.2 DESIGNING THE STUDY

2.2.1 The Exposure–Disease Association

A common objective of biomarker studies is to investigate the association between an "exposure" (e.g., a hypothesized risk factor for a disease, a characteristic or behavior thought to protect against disease, etc.) and a "disease" (e.g., presence of a certain disease, death, or, more generally, any health characteristic or outcome). Although the exposure and disease can be quantified using any level of measurement, treating both as a dichotomous variable (e.g., either "present" or "absent") is a frequently encountered scenario in biomarker research. In such a situation, one will need to decide which study design to use to investigate the exposure–disease (E-D) association. (Note that, although the E-D association is of primary interest, it is often advantageous to collect data on other covariates to determine if adjustment for these factors alters the primary E-D association of interest.) All studies of the E-D association must include subjects that are both exposed and unexposed and subjects that do and do not have the disease; otherwise, none of the statistical methods that we describe can be properly applied.

A number of study designs could be used, each having advantages and disadvantages. The choice of study design generally involves a tradeoff between *feasibility* (i.e., the ability to complete the study and successfully address the research question(s), taking into account investigator time and resource constraints) and *validity* (i.e., arriving at the correct answer to the research question that is then generalizable to the target population). A study design emphasizing validity over feasibility usually requires more time and resources, whereas a study design that is easier to accomplish can be susceptible to *bias* (inaccurate estimation of the E-D association due to imperfect measurement of study variables or selection bias that yields a study sample that is not representative of the target population) and/or *confounding* (inaccurate estimation of the E-D association due to the influence of other risk factors that are not accounted for in the study).

When considering how to examine an E-D association for the first time, a rational approach to choosing the study design is to begin with the most feasible strategy available to address the research question. The information obtained from such a preliminary study can then be used to determine whether further research is merited and, if so, the preliminary results can be used to inform the study design (e.g., provide parameter estimates for power analyses, suggest which variables are or are not worthy of future consideration, etc.) of a future investigation utilizing a more rigorous study design. In the discussion that follows, commonly used study designs for biomarker research are described in increasing order of validity (Knapp and Miller 1992, p. 121).

2.2.2 Cross-sectional Studies

The exposure and disease status (and values of other covariates of interest) for each subject are assessed at a single point in time in a *cross-sectional study*. Associations between subject characteristics and the disease state can be quantified, but causality cannot be inferred since the cross-sectional study does not establish that the exposure precedes the onset of disease. To conduct a cross-sectional study, the investigator begins by selecting a sample of subjects that is representative of the target population. Then, exposure and disease status are ascertained on all subjects simultaneously. The validity of results obtained from a cross-sectional study is lower than all other studies described below; however, this type of study can usually be completed quickly with relatively little effort. Thus, a cross-sectional study can serve as a useful prelude to a more rigorous follow-up study.

Example 2.1 Cross-sectional Biomarker Study

Miller et al. (2006) used a cross-sectional design to investigate the association of salivary biomarkers of inflammation, collagen degradation, and bone turnover with clinical features of periodontal disease. They concluded that the mean levels of interleukin-1 beta and matrix metalloproteinase were significantly higher in patients with moderate-to-severe periodontal disease compared to subjects without periodontal disease.

2.2.3 Case–Control Studies

The investigator begins a *case–control* study by identifying *cases*, that is, subjects who have the disease of interest. Then a comparable sample of subjects who are free of disease, known as *controls*, is identified, and the exposure status of the cases and controls is assessed retrospectively. In some case–control studies, each case is "matched" to one or more controls; in other words, only those subjects without the disease who are similar in some way to one of the cases is eligible for inclusion in the study. The pre-specified case–control matching criteria can consist of one or more of the "Big 3" confounders (age, race, and sex), or they may include previously established risk factors for the disease under investigation. The purpose of matching is to control for the confounding effect of the matching criteria so that the cases and controls that are selected have roughly the same risk of disease in terms of known risk factors. The intention is to facilitate valid estimation of the E-D association for the primary risk factor of interest, controlling for the effects of the confounding variables. Matching each case with a single control (i.e., 1:1 matching) is most common, but each case can be matched with multiple controls, and sometimes more than one control group is used with different matching criteria for each group. If matching is used, the resulting dependence between cases and controls must be taken into account in the statistical analysis of the study data; methods for doing this are described in Sections 4.4.2 and 4.4.3.

Great caution should be used when identifying the control group in a case–control study. Consider a study with controls defined to be inpatients from the same hospital who are of the same age and gender as the cases. The possibility of a biased estimate of the E-D association arises if, as is commonly the case, the hospital treats a large number of patients with a certain disease other than the disease being studied. The other disease might have some risk factors in common with the disease of interest, so that when examining the E-D association, the investigator might erroneously conclude that the risk factors for the other disease are protective against the disease being studied since the risk factor is more commonly present in controls than in cases. The reason for this spurious association is that the proportion of control subjects having the risk factor is not representative of the true proportion having the risk factor in the target population of disease-free individuals. A simple way to avoid this problem would be to obtain a random sample of subjects from the target population rather than matching cases with controls. But in situations when a rare disease is being studied and there are time and resource limitations, using a random sample might not provide enough diseased subjects to facilitate estimation of the E-D association with sufficient precision.

Once all the data on exposure status have been collected for the cases and controls, the odds ratio (OR) (see Sections 3.10.2 and 4.9.1.1) is used to measure the E-D association. In a case–control study, disease prevalence cannot be estimated due to the lack of a representative sample from the target population (especially if matching was used), so the relative risk is not appropriate (see Sections 2.3.1.1 and 4.9.1).

Since subjects with prevalent (existing) disease are selected as cases, disease incidence (i.e., the rate of conversion from a disease-free to a diseased state) cannot be estimated from a case–control study. Also, it can be difficult to establish that the exposure preceded the onset of disease in a case–control study because, for exposed and diseased subjects, one does not know when the exposure and disease initially occurred; one might only know when the exposure and disease status were assessed for the study sample. However, an advantage of the case–control study is that the E-D association for multiple exposures can be examined.

Example 2.2 Case–Control Biomarker Study

Van Winden et al. (2009) used a case–control design to investigate the relationship between serum protein biomarkers and breast cancer. Previously collected serum samples of cases and controls were obtained from a serum bank and analyzed by surface-enhanced laser desorption/ionization time-of-flight mass spectrometry. Each of the 48 breast cancer cases were matched with a cancer-free control on the basis of age and storage duration of the serum sample. Van Winden et al. concluded that subjects categorized as having a "low intensity" peak for *m/z* 4276 and *m/z* 4292 had significantly higher odds of breast cancer compared to subjects with a "high intensity" peak for these biomarkers.

2.2.4 Retrospective Cohort Studies

The investigator begins a *retrospective cohort* study by identifying a sample of study subjects (i.e., the *cohort*) for whom the data to be analyzed have already been collected. (Usually, these data are obtained from a medical records database or similar repository.) Next, using the previously obtained information, the investigator obtains data on the baseline exposure status (and other covariates) for all study subjects and then the subsequent disease status is determined. Since subjects are initially defined in terms of their exposure status, it is possible to examine the relationship between the exposure and any disease outcome for which data are available. As with a case–control study, the ability to infer causal relationships is limited in a retrospective cohort study since the temporal sequence of exposure and disease is generally not readily established. However, a retrospective cohort study can provide a convenient approach for obtaining a large data set in a relatively short period of time so that one can estimate the E-D association of interest with a reasonable amount of precision.

Example 2.3 Retrospective Cohort Biomarker Study

Tian et al. (2009) conducted a retrospective cohort study using laboratory data on 6033 patients from a hospital's electronic medical record database. They concluded that patients suffering from acute kidney injury "with a serum creatinine level that returned to normal within 48 hours had substantially greater mortality rates (14.2%) than those who initially presented with an increased serum creatinine level on admission and subsequent serum creatinine level decrease of 0.3 mg/dL or greater to normal within 48 hours."

2.2.5 Prospective Cohort Studies

A *prospective cohort* study begins with subjects who are initially free of disease. All persons with a prevalent case of the disease are excluded when screening potential subjects for study eligibility. Upon enrollment into the study, each subject's exposure status for the primary risk factor of interest is ascertained and baseline data on relevant covariates (including other risk factors for the disease of interest) are obtained. Then all subjects are followed prospectively for development of the disease. Exposed and unexposed subjects are then compared in terms of disease incidence at the end of the study using the *relative risk*, also known as the *risk ratio* (RR). The RR is an appropriate measure of the E-D association for both prospective and retrospective cohort studies as long as the study data provide an accurate estimate of the incidence of the disease (see Sections 2.3.1.1 and 4.9.1.2).

In a prospective cohort study, potential study subjects are not eligible unless they are determined to be free of disease prior to enrollment. Then exposure status at baseline is determined and subjects are followed over time in order to estimate the disease incidence for both the exposed and unexposed groups. Thus, the prospective cohort study provides a remedy for the compromised validity in retrospective and cross-sectional studies resulting from their lack of evidence for the temporal sequence of exposure and disease occurrence. However, the prospective cohort study is often not feasible since the large sample size required to provide reasonably precise estimates of the E-D association might require an exceedingly long period of time and consume an excessive amount of resources in order to prospectively ascertain the disease status of all study subjects with a high degree of accuracy. These issues are especially problematic when studying relatively rare diseases. Sample size estimates derived from an *a priori* power analysis can help the investigator decide if the study will be feasible given the time and resources required, including efforts necessary to minimize loss to follow-up. A variety of resources are available to perform sample size and power calculations for both case–control and cohort studies. (See Section 2.3.3.)

Example 2.4 Prospective Cohort Biomarker Study

The fasting plasma glucose levels of 64,597 subjects with no previous history of cancer were measured as part of a prospective cohort study associated with the Västerbotten Intervention Project in northern Sweden. Stattin et al. (2007) found that subjects with baseline fasting glucose levels in the highest quartile had a significantly higher risk of subsequently developing cancer compared to subjects with baseline fasting glucose levels in the lowest quartile (RR = 1.26, 95% CI 1.09–1.47).

2.2.6 Observational Studies

All of the study designs described up to this point are examples of *observational studies*, in which data on the subjects' exposure, disease, and covariate status are merely recorded and analyzed, but the study subjects undergo no intervention. The results obtained from observational studies are of lower validity than results from an intervention study (see Section 2.2.7), but there are things the researcher can do to improve the validity of an observational study. For example, exposure status should be verified by multiple sources whenever possible, and disease status should be ascertained using the gold standard test, if available. *Masking* (also known as *blinding*) should be used whenever possible; for example, in a cohort study, the investigator who is assessing disease status should be unaware of the subject's exposure status.

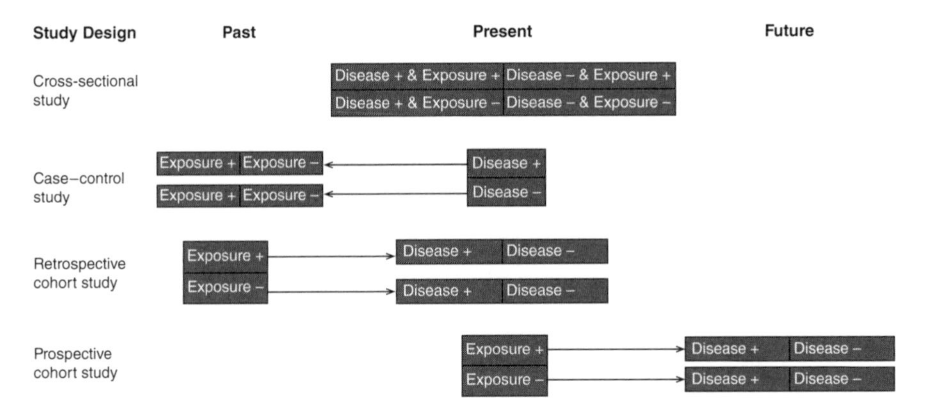

FIGURE 2.1 Schematic representation of four types of observational studies.

Similarly, in a case–control study, the investigator assessing exposure status should be unaware of the subject's disease status.

When deciding which type of observational study to use, the researcher should always consider time and resource limitations. Cross-sectional and retrospective cohort studies are generally much faster and easier to conduct than a prospective cohort study since the data are already available, typically in a medical records database or similar repository. However, data integrity can be comprised since the data were not originally collected specifically for the research study. Case–control studies are ideal for rare diseases and are suitable for situations when the investigator wishes to examine the associations of more than one exposure with the disease of interest. On the other hand, cohort studies allow researchers to investigate the associations of the exposure of interest with more than one disease outcome. The prospective cohort study is most appropriate when accurate assessment of exposure status and estimation of disease incidence is of primary concern, especially if one wishes to establish that the exposure preceded the disease. However, as mentioned previously, this study design requires more time and resources than other observational studies, especially when studying diseases that are relatively rare. Figure 2.1 depicts the basic design features of the four types of observational studies that we have described.

2.2.7 Randomized Controlled Trials

In an observational study, there is no manipulation of the study conditions (or the study subjects); data are recorded on subjects as they behave "in the usual way." As discussed above, observational studies are susceptible to problems with confounding since the observed E-D association might be due to the effect of a third variable not considered in the analysis that is related to both the exposure and disease. By way of contrast, in an *intervention (experimental)* study, some of the study subjects (usually half) are assigned to an intervention as part of the study design, whereas the other subjects do not receive the intervention. These latter subjects serve as the *control group* for the sake of comparison with those in the intervention group. (Note the distinction between the "control group" in an intervention study and the previously described "controls" in a case–control study, who are those study subjects without the disease. This is an unfortunate choice of terminology, as the term "control" has a completely different meaning within the two study types.)

Ideally, subjects in an intervention study should be randomly assigned (i.e., *randomized*) to treatment groups (e.g., either "intervention group" or "control group"). By using this mechanism, the effects of any variables that might confound the E-D association in an observational study should be balanced across treatment groups, provided that a valid randomization process is used. This is the rationale for referring to such a study as a *randomized controlled trial* (RCT) or *randomized clinical trial*. The double-blind RCT is the most common type of intervention study and is considered to be the gold standard of study designs in terms of the validity of results. Examples of other types of intervention studies include nonrandomized studies in which the "best treatment available" principle is used to determine the treatment that each study subject receives, and "time series" studies, in which a single group of study subjects is observed first under the control condition and then under the intervention.

RCTs are prospective studies that begin by randomly allocating subjects, all of whom typically have the "disease" of interest, to treatment groups. If possible, study participants should be *blinded* to their treatment group assignment; in other words, the subjects should not know to which treatment group they have been assigned. In addition, whenever possible, the investigators who are assessing study subjects in terms of baseline characteristics and treatment outcomes or are responsible for data collection should be blinded to the subjects' treatment group assignment. *Double blinding* refers to an RCT in which neither the study subjects nor the investigators observing the study subjects know the treatment group assignment of the subjects. Blinding is used to avoid biases in study results that might occur due to subjects or investigators having knowledge of the treatment group assignments.

Consider a hypothetical study in which a new synaptic serotonin reuptake inhibitor (SSRI) available in pill form is being evaluated for treatment of depression. Subjects who are told that they are taking a *placebo*, a pill that in all other ways resembles the new SSRI but has no active ingredients, might show no improvement on average, whereas subjects who are blinded to the fact that they are receiving a placebo might show improvement in their depression levels due to a psychological boost, called the "placebo effect," which study participants derive from the belief that they are receiving an active treatment. (In most modern RCTs, the *standard of care*, i.e., the usual course of treatment, is considered to be a more appropriate control condition than a placebo.) If subjects in the SSRI and placebo groups are all blinded to their treatment group assignment, the placebo effect should be the same for both groups. Similarly, investigators who are assessing study subjects' depression symptoms could be subconsciously biased by their knowledge of the subjects' treatment group assignment, but no such bias should occur if the investigators are blinded. The randomization and double blinding typically employed in RCTs should prevent any systematic differences between treatment groups other than those that can be attributed to the differences between the treatments being compared. There are other unique aspects of the RCT study design in addition to random assignment of study subjects to treatment groups and the use of blinding. For example, there are variations on the simple two-group randomization scheme described above. For example, in a *crossover* study, each subject is observed under both the control condition and the intervention; half of the study subjects receive the control first, and half receive the intervention first. (Most crossover studies include a *washout period* to allow time for the effect of the previously received treatment to fade.) Another variation is the *cluster randomized* trial, in which entire groups (or *clusters*) of study subjects are randomized to receive either the control or the intervention. (See Section 4.6.) We highly recommend the textbooks by Piantadosi (2005) and Chow and Liu (2013) for thorough discussions of various aspects of RCTs.

Example 2.5 Randomized Controlled Clinical Trial Involving Biomarkers

Steigen et al. (2006) randomized patients with coronary artery bifurcation lesions to treatment with either stenting both the main vessel and the side branch or stenting the main vessel only. They found that patients treated by stenting the main vessel only were significantly less likely to have procedure-related elevation of creatine kinase MB or troponin levels.

2.3 DESIGNING THE ANALYSIS

Designing the statistical analysis for a research study is an important, but often overlooked, component of the overall study design. A careful description of the statistical methods to be used in a study is often sacrificed since most of the attention during the planning stage is focused on determining the minimally acceptable n. However, one cannot perform the correct sample size calculation for the study that is being planned unless one knows exactly what statistical method will be used to analyze the study data once they are collected. We have found it useful to write a detailed statistical analysis plan *before any data are collected*, just as one would do as part of the Research Methodology section of a grant proposal. One can then use this analysis plan as a preliminary draft of the Statistical Analysis section that is typically included in the Methods section of any manuscript based on the study results. Even though it may seem unnecessarily tedious, we have found that putting together a detailed description of the statistical methods that will eventually be used to analyze the study data can be extremely useful in helping to identify important data elements that had not been identified previously. For example, it might be that carefully describing the analyses that will eventually be used to adjust for the effects of confounding variables will remind the investigator that he or she needs to include a biomarker for exposure to second-hand cigarette smoke among the study variables. To us, it is just as important to the validity of the study to develop a detailed statistical analysis plan prior to collecting the study data as it is to develop a detailed data collection protocol prior to beginning recruitment of study subjects. Our strong recommendation is that one adopt the model that is commonly used when a research team is developing a competitive proposal for extramural funding support; namely, clearly describing how the study data will be analyzed is just as important as clearly describing how the study data are to be collected.

Of course, it is a reality of scientific research that, once the study data are available for analysis, it may be necessary to modify the data analysis protocol that was previously specified, just as it may be necessary to modify the data collection protocol while a study is underway. The extent of these modifications should be minimized to the greatest extent possible; on the other hand, an experienced analyst can usually develop a valid statistical analysis plan for almost any set of data, even if the original research protocol had to be modified extensively. Our feeling is that data analysts should strive to develop the ability to adapt their data analysis plan to handle whatever modifications might be made to the original study design or data collection procedures.

Issues that arise when trying to determine the appropriate statistical method(s) for analyzing data from research studies involving biomarkers are the same issues that must be dealt with in any type of research that involves the quantitative evaluation of data. Regardless of the field of inquiry, after one has carefully formulated the research question (or research hypothesis), one must then identify the measurable entities that are most pertinent to the research, and then clearly describe how the entities are to be measured. In this chapter, we will use the generic terms *predictor* and *outcome* to refer to the two measurable entities that are to be examined. *Predictor* will typically be used to refer to the entity that occurs first chronologically. (In this context, the "predictor" is equivalent to the independent variable and the "outcome" is equivalent to the dependent variable. In epidemiological research, the "predictor" would be exposure to the risk factor of interest and the "outcome" would be the disease being studied. See Section 2.2.1 for further discussion.) Of course, in studies involving biomarkers, either the predictor or the outcome (or both) will be the observed value of a biomarker, perhaps a biomarker of exposure to a potentially harmful agent. A given biomarker may serve as the "outcome" in one phase of the research and the "predictor" in another phase.

For example, Cook et al. (1993) examined the association between passive smoking and spirometric indices in children as part of their evaluation of salivary cotinine as a biomarker for second-hand smoke. In the validation phase of their research, they examined the association between the "true" level of passive smoking, as measured by the number of smokers to whom the child was exposed (the *predictor*), and the potential biomarker, salivary cotinine (the *outcome*). In the experimental phase, they examined the association between salivary cotinine (the *predictor*) and lung function (the *outcome*), as measured by various spirometric indices.

To design (and eventually carry out) a proper statistical analysis of the data collected from a research study such as that described in Cook et al., one must complete the following steps (in this order): (1) choose the appropriate numerical measure(s) to be used to describe the association between the predictor and the outcome, (2) choose the appropriate statistical method(s) to apply when analyzing the data that will ultimately be obtained from the study, and (3) determine the appropriate sample size to be used in the study. *Data collection should not begin until each of these steps has been completed.* We describe and illustrate each of these steps separately in the following three sections.

TABLE 2.1 Determining Which Measure of Association to Use

	Outcome Variable		
Predictor Variable	Dichotomous	Ordinal	Continuous
Dichotomous	Odds ratio (OR)[a] Phi coefficient[b]	Spearman's r_s Kendall's t_b	Point biserial r or Spearman's r_s[c]
Ordinal	Spearman's r_s	Spearman's r_s Kendall's t_b	Spearman's r_s
Continuous	Point biserial r or Spearman's r_s[c]	Spearman's r_s Kendall's t_b	Pearson's r or Spearman's r_s[c]

[a]The risk ratio (RR) should be used for cohort and intervention studies.
[b]Used as an alternative to Pearson's r. See Helsel (2012, pp. 219–221).
[c]Use the measure listed first if the continuous variable(s) is(are) normally distributed. Use the measure listed second if the continuous variable(s) is(are) not normally distributed.
Source: Adapted from Table 2 of Looney and Hagan (2006b). Reproduced with permission of Taylor & Francis Group LLC in the format Republish in a Book via Copyright Clearance Center.

2.3.1 Choosing the Appropriate Measure of Association

Table 2.1 can provide assistance in selecting the appropriate measure of association between predictor and outcome to use in a research study. It is often the case in research studies involving biomarkers that both the predictor and the outcome are dichotomous. The predictor might be exposure to a hazardous substance, classified as "high" or "low" according to the observed value of a particular biomarker, and the outcome might be the presence or absence of a disease or condition. For example, in a cross-sectional study, Tunstall-Pedoe et al. (1995) examined the association between the level of serum cotinine (a biomarker for passive smoking) and the presence or absence of several adverse health outcomes (chronic cough, CHD, etc.). Serum cotinine level was grouped into four ordinal categories: "non-detectable," 0.01–1.05 ng/mL, 1.06–3.97 ng/mL, and 3.98–17.49 ng/mL. As indicated in Table 2.1, the authors correctly used the OR in their comparisons of each serum cotinine category versus the referent category of "non-detectable" in terms of the odds of each adverse health outcome in that serum cotinine category. This example is considered further in Section 4.9.5.1 and in Example 4.36.

2.3.1.1 Odds Ratio versus Risk Ratio The RR (also known as relative risk) is an appropriate measure of the association between exposure and disease in an epidemiological research study only if the estimated prevalence (or incidence) of disease from the study is based on a representative sample of exposed and unexposed subjects. For example, in a *case–control study* (Section 2.2.3), subjects with disease (cases) are often matched with subjects without disease (controls). If 1:1 matching is used, the estimated prevalence of disease based on the sample of cases and controls is 50%, which in general will not be a valid estimate of the true prevalence (or incidence) of the disease in the population. In fact, due to the inherent nature of the design of any case–control study, estimates of the prevalence (or incidence) of disease obtained from a case–control study data usually cannot be treated as valid, so a measure of association other than relative risk is needed. (See Section 4.9.1.2.)

The most commonly used alternative to the RR for measuring association is the OR, which is an appropriate measure of association under a wide variety of research scenarios (see Table 2.1). (For further discussion of the OR, see Sections 3.10.2 and 4.9.1.1.)

For example, in a case–control study, Hobbs et al. (2005) examined the association of low plasma methionine level (<24.17 μmol/L) in pregnant women with presence of congenital heart defects in their offspring. Of the 223 mothers whose infants had a congenital heart defect (the cases), 103 (46.2%) had a low plasma methionine level; of the 90 mothers whose infants did not have a heart defect (the controls), 27 (30.0%) had a low level, yielding an OR of 2.00. The (invalid) estimated RR based on these results would be 1.21, giving the impression of a much weaker association between having a low plasma methionine level during pregnancy and giving birth to a baby with a congenital heart defect. This study illustrates why the relative risk is not a valid measure of association for a case–control study: the true proportion of babies born with a congenital heart defect in the general population (i.e., the prevalence) is much lower than the estimated prevalence of 223/(223 + 90) = 71.2% obtained from the study data. For further consideration of this study, see Section 4.9.1.2.

2.3.1.2 Consequences of Not Choosing the Appropriate Measure of Association

Not using the correct measure of association can lead to any one of the following adverse consequences: (1) Loss of statistical efficiency (in terms of coverage probability of confidence intervals (CIs) and power of statistical tests) by failing to make the greatest possible use of the information contained in the study data; for example, failure to take advantage of the fact that either the predictor or the outcome (or both) are ordinal by treating both of them as nominal. (See Table 2.1.) (2) Using a measure of association that is inappropriate for the study design that was used; for example, using the relative risk as the measure of association in a case–control study. This can lead to incorrect conclusions about the strength of association (i.e., clinical significance), as well as statistical significance. (3) Using a measure of association when the underlying assumptions are violated; for example, using Pearson's correlation when either the predictor or the outcome is not normally distributed. This can lead to incorrect inferences concerning the true association between the predictor and outcome. See Section 4.5.1 for examples and further discussion of this issue.

2.3.2 Choosing the Appropriate Statistical Analysis

Once one has selected the appropriate measure of association, one must then use the appropriate statistical method(s) to determine if the study result is statistically significant. Table 2.2 can provide assistance in determining the correct statistical method to use when evaluating the observed association between predictor and outcome for statistical significance. For example, in the study described in the previous section, Tunstall-Pedoe et al. (1995), correctly used logistic regression to find CIs and p-values for the OR in their study (see Table 4.42). An advantage of using logistic regression to analyze the data when the OR has been chosen as the measure of association is that adjustment for the effects of confounding variables

TABLE 2.2 Determining Which Method of Statistical Analysis to Use

Predictor Variable	Outcome Variable			
	Dichotomous	Nominal	Ordinal	Continuous
Dichotomous	Logistic regression or Fisher's exact test[a]	Fisher–Freeman–Halton test	Mann–Whitney–Wilcoxon test	*t*-test or Mann–Whitney–Wilcoxon test[b]
Nominal	Fisher–Freeman–Halton test	Fisher–Freeman–Halton test	Kruskal–Wallis test	ANOVA or Kruskal–Wallis test[b]
Ordinal	Cochran–Armitage test for trend	Fisher–Freeman–Halton test	Linear-by-linear association test	Linear-by-linear association test
Continuous	Logistic regression	Polytomous logistic regression	Spearman's r_s	Pearson's r or Spearman's r_s[b]

[a]Use logistic regression if the odds ratio is being used as the measure of association. Use Fisher's exact test for testing the equality of binomial proportions.
[b]Use the statistical method listed first if the continuous variable(s) is(are) normally distributed. Use the method listed second if the continuous variable(s) is(are) not normally distributed.
Source: Adapted from Table 3 of Looney and Hagan (2006b). Reproduced with permission of Taylor & Francis Group LLC in the format Republish in a Book via Copyright Clearance Center.

is straightforward (Kleinbaum et al. 1982), thus enabling the analyst to determine if there is an "independent effect" of the main predictor of interest. For example, Tunstall-Pedoe et al. adjusted their OR for the effects of age, housing tenure, cholesterol, and diastolic blood pressure and concluded that there was a significantly increased odds of diagnosed CHD in the high passive smoking exposure group, as defined by a serum cotinine level between 3.98 and 17.49 ng/mL.

2.3.3 Choosing the Appropriate Sample Size

Once one has designed the statistical analysis for a study, the next step is to determine the appropriate sample size to be used. *Both of these steps should be performed prior to beginning data collection.* Sample size determination is specific to the statistical method that is to be used to analyze the study data once they have been collected. There are many textbooks that provide extensive descriptions of methods that can be used to determine the sample size required for a particular statistical method. The classic text in this area is Cohen (1988), which provides extensive tables for determining the required sample size for many of the statistical methods described in this book. Fleiss et al. (2003) devote their entire Chapter 4 (pp. 64–85) to a discussion of sample size determination when comparing two population proportions. Aberson (2010) describes methods that can be used for sample size and power calculations for many commonly used statistical methods.

Software for performing sample size and power calculations is also readily available; for example, many of the sample size methods described by Fleiss et al. have been implemented in the freely available Epi Info software, which can be downloaded from http://wwwn.cdc.gov/epiinfo/7/. Internet-based tools available on the OpenEpi website http://www.openepi.com/v37/Menu/OE_Menu.htm can be used to perform sample size calculations for the study designs we discussed in Section 2.2. Aberson (2010) provides SPSS syntax for carrying out the sample size methods covered in his book. StatXact has extensive capabilities for determining the appropriate sample size to use when applying various methods for analyzing categorical data, and is especially helpful when it is anticipated that the sample size of the study that is being planned will have to be small because of budget or time constraints, availability of experimental material, etc. In this text, we emphasize the use of SAS for carrying out most of the statistical analyses we describe. With each new release of SAS, more and more capabilities for sample size and power calculations are added to the POWER procedure. The freely available R software, which can be downloaded from http://cran.r-project.org/, contains several packages that can be used to perform sample size and power calculations for the methods we describe in this book.

From a more general perspective, we recommend Goldsmith (2001) for good practical advice on performing sample size calculations and statistical power analyses; this author also provides an extensive list of valuable references related to these issues. Goldsmith also provides very useful advice on determining the appropriate statistical package(s) to use for sample size calculations for many of the statistical procedures described in this book. Throughout this book, we provide details on how to perform sample size calculations for many of the statistical methods that we describe.

The Methods section of any manuscript based on a study in which biomarker data were collected and analyzed should always include a justification for the sample size that was used. Unfortunately, published biomarker studies to date have generally been deficient in this regard. For example, in the study by Tunstall-Pedoe et al. (1995) described above, the authors gave no justification at all for their sample size. However, not all authors have ignored this important aspect of describing their research methodology. For example, Lagorio et al. (1998) provided graphical displays that one could use to determine the sample size required for obtaining precise estimates of the population mean concentration of biomarkers based on urinary benzene and urinary *t*, *t*-muconic acid. In their study of three biomarkers for early detection of renal injury, Stengel et al. (1999) provided tables that one could use to examine the effect that the number of repeated measurements had on sample size and power in their study.

2.4 PRESENTING STATISTICAL RESULTS

After the research study has been completed, all study data have been collected, entered into the study database and "cleaned," and all appropriate statistical analyses have been completed, the next step is to prepare the presentation of the statistical results. As a general rule, each of the following items should be included in the presentation of the results of *any* statistical analysis: summary measures of central tendency and variability (or other relevant numerical summaries), test statistic (if different from the summary measure(s)), degrees of freedom associated with the test statistic (if appropriate), p-value of the relevant hypothesis test (if any), and CI for the parameter of interest (Lang and Secic 2006). In most published biomarker studies, p-values are emphasized, and p-values certainly have their place, especially with regard to determining statistical significance. However, it is generally preferable to present both the p-value for the appropriate hypothesis test *and* the corresponding CI. (See Section 3.6 for a general description of statistical inference.)

Without the CI, the reader has no direct way to ascertain the precision of the sample result, or to get an idea of what reasonable lower and upper bounds might be for the true value of the unknown parameter. Without the p-value, the reader is unable to ascertain the strength of evidence against the null hypothesis. Of course, CIs are always appropriate, regardless of whether it is of interest to test any particular hypothesized value or not.

Consider the study by Pérez-Stable et al. (1995), who examined the associations of several biochemical, physical examination, and depression assessments with serum cotinine levels (as a biomarker for cigarette smoking). The Pearson correlation coefficient (r) was used to measure these associations. Table 3 of their article provides the value of r and an asterisk ($*$) is used to indicate statistical significance if the p-value is less than 0.01; a cross (†) is used if $p \leq 0.05$. However, using these symbols to indicate significance provides no information about the strength of evidence against the null hypothesis H_0: $\rho = 0$, where ρ denotes the population correlation coefficient: a p-value of 0.049 is treated the same as 0.011. In addition, CIs were not provided, so there is no information on how precise these correlation estimates were (and hence how useful they were in contributing to the body of knowledge in this field of research). In another example, Henderson et al. (1989), in their study of exposure to second-hand smoke among preschool children, found a correlation of $r = 0.68$ ($p = 0.005$) between urinary cotinine/creatinine ratio (the potential biomarker) and home air nicotine level in a sample of 15 children who lived with at least one smoker. For these data, a 95% CI for the population correlation is (0.26–0.88), that is, it is likely that the population correlation is somewhere between 0.26 and 0.88. A CI this wide tells us that the estimate of the population correlation (0.68) is not very precise, indicating that this study contributes very little definitive information about the association of interest. Preferred methods of analysis for correlation coefficients are described in greater detail in Section 4.5.2.

There are several issues that one must keep in mind when presenting both CIs and the results of hypothesis tests. One is that the analyst must make sure that the CI procedure they use will yield a conclusion that is consistent with the conclusion from the hypothesis test that they perform. For example, if one uses an exact hypothesis test (e.g., for a binomial proportion), then one must also use the exact CI. Otherwise, the conclusions concerning some hypothesized value for the true proportion could be quite different. Another possible inconsistency could occur when a one-tailed hypothesis test is used (i.e., only the upper- or lower-tailed p-value is reported), but a two-sided CI is used. In this case, the one-sided CI corresponding to the one-tailed hypothesis test should be used instead of the two-sided CI.

PROBLEMS

2.1. Match each of the following possible configurations of row and column variables in a two-way contingency table to the appropriate analysis strategy. Note that for some configurations, it may be that ***none*** of the listed analysis strategies are appropriate, or that ***more than one*** of the strategies are appropriate. It is not necessary to use all of the analysis strategies.

Configuration		Analysis Strategy
>2 nominal rows, >2 nominal columns	_______	A. Test for linear association
>2 ordinal rows, >2 ordinal columns	_______	B. Mann–Whitney–Wilcoxon
2 rows, >2 nominal columns	_______	C. Pearson's correlation
2 rows, >2 ordinal columns	_______	D. Spearman's rho
>2 nominal rows, 2 columns	_______	E. Fisher's exact test
>2 ordinal rows, 2 columns	_______	F. *t*-test
2 rows, 2 columns	_______	G. Fisher–Freeman–Halton test
		H. Cochran–Armitage test
		I. Permutation test for trend
		J. Shapiro–Wilk test

3

ELEMENTARY STATISTICAL METHODS FOR ANALYZING BIOMARKER DATA

3.1 INTRODUCTION

In this chapter, we briefly review basic statistical methods that are commonly used in the analysis of biomarker data, and illustrate each one with examples taken from the biomarker literature. Some of the methods we discuss, though commonly used, are not necessarily optimal and alternative tests and guidelines on when to use them are presented in Chapter 4. In this chapter, no claim is made as to completeness of coverage of elementary statistical methods and, out of necessity, many of the technical details are omitted. We strongly encourage the interested reader to refer to an introductory biostatistics textbook for more detail concerning computational formulas, model assumptions, etc., especially if they are inexperienced in the application of basic statistical methods. Examples of such textbooks include Rosner (2011) and Triola and Triola (2005).

3.2 GRAPHICAL AND TABULAR SUMMARIES

After the data have been collected, there are numerous ways one can summarize the study results. Graphs and tables are useful for providing readers with a quick summary of study results that convey salient characteristics of the data. Effective graphs and tables should stand alone, apart from the text, and be easy for the reader to interpret. The appropriate choice of graphical and tabular summaries depends largely on the measurement scale used. *Dichotomous* (or *binary*) variables can assume two

Analysis of Biomarker Data: A Practical Guide, First Edition. Stephen W. Looney and Joseph L. Hagan.

possible values, such as a positive or negative result on a diagnostic test. *Nominal* variables fall into categories (or *levels*) with no inherent order, such as type of leukemia: acute lymphoblastic leukemia, chronic lymphocytic leukemia, acute myelogenous leukemia, and chronic myelogenous leukemia. *Ordinal* variables, such as tumor stage (I, II, III, and IV), do have an inherent order but the distance between levels has no intrinsic meaning. *Continuous* variables, such as serum concentration of the inflammation biomarker C-reactive protein, can take on any of a range of values (e.g., 1.28 mg/L, 1.29 mg/L, etc.). Continuous variables can be measured on an *interval scale* for which the 0 point is arbitrary (e.g., temperature in degrees Fahrenheit) or a *ratio scale* for which the 0 point is not arbitrary (e.g., temperature in degrees Kelvin, with the value of 0 corresponding to absolute zero). Dichotomous, nominal, and ordinal data are often summarized in tabular form via frequencies and percentages whereas continuous data are commonly summarized using sample means and standard deviations or other measures of location and variability (see Section 3.3). In addition, continuous variables are sometimes summarized in a frequency table (i.e., as grouped data), in which the range of observed data is divided into intervals and the frequency and percentage of observations falling into each interval are displayed.

The appropriate choice of a graphical method to summarize the data also depends on the variable's measurement scale. For continuous variables, the *histogram* is a graphical method analogous to a frequency table where, again, the range of observed data is divided into intervals. Rectangles are displayed with the location of the base on the horizontal axis corresponding to that data interval, and the height of the rectangle being proportional to the number of observations in the interval. (Alternatively, each rectangle can be constructed so that its area is proportional to the percentage of observations falling into that interval.) For example, Muscat et al. (2005) used a histogram to portray ethnic differences in the ratio of cigarette smoke carcinogen urinary metabolites (Figure 3.1).

A *bar chart* (or *bar graph*) is a graphical method similar to a histogram that can be used with nominal or ordinal data. Unlike a histogram, in which each bar corresponds to an interval of data, each bar in a bar chart represents a discrete value of the observed data, and the height of the bar is proportional to the number or percentage of observations having that value. Bar charts can also be used to help visualize comparisons among groups in terms of a continuous variable, with the height of the bar proportional to some summary statistic for the continuous variable such as the sample mean. Error bars can be added to represent the amount of variability in the continuous variable for each group, where the length of the error bar typically corresponds to the standard deviation or standard error in that group (see Section 3.3). For example, Duncan et al. (2009) used bar charts to display the intracellular expression levels of various biomarkers in macrophages infected with several genetic strains of *Leishmania donovani* (Figure 3.2).

A *box plot* (sometimes called a *box-and-whisker plot*) is another way to graphically compare groups in terms of a continuous variable, in which descriptive statistics based on percentiles (see Section 3.3) are used to summarize the data. For example, the

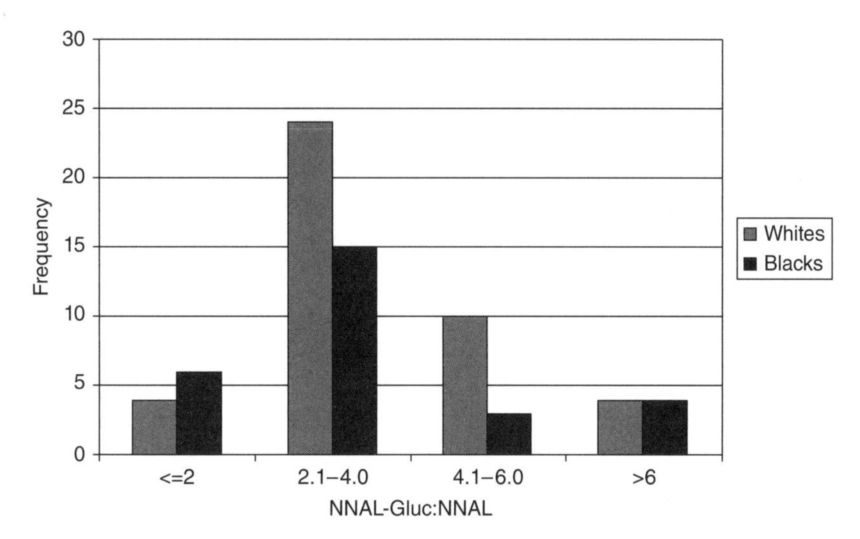

FIGURE 3.1 Histogram comparing white and black male subjects in terms of the ratio of two cigarette smoke carcinogen urinary metabolites. Reprinted from Figure 3 of Muscat et al. (2005, p. 1424) with permission from John Wiley & Sons.

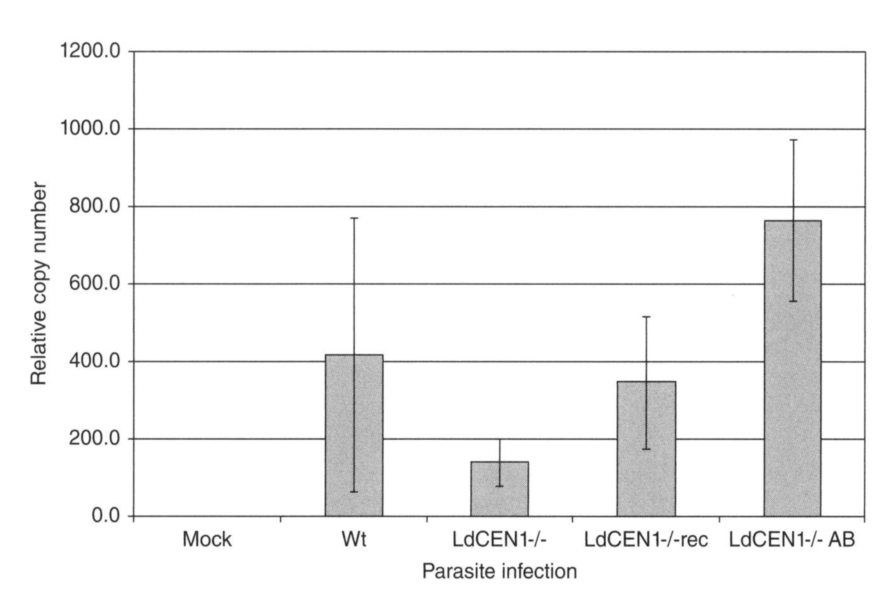

FIGURE 3.2 Bar chart of the intracellular P27 expression levels in macrophages infected with several genetic strains of *Leishmania donovani*. Reprinted from Figure 4a of Duncan et al. (2009, p. 21) with permission of Robert Duncan.

median (50th percentile) is used as the measure of location and the inter-quartile range (IQR = 75th percentile minus 25th percentile) is used to measure variability. A box plot consists of a rectangle which can be oriented either vertically or horizontally. For a vertical box plot, the bottom of the box represents the location of the first quartile (25th percentile) and the top of the box represents the third quartile (75th percentile). A horizontal line inside the box represents the second quartile (median). The "whiskers" extending outward from the top and the bottom of the box represent the minimum and maximum observations unless an extreme observation is present; such a value is depicted as a point beyond the whisker using a special symbol, typically an asterisk. In this case, the length of the whisker is usually 1.5 times the IQR. Box plots can be helpful in the visual identification of observations that are potential *outliers* (also called *discordant observations*; see Section 4.7). Continuous variables with symmetrical distributions will tend to yield box plots with approximately equal distances between quartiles, whereas *skewed* distributions (see Section 3.3) will have unequal distances between quartiles. Side-by-side box plots provide an effective way to compare groups in terms of the location, variability, and symmetry of a sample of continuous data values. For example, Kim et al. (2007) used side-by-side box plots to compare gene expression levels in adenocarcinoma (ADC) samples and squamous cell carcinoma (SCC) samples (Figure 3.3).

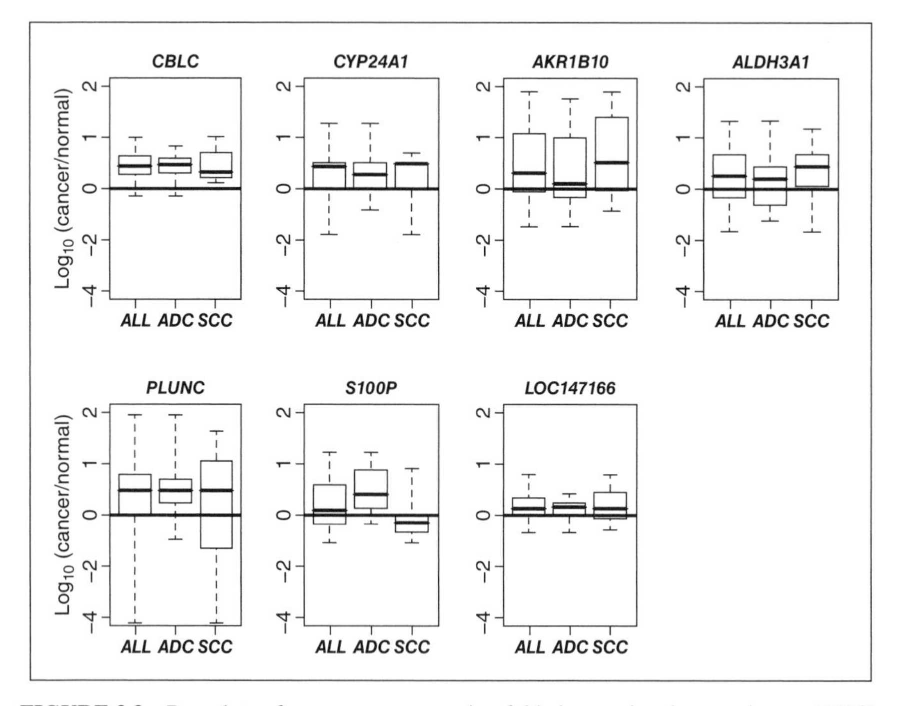

FIGURE 3.3 Box plots of seven gene expression fold changes in adenocarcinoma (ADC), squamous cell carcinoma (SCC), and all cancer patient (ALL) samples compared to normal patient samples. Reprinted from Figure 3 of Kim et al. (2007) with permission from AACR.

A scatter plot is a graphical device that is useful for showing the relationship between two continuous variables. Scatter plots simultaneously display values of two variables using Cartesian coordinates, with one variable (usually denoted by Y) plotted on the vertical axis and the other variable (usually denoted by X) plotted on the horizontal axis. The observed data are represented as points on the scatter plot where the values of the two variables (x, y) observed for each specimen or subject provide the coordinates which determine the corresponding position of the point in the Cartesian plane. Often, one of the two variables is considered to be the *independent variable* (IV, sometimes called the *predictor* or *explanatory* variable), which is manipulated or controlled by the researcher in an experimental study and hypothesized to have an effect on the *dependent variable* (DV, sometimes called the *outcome* or *response* variable). The convention is to let the horizontal x-axis represent the IV and the vertical y-axis represent the DV. For example, Joseph et al. (2005) used a scatter plot to display the relationship between urinary 4-(methylnitrosamino)-1-(3-pyridyl)-1-butanol (NNAL) concentration, a biomarker for tobacco toxin exposure (Y), and the number of cigarettes smoked per day (X) for subjects from four different studies. A different plotting symbol was used to represent subjects from each of the four studies (Figure 3.4).

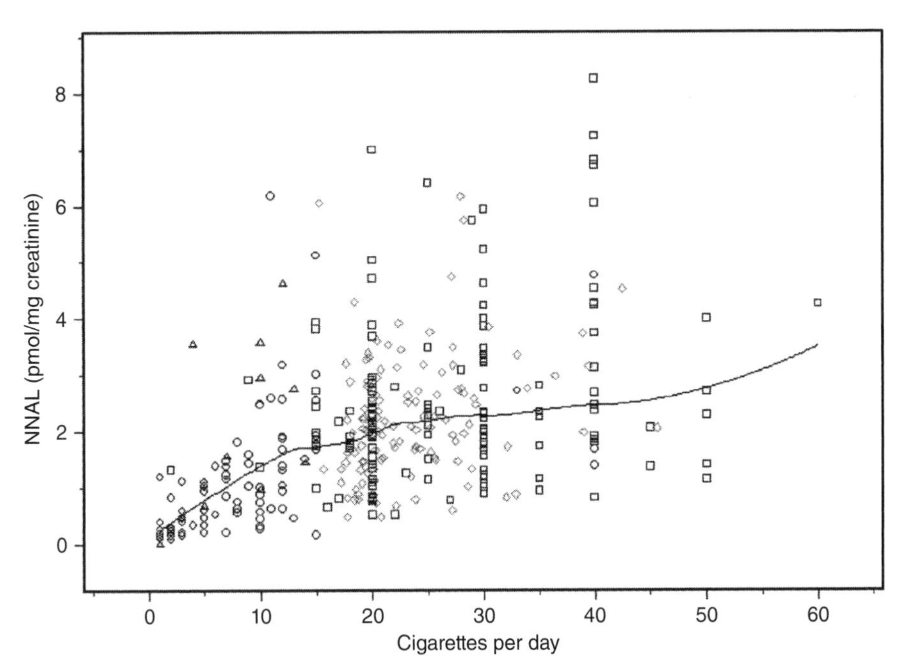

FIGURE 3.4 Scatter plot showing the relationship between NNAL concentration and the number of cigarettes smoked per day for subjects from four different studies, with a different symbol used to represent subjects from each study. Reprinted from Figure 2 of Joseph et al. (2005) with permission from AACR.

3.3 DESCRIPTIVE STATISTICS

It is usually informative to quantify the location of the center of a sample of data. The most commonly used measures of central tendency are the arithmetic mean, the median, and the mode. The arithmetic mean, usually referred to as the *sample mean* by statisticians, is simply the numerical average of the observations, computed by summing all the data values and dividing this sum by the number of data values in the sample:

$$\bar{x} = \frac{\sum_{i=1}^{n} x_i}{n}. \tag{3.1}$$

An alternative measure of central tendency we mentioned in the context of box plots is the sample *median* (denoted by m), which is obtained by arranging the n data values in order from smallest to largest and then selecting the observation "in the middle." Since there will be no single observation in the middle when n is an even number, the convention is to define the median to be the average of the two observations in the middle of the sorted data. When n is an odd number, the median is defined to be the single middle value. More formally, when n is odd, the median is the $(\frac{n+1}{2})$th largest observation; when n is even, the sample median is the average of the $(\frac{n}{2})$th and $(\frac{n}{2}+1)$th largest observations.

Example 3.1 Computing the Sample Mean and Median

In a study of potential biomarkers for severity of manic-depressive disorder (Naylor et al. 1976), sodium–potassium activated ATPase (Na–K ATPase) was measured in 11 patients with bipolar illness on placebo and 10 bipolar patients who were being treated with lithium. The Na–K ATPase levels (in mmol PO_4/L RBC, h) of the 11 patients on placebo (ordered from smallest to largest) and their ranks were as follows:

0.284	0.297	0.339	0.364	0.407	0.453	0.680	0.688	0.841	0.888	0.945
1	2	3	4	5	6	7	8	9	10	11

Since the number of observations ($n = 11$) is odd, the median is given by the $(\frac{11+1}{2}) = 6$th largest observation: $m_1 = 0.453$ mmol PO_4/L RBC, h.

The Na–K ATPase levels (in mmol PO_4/L RBC, h) of the 10 patients on lithium (ordered from smallest to largest) and their ranks were as follows.

0.550	0.568	0.586	0.616	0.666	0.797	0.828	0.833	1.151	1.307
1	2	3	4	5	6	7	8	9	10

Since the number of observations ($n = 10$) is even, the median is given by the average of the $(\frac{10}{2}) = 5$th and $(\frac{10}{2} + 1) = 6$th largest observations: $m_2 = (0.666 + 0.797)/2 = 0.732$ mmol PO_4/L RBC, h.

By way of contrast, the sample mean for the 11 bipolar patients on placebo is $\overline{x_1} = 0.562$ mmol PO_4/L RBC, h, and, for the 10 patients on lithium, $\overline{x_2} = 0.790$ mmol PO_4/L RBC, h. Thus, regardless of which summary measure of central tendency is used, patients on lithium tend to have higher Na–K ATPase levels.

SAS code that can be used to compute the sample mean and median Na–K ATPase level for patients on lithium and placebo is given below. This SAS code, as well as the SAS code for all of the examples in this chapter, is provided on the companion website.

```
OPTIONS FORMCHAR="|----|+|---+=|-/\<>*";

proc format;
value groupfmt
      1='placebo'
      2='lithium';
data placebo;
input NaK_ATPase @@;
datalines;
0.284 0.297 0.339 0.364 0.407 0.453 0.680 0.688 0.841 0.888 0.945
;
run;

data lithium;
input NaK_ATPase @@;
datalines;
0.550 0.568 0.586 0.616 0.666 0.797 0.828 0.833 1.151 1.307
;
run;

data placebo;
set placebo;
group = 1;

data lithium;
set lithium;
group = 2;

data ATPase;
set placebo lithium;

proc means data=ATPase mean median;
format group groupfmt.;
class group;
```

```
var NaK_ATPase;
title 'Na-K ATPase mean and median for bipolar patients';
run;
```

The *mode* is the data value that occurs most frequently in the sample. There could be two or more modes in a sample if more than one value is tied for the most frequently occurring, or no mode if all values in the sample occur only once.

Example 3.2 Computing the Mode

In a study of bone turnover in spondyloarthropathies (a joint disease of the vertebral column), Lata et al. (2010a) measured erythrocyte sedimentation rate (ESR) in 18 psoriatic arthritis patients (Table 3.1). The mode for this sample is 4 mm/h.

SAS code for computing the mode for the data in Table 3.1 is provided below:

```
OPTIONS FORMCHAR="|----|+|---+=|-/\<>*";

data PA;
input ESR  @@;
datalines;
63 23 9 4 1 53 22 4 4 12 6 17 2 4 14 27 38 2
;
run;

proc means data=PA mode;
var ESR;
title 'ESR mode for Psoriatic Arthritis patients';
run;
```

The decision as to which measure of central tendency is most appropriate for a given sample of data depends on the characteristics of the data. Extremely large or small values (outliers) exert a large degree of influence on the value of the sample mean, especially if n is small. This is a commonly encountered issue with data such as serum or urinary biomarker concentrations, many of which exhibit a *right-skewed* distribution, that is, data values above the median are generally further removed from

TABLE 3.1 Erythrocyte Sedimentation Rate (mm/h) in Psoriatic Arthritis Patients

63	23	9	4	1	53
22	4	4	12	6	17
2	4	14	27	38	2

Source: Data courtesy of Dr. Luis Espinoza.

the median than data values below the median. (See Section 3.4.) Since extremely high (or low) values can increase the mean disproportionately, the median is generally preferred as a measure of central tendency for skewed data (i.e., data exhibiting an asymmetric distribution).

For example, in a study by Susanto et al. (2012), the authors considered periodontal inflamed surface area (PISA) as a biomarker for impaired blood glucose control (as measured by HbA1c). Presumably because of the extreme skewness in the data, the authors used the median as a summary statistic for the PISA levels in a sample of 132 healthy controls ($m_1 = 83.9$ mm^2) and 101 patients with Type 2 diabetes mellitus ($m_2 = 170.4$ mm^2).

Measures of *dispersion* (also known as *variability*) represent another important class of descriptive statistics that complement measures of central tendency. A very simple and intuitive measure of dispersion is the *range*, which is the difference between the largest and smallest data values. A drawback of the range is that only two observations contribute to its calculation. A more appealing (but less intuitive) measure of dispersion, to which all observations contribute, is based on the concept of the average squared difference of each observation from the mean. (For finite populations, this is referred to as the *population variance*.) For samples, especially when n is small, the average squared difference from the sample mean generally underestimates the true variability in the population. To adjust for this, the *sample variance* is computed by dividing the sum of squared deviations from the sample mean by $n - 1$ instead of n:

$$s^2 = \frac{\sum_{i=1}^{n} (x_i - \bar{x})^2}{n - 1}. \tag{3.2}$$

(Adjusting the sample variance in this way also results in an *unbiased* estimate of the population variance.)

An equivalent formula for calculating s^2, sometimes called the "computational formula" because it is generally considered to be easier to use with a hand-held calculator, is given by

$$s^2 = \frac{\sum_{i=1}^{n} x_i^2 - n(\bar{x})^2}{n - 1}. \tag{3.3}$$

Regardless of whether Equation (3.2) or (3.3) is used, the numerical result for s^2 should be the same, to within round-off error.

The most commonly used measure of dispersion is the *sample standard deviation,* which is given by the square root of the sample variance: $s = \sqrt{s^2}$, where s^2 is given by Equation (3.2) or (3.3). An appealing characteristic of the standard deviation is that it is in the same units as the original data. The sample variance and standard deviation generally perform well as measures of variability as long as the distribution of the data is fairly symmetrical. For the 11 bipolar patients on placebo in Example 3.1,

$s_1 = 0.252$ mmol PO_4/L RBC, h, and, for the 10 patients on lithium, $s_2 = 0.257$ mmol PO_4/L RBC, h, thus indicating a slightly higher degree of variability for the patients on lithium. The estimated *standard error of the mean* (SEM), a measure of variability that is used in constructing confidence intervals (CIs) and calculating test statistics (Sections 3.6.1 and 3.6.2), is given by $\widehat{\text{SEM}} = (\frac{s}{\sqrt{n}})$.

Another measure of dispersion, the *coefficient of variation* (CV), is obtained by dividing the sample standard deviation by the sample mean and multiplying by 100%:

$$\text{CV} = \frac{s}{\bar{x}} \times 100\%. \tag{3.4}$$

For the data in Example 3.1, CV = (0.252/0.562) × 100% = 45% for patients on placebo and CV = (0.257/0.790) × 100% = 33% for the patients on lithium. Note that, because of the higher mean level of Na–K ATPase level for the patients on lithium, the CV indicates a higher degree of variability for the patients on placebo.

In contrast to the standard deviation, which is unit dependent and is expected to increase as the mean increases, the CV is unit free, thereby allowing for comparison of variability across different samples or between different variables. The CV is commonly used to compare the precision or reproducibility of different laboratories, assays, etc. For example, Blankenberg et al. (2010) used the CV to assess the intra-assay and inter-assay precision of measurements of 30 biomarkers related to cardiovascular health.

Guidelines for interpreting the CV are not clear-cut, but generally $\leq$5% is considered good and $\geq$10% is considered bad, with the caveat that a high CV is not very informative when the mean concentration is very low (Zady 2009). Depending on the field of application, different cutoffs may be used for acceptable values of the CV. In the study by Blankenberg et al. (2010), intra-assay precision ranged from 0.09% for creatinine to 8.17% for Vitamin B12; inter-assay precision ranged from 0.83% for C-reactive protein to 16.68% for adiponectin.

Another measure of variability that is sometimes used to summarize highly skewed data is the IQR, which is equal to the 75th percentile ($p_{0.75}$) minus the 25th percentile ($p_{0.25}$). As discussed in Section 3.2, the IQR is used in the construction of box plots. The IQR is generally considered to be preferable to the range as a measure of variability for skewed data. For such data, we recommend that the median be used as a summary measure of location and that the IQR be used as a summary measure of variability, unless other descriptive statistics are thought to be more appropriate for the problem at hand.

In the study by Susanto et al. (2012) that examined the use of PISA as a biomarker for impaired blood glucose control, the authors used the IQR as a summary measure of variability. In their sample of 132 healthy controls, $p_{0.75} = 206.4$, $p_{0.25} = 35.2$, and IQR = 171.2 mm^2. In their sample of 101 patients with Type 2 diabetes mellitus, $p_{0.75} = 392.6$, $p_{0.25} = 91.5$, and IQR = 301.1 mm^2, indicating a higher degree of variability for the diabetic patients.

SAS code that can be used to compute the measures of variability for Na–K ATPase level for the patients on lithium and placebo in Example 3.1 is given below:

```
proc means data=ATPase mean var std stderr cv p25 p75 ;
format group groupfmt.;
class group;
var NaK_ATPase;
title 'Measures of variability for Na-K ATPase for bipolar
patients';
run;
```

3.4 DESCRIBING THE SHAPE OF DISTRIBUTIONS

In Section 3.3, we mentioned that the choice of an appropriate measure of central tendency or variability often depends on the shape of the distribution of the data. Theoretical distributions of data (i.e., for the population from which the sample data were obtained) can be symmetrical, skewed left, or skewed right. Figure 3.5 illustrates

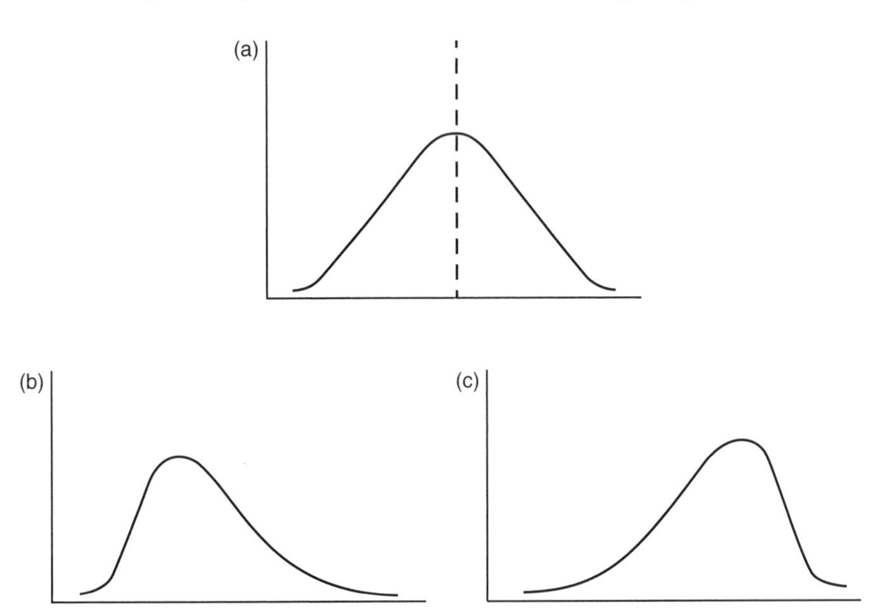

FIGURE 3.5 (a) Example of a symmetrical distribution. The dashed line indicates the location of the mean, median, and mode of the distribution. Reprinted from Figure 1-4 (a) of Knapp and Miller (1992, p. 7) with permission from Lippincott Williams & Wilkins. (b) Example of a right-tailed distribution. The distribution is said to be *skewed right*. Reprinted from Figure 1-4 (b) of Knapp and Miller (1992, p. 7) with permission from Lippincott Williams & Wilkins. (c) Example of a left-tailed distribution. The distribution is said to be *skewed left*. Reprinted from Figure 1-4 (c) of Knapp and Miller (1992, p. 7) with permission from Lippincott Williams & Wilkins.

TABLE 3.2 Semaphorin Concentration (per pg/mg Urinary Creatinine) for Children without Acute Kidney Injury Following Coronary Artery Bypass Surgery (CABG)

310.0	185.0	237.0	166.5	328.5	319.5
739.5	149.3	168.0	159.8	153.0	322.9
430.5	353.0	130.0	88.0	32.0	121.5
662.5	199.5	388.5	139.0	146.0	269.0
433.0	570.0	173.0	66.0	104.0	170.0
146.0	605.0	370.0	194.0		

Source: Data courtesy of Dr. Ganesan Ramesh.

each of these shapes. Highly skewed data are often transformed in the hope that the newly transformed data values will look more like a normal distribution (or at least be closer to symmetrical).

Example 3.3 Log-Transformations and Distributional Shape

Consider the data in Table 3.2 taken from Jayakumar et al. (2013). In this study, urinary semaphorin 3A concentration (measured in pg per mg urinary creatinine) was evaluated as a biomarker for use in diagnosing acute kidney injury (AKI) in children who had undergone coronary artery bypass graft (CABG) surgery. The data in Table 3.2 are the semaphorin concentrations measured at 12 hours following CABG for the 34 children who did not develop AKI. Figure 3.6 contains a histogram of these data with the graph of a log-normal distribution superimposed. The log-normal is a theoretical distribution that is often used when analyzing biomarker data. If, after applying a logarithmic transformation to each of the original data values, the transformed values follow a normal distribution, then the original data are said

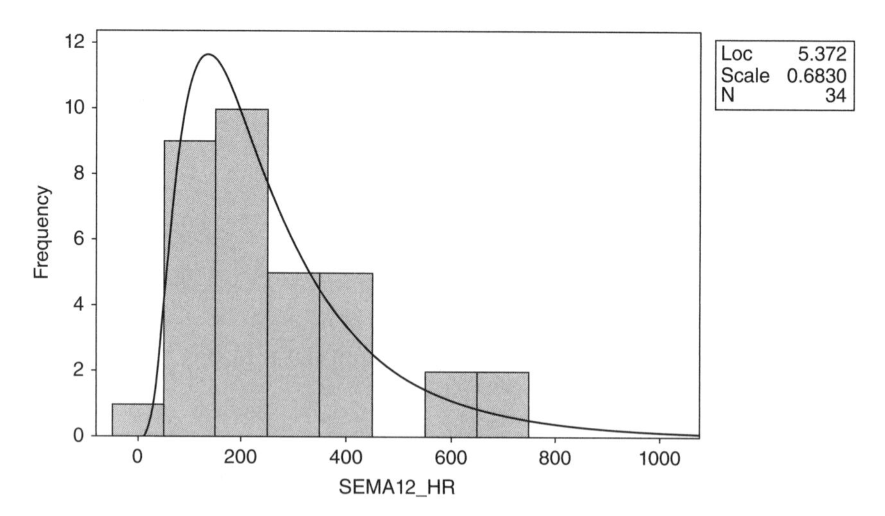

FIGURE 3.6 Histogram of semaphorin concentrations for 34 children who did not develop AKI following CABG with the graph of a log-normal distribution superimposed.

TABLE 3.3 Log Semaphorin Concentration for Children without AKI Following CABG

5.7	5.2	5.5	5.1	5.8	5.8
6.6	5.0	5.1	5.1	5.0	5.8
6.1	5.9	4.9	4.5	3.5	4.8
6.5	5.3	6.0	4.9	5.0	5.6
6.1	6.3	5.2	4.2	4.6	5.1
5.0	6.4	5.9	5.3		

to follow a *log-normal* distribution. Based on a visual inspection of Figure 3.6, the log-normal distribution appears to fit the data quite well.

The data in Table 3.3 are the transformed semaphorin concentrations after taking the natural logarithm ("log base e") of each value in Table 3.2. Figure 3.7 contains a histogram of the transformed values with the graph of a normal distribution superimposed. Based on visual inspection, the normal distribution appears to fit the transformed data quite well. The transformed values can now be analyzed using statistical techniques that are based on the assumption that the data are normally distributed (e.g., *t*-test, Pearson correlation). The issues of formally testing data for normality and identifying a possible transformation are discussed in Section 4.2.

3.5 SAMPLING DISTRIBUTIONS

The descriptive statistics discussed in the previous sections are all calculated from a single sample of data, which is usually drawn, ideally at random, from a larger population. Statistics computed from a sample of data are observed values of a

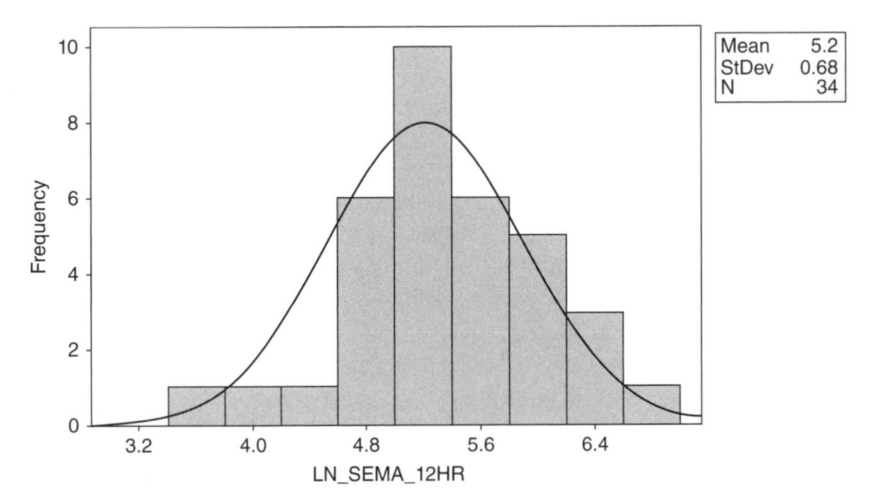

FIGURE 3.7 Histogram of log-transformed semaphorin concentrations for 34 children who did not develop AKI following CABG with the graph of a normal distribution superimposed.

random variable, because the realized value of the statistic will vary with each distinct sample. The *sampling distribution* of a statistic is described by the theoretical *probability density function* (pdf) of this random variable, and it describes, over all possible samples of a particular size, the relationship between the possible values of the statistic and the probability of assuming those values, or a particular interval of these values. For example, the distribution of the sample mean over all possible samples of size n is referred to as the "sampling distribution of the sample mean." In general, the standard deviation of a statistic over all possible samples of size n is referred to as the *standard error* of that statistic. For example, the standard deviation of the sample mean is referred to as the SEM and is estimated from a sample of data by

$$\widehat{\text{SEM}} = \left(\frac{s}{\sqrt{n}}\right). \tag{3.5}$$

When the pdf of a continuous random variable is plotted (as in Figure 3.5), the x-axis represents the value of the random variable and the y-axis represents the "density" corresponding to that value of x. The probability that a continuous random variable will assume a value within some specified interval can be computed by finding the proportion of the total area under the curve that falls between the two points on the x-axis that represent the upper and lower bounds of the interval. The *normal distribution* is a continuous distribution that is the most commonly used distribution in statistical analysis because many variables in nature are approximately normally distributed and the properties of this distribution are well understood. The graph of the pdf of any normal distribution resembles a "bell-shaped" curve that is symmetrical, with the mean, median, and mode all occurring at the peak in the center of the curve as in Figure 3.5a. For all normal distributions, regardless of the mean and variance, approximately 95% of the total area under the curve will lie within two standard deviations of the mean. According to the *central-limit theorem*, sample means obtained from repeated random samples will have an approximate normal distribution even if the distribution of the individual observations in the population from which the samples are obtained is not normal. This property can be exploited for the purposes of statistical inference. For example, hypothesis tests and CIs for a binomial proportion can be based on the normal approximation to the binomial. Figure 3.8 shows how closely the normal approximation approximates the binomial distribution when $n = 10$ and $p = 0.5$.

3.6 INTRODUCTION TO STATISTICAL INFERENCE

3.6.1 Point Estimation and Confidence Interval Estimation

Usually the value of a sample statistic is not of direct interest, but instead it is used to estimate the value of a population parameter (also called the "true value").

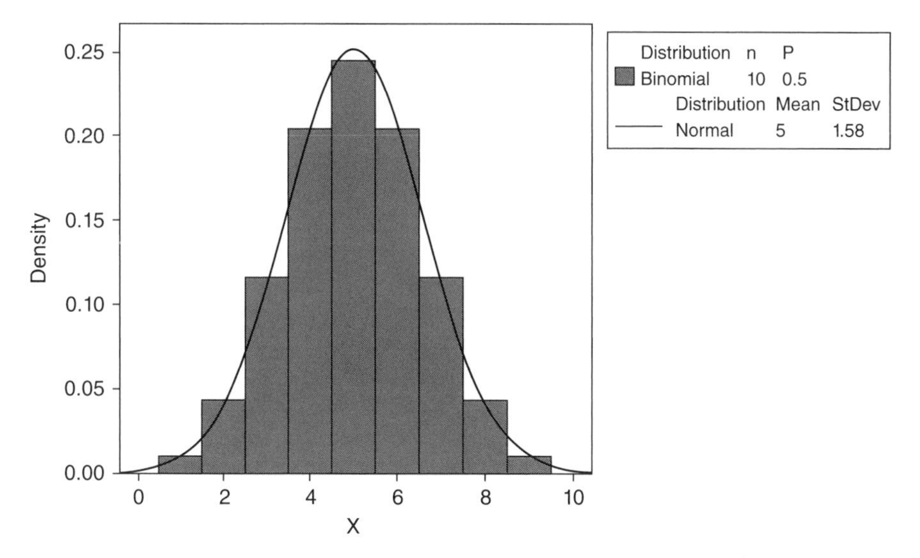

FIGURE 3.8 Normal approximation to the binomial.

Throughout this textbook, we will follow standard statistical practice and use Greek letters to denote unknown population parameters.

For example, a study might be undertaken with the intention of estimating the true mean plasma glucose level of pregnant women 1 hour after a 50 g oral glucose challenge. The true mean plasma glucose of all pregnant women 1 hour after a 50 g oral glucose challenge, denoted by the Greek letter μ, is a population parameter that can never be known exactly, since it would be infeasible (or physically impossible) to measure the plasma glucose level of all pregnant women. Instead, data values (i.e., glucose levels) obtained from a sample of pregnant women chosen in some appropriate manner are used to calculate an estimate of this parameter value; namely, the sample mean, denoted by $\bar{x}$. In such a situation, the mean plasma glucose value obtained from a single sample of pregnant women represents a *point estimate* of the population parameter. But realizing that each new sample of pregnant women would provide a different estimate, it would be useful to obtain a plausible interval of values that is likely to contain the true value of the mean glucose for all pregnant women. Such an interval is called a CI. The *confidence level*, a number between 0% and 100%, describes how confident we are that the CI contains the true value of the parameter. Assuming that the sample observations are normally distributed, an exact 95% CI (i.e., a CI with a confidence level of 95%) for the population mean (μ) is given by

$$\bar{x} \pm t_{\alpha/2,n-1}\left(s/\sqrt{n}\right), \tag{3.6}$$

where $t_{\alpha/2,n-1}$ is the upper $\alpha/2$-percentage point from a Student's t-distribution with $n-1$ degrees of freedom (*df*). Values such as $t_{\alpha/2,n-1}$ (which are typically found in the

"t-table" in any standard introductory statistics book) are also called *critical values* and can be obtained from many standard software packages, including Excel, SAS, R, etc.

As noted previously, an assumption underlying the CI in (3.6) is that the sample was drawn from a parent population in which the random variable of interest is normally distributed. If this assumption cannot be verified (see Section 4.2.2) and n is "large enough" (generally taken to be $n \geq 30$), the central limit theorem allows us to construct an approximate CI by replacing the critical value from the t-distribution in (3.6) with the corresponding critical value from the standard normal, $z_{\alpha/2}$. (A "standard normal" distribution has a mean of 0 and a standard deviation of 1.) However, for sufficiently large n, there will be very little difference between the t-based and z-based CIs.

The most commonly used confidence level in biomarker studies is 95%; this means that approximately 95% of the CIs computed from repeated random samples from the same population will contain the true population mean. The width of the CI can also be thought of as a measure of the precision of the estimate of the population parameter. In order to increase the precision of the estimate, the researcher can increase the number of observations in the sample of data and hence decrease the width of the CI.

As an illustration of the use of CIs in biomarker studies, consider the study by England et al. (2004). The authors provided CIs for the true mean plasma glucose level among pregnant women 1 hour after a 50 g glucose challenge for never smokers (106.7 mg/dL [95% CI, 105.7–107.6]) and for current smokers (115.2 mg/dL [95% CI, 112.9– 117.5]).

For a dichotomous variable (e.g., subjects' disease status, categorized as "disease" or "no disease"), the *binomial proportion, π,* is estimated from a sample of data as the number of "events" (e.g., subjects with disease) divided by n, the total number subjects in the sample. The standard terminology for the binomial is to refer to one of the outcomes (usually the one of most interest) as a "success" and the other outcome as a "failure."

For large samples, an approximate $100(1 - \alpha)\%$ CI for the proportion of subjects with the disease in the population can be obtained using the normal approximation to the binomial, yielding the familiar "Wald interval":

$$p \pm z_{\alpha/2} \sqrt{p(1-p)/n}, \tag{3.7}$$

where p is the sample proportion, $z_{\alpha/2}$ is the upper $\alpha/2$-percentage point of the standard normal distribution and $\sqrt{p(1-p)/n}$ is the estimated standard error of the sample value of the binomial proportion.

Example 3.4 Confidence Intervals for a Binomial Proportion

As an example of the use of a CI to estimate a binomial proportion in a study involving biomarkers, consider the study by Subar et al. (2003), who assessed dietary measurement error by comparing self-reported information on a food frequency questionnaire (FFQ) to the study subjects' actual intake estimated from "unbiased biomarkers." In particular, the authors used urinary nitrogen to estimate true protein intake, and then compared the biomarker results to self-reported results to determine what proportion of subjects were below a certain threshold defined to indicate underreporting. Using data obtained from 261 male subjects and 223 female subjects, Subar et al. concluded that 39% of the men (95% CI: 33%, 45%) and 29% of women (95% CI: 23%, 35%) underreported protein intake on the FFQ.

An *exact* CI for a binomial proportion can be obtained using the binomial distribution, but such an interval will usually differ very little from the Wald interval calculated using the same data, as long as n is sufficiently large and p is not too close to 0 or 1. The generally accepted rule of thumb is that the approximate interval can be used as long as both np (the number of "successes" in the sample) and $n(1 - p)$ (the number of "failures") are greater than or equal to 5. For the data in Example 3.4, there were 102 "successes" among the men and 159 "failures." Among the women, the numbers of successes and failures were 65 and 158, respectively. Therefore, the Wald intervals should differ very little from the exact. In fact, the intervals are identical to the nearest whole percent.

The FREQ procedure in SAS can calculate both approximate and exact CIs for π. SAS code that can be used to analyze the data in Example 3.4 is provided below:

```
data Men;
input under$ count;
datalines;
Y 102
N 159
;
run;

title1 'Exact and Approximate Confidence Intervals for the
Binomial Proportion';

proc freq data=Men order=data;
tables under / binomial;
weight count;
title2 'Proportion of Men Underreporting Protein Intake';
run;

data Women;
input under$ count;
datalines;
Y 65
N 158
;
run;
```

```
proc freq data=Women order=data;
tables under / binomial;
weight count;
title2 'Proportion of Women Underreporting Protein Intake ';
run;
```

3.6.2 Hypothesis Testing

One or more research questions will be the impetus for undertaking a biomarker study. (See Section 2.1.) From a statistical perspective, each research question is translated into a *null hypothesis* and an *alternative hypothesis*. In general terms, the null hypothesis usually posits that there is no association between the independent and DVs, whereas the alternative hypothesis posits that there is such an association. An appropriate statistical method is then applied to the experimental data to determine the probability that a sample result this "extreme" (in terms of the null hypothesis) would be obtained simply by random chance if the null hypothesis were really true. This probability is called the *p-value*. Based on the p-value, a decision is made about whether or not to reject the null hypothesis. If the p-value is below a predetermined cutoff called the *significance level* (α), almost always 0.05 in biomarker studies, the null hypothesis is rejected in favor of the alternative hypothesis. However, because of sampling error (attributed to the fact that one is attempting use a sample of data to draw a conclusion about the entire population), it is possible to get a small p-value and reject the null hypothesis, even when the null hypothesis is actually true. Such a mistake is called a *Type I error*, and the hypothesis test is designed such that the probability of a Type I error is equal to α, the preselected significance level. On the other hand, when the alternative hypothesis is true, it is possible, again because of sampling error, to get a p-value larger than the significance level and therefore decide not to reject a null hypothesis that is actually false. Such a mistake is called *Type II error*, occurring with probability β. The complementary event, that of making the correct decision and rejecting a null hypothesis that is, in fact, false, has a probability of $1 - \beta$; this value is called the *statistical power* of the test. There is a trade-off between Type I and Type II error. Decreasing the significance level in an effort to avoid erroneously rejecting a true null hypothesis will increase the probability of a Type II error, thereby reducing the power of the hypothesis test to detect an alternative hypothesis that is true.

The above concepts can be more easily understood by examining Figure 3.9. The "true state of nature" (similar to the gold standard result in diagnostic testing) is dichotomized according to whether the null hypothesis is true or not. The conclusion from the hypothesis test is dichotomized in the same way. Each of the four possible combinations of rows and columns in the figure defines one of the possible outcomes of the hypothesis test.

The *one-sample t-test* is an example of a statistical method used to perform a hypothesis test. This method is used to test the null hypothesis (H_0) that a population mean (μ) is equal to some prespecified value (μ_0) under the null hypothesis versus

		True state of nature	
		H_0 is false	H_0 is true
Conclusion from hypothesis test	Reject H_0	***No error***	***Type I error***
	Fail to reject H_0	***Type II error***	***No error***

FIGURE 3.9 Representation of types of error in hypothesis testing.

the two-sided alternative hypothesis (H_a) that the population mean is not equal to this value, or symbolically:

$$H_0 : \mu = \mu_0 \text{ vs. } H_a : \mu \neq \mu_0$$

Assuming that the sample observations can be assumed to follow a normal distribution, the first step in the hypothesis testing procedure is to calculate the test statistic for the one-sample t-test using the sample data:

$$t_0 = \frac{\bar{x} - \mu_0}{s/\sqrt{n}}. \tag{3.8}$$

The absolute value of this test statistic is compared with the appropriate critical value t^*; namely, the upper $\alpha/2$-percentage point from the Student t-distribution with $(n - 1)$ degrees of freedom, denoted by $t^* = t_{\alpha/2,n-1}$. If $|t_0| > t^*$, the null hypothesis is rejected in favor of the alternative hypothesis. Otherwise the null hypothesis is not rejected. Note that this is the same t-value as that used in the formula for the CI given in Equation (3.6). This relationship implies that conclusions concerning a population parameter (mean, proportion, variance, etc.) will be the same, regardless of whether a CI or hypothesis test is used. This concept is illustrated further with an example in the discussion below.

Example 3.5 Statistical Inference for a Population Mean

To illustrate the concepts of hypothesis testing and CI estimation, consider the study by Faupel-Badger et al. (2006). The investigators considered the research question "Does the breast cancer prevention drug raloxifene affect the serum estradiol levels of premenopausal women at high risk for developing breast cancer?" To address this question, the researchers measured the serum estradiol levels of premenopausal women at baseline upon enrollment into their study, and then again after taking 60 mg raloxifene daily for 12 months. In the context of their study design, the research question can be translated into the null hypothesis, "On average, *there is no change* in the serum estradiol levels of premenopausal women at high risk for developing breast cancer taking 60 mg raloxifene daily for 12 months." The corresponding alternative hypothesis is, "On average, *there is a change* in the serum estradiol levels of premenopausal women at high risk for developing breast cancer taking 60 mg raloxifene daily for 12 months." For this example, $\mu_0 = 0$ because, under the null hypothesis, there is no change in estradiol levels after taking raloxifene. Symbolically, these hypotheses could be expressed as $H_0 : \mu = 0$ versus $H_a : \mu \neq 0$, where μ represents the true mean change in estradiol levels in the population of all premenopausal women at high risk for developing breast cancer who take 60 mg raloxifene daily for 12 months. The basic concepts of hypothesis testing depicted in Figure 3.9 are illustrated for the study by Faupel-Badger et al. in Figure 3.10.

In their study, Faupel-Badger et al. measured the serum estradiol levels of 15 premenopausal women at high risk for developing breast cancer before and after 12 months of taking raloxifene. They calculated the change (after – before) in serum estradiol levels for the 15 women and found a mean increase of 42 pg/mL with a 95% CI of (1–84). Since $\mu = 0$ pg/mL (i.e., no mean change) is not included in the 95% CI, it can be concluded that, at the 0.05 significance level, there is a statistically significant change (specifically an increase, since the entire CI is above 0) in the serum estradiol levels of premenopausal women at high risk for developing breast cancer taking 60 mg raloxifene daily for 12 months. Furthermore, the one-sample

		True state of nature	
		Raloxifene affects serum mean estradiol level (H_0 is false)	Raloxifene does not affect mean serum estradiol level (H_0 is true)
Conclusion from hypothesis test	Raloxifene affects mean serum estradiol level (H_0 is rejected)	***No error***	***Type I error***
	Raloxifene does not affect mean serum estradiol level (H_0 is not rejected)	***Type II error***	***No error***

FIGURE 3.10 Types of error in hypothesis testing illustrated using the hypotheses in Faupel-Badger et al. (2006).

t-test described above yields a p-value of 0.045, which also leads to the decision to reject the null hypothesis that the mean change in estradiol levels is 0 pg/mL since the p-value is less than the significance level of 0.05. It should be noted that performing a one-sample t-test on the mean change (after − before) in serum estradiol levels yields exactly the same result as using the paired t-test (Section 4.4.2.1) to compare subjects' serum estradiol levels before and after taking raloxifene. Note also that the CI and hypothesis testing results yield the same conclusions regarding the mean change in serum estradiol levels; this will always be the case if the appropriate CI and hypothesis testing procedures are used.

In Example 3.5, the one-sample t-test would generally be considered to be the appropriate way to address the research question and test the corresponding null hypothesis, assuming that the change in serum estradiol level follows a normal distribution. (This assumption could be verified using the methods described in Section 4.2.2.) But different research questions and data structures call for different statistical methods. Regardless of the specific statistical method used, a test statistic is calculated using the sample data. In many hypothesis testing situations, the test statistic k_0 will have the general form

$$k_0 = \frac{\hat{\theta} - \theta_0}{\mathrm{SE}(\hat{\theta})}, \tag{3.9}$$

where $\hat{\theta}$ denotes the sample estimate of the unknown parameter θ, θ_0 denotes the hypothesized value of θ, and $\mathrm{SE}(\hat{\theta})$denotes the estimated standard error of $\hat{\theta}$. When testing a "two-sided" hypothesis of the form $H_0 : \theta = \theta_0$ versus $H_a : \theta \neq \theta_0$, larger values of the test statistic (in absolute value) provide stronger evidence that H_0 is false and should be rejected. The sampling distribution of the test statistic is assumed to be known under the assumption that H_0 is true; this probability distribution is referred to as the "null distribution" of the test statistic. (For example, the commonly used "Wald method" is based on the assumption that the test statistic in (3.9) follows a standard normal distribution.) Therefore, under the assumption that the null hypothesis is true, one can calculate the p-value, which is the probability that a random sample of data would yield a test statistic as large as or larger in magnitude than the value of the test statistic calculated from the observed data. The p-value is then compared with the prespecified significance level (α). Alternatively, one can compare the calculated value of the test statistic with the critical value corresponding to α, which is obtained from the null distribution of the test statistic. If the absolute value of the test statistic is greater than or equal to the critical value, H_0 is rejected. This is equivalent to the p-value being less than or equal to the significance level. On the other hand, if the absolute value of the test statistic is less than the critical value, the null hypothesis is not rejected; this is equivalent to the p-value being greater than the significance level.

The decision to either reject or fail to reject a particular hypothesized value of the unknown parameter should be the same, regardless of whether the decision was reached by testing $H_0 : \theta = \theta_0$ vs. $H_a : \theta \neq \theta_0$ using significance level α, or by constructing a $100(1 - \alpha)\%$ CI for the unknown parameter θ. If the p-value for the test of $H_0 : \theta = \theta_0$ is less than or equal to α (leading to rejection of H_0), then the $100(1 - \alpha)\%$ CI for θ will exclude the null value θ_0. Similarly, if the p-value for the test of $H_0 : \theta = \theta_0$ is greater than α (leading to failure to reject H_0), then the $100(1 - \alpha)\%$ CI for θ will include the null value θ_0.

Example 3.5 Continued

In the study by Faupel-Badger et al. (2006) discussed previously, the p-value for the test of $H_0 : \theta = 0$ was 0.045, and the 95% CI for the true value of θ was (1–84) pg/mL. Both analyses result in the decision to reject the null hypothesis and conclude that there is a significant change in the serum estradiol levels of premenopausal women at high risk for developing breast cancer after taking raloxifene. This conclusion can be reached because the 95% CI for the mean change in estradiol levels did not include the "null value" of 0 pg/mL, and the hypothesis test rejected the null hypothesis of no change in serum estradiol level $H_0 : \theta = 0$ since $p < 0.05$. Note, however, that the equivalence between hypothesis testing and CI estimation is dependent on two conditions: (1) the equivalent hypothesis testing and CI procedures are used, and (2) the "directions" of the hypothesis test and CI are the same. With regard to (1), if a test statistic of the form in Equation (3.9) is used, for example, then the correct CI formula would be $\hat{\theta} \pm k^* SE(\hat{\theta})$, where k^* is the appropriate critical value for a $100(1 - \alpha)\%$ CI for θ. (If the Wald method is being used, then $k^* = z_{\alpha/2}$.) Thus, one could not necessarily expect to obtain the same conclusions concerning a binomial proportion if an exact hypothesis test were used, but a Wald CI was calculated. With regard to condition (2), there are "one-sided" CI procedures corresponding to "one-sided" hypothesis tests; that is, those with alternative hypotheses of the form $H_a : \theta > \theta_0$ or $H_a : \theta < \theta_0$. If a one-sided alternative hypothesis is used, then it is necessary to use the corresponding one-sided CI in order to obtain equivalent conclusions. One-sided CIs are beyond the scope of this text; however, they are covered in most standard introductory biostatistics textbooks (e.g., Rosner 2011, pp. 193–195).

Examination of the formula for the CI for the population mean in (3.6) reveals that the CI tends to become wider when the sample size decreases or the variability (as measured by s) increases. Thus, either of these changes would decrease the statistical power to detect, for example, a change in estradiol level. The width of the CI also varies with the level of confidence that the true value of the population mean lies within the interval; the higher the confidence coefficient, the wider the CI will be. (Note that a larger confidence coefficient corresponds to a smaller significance level since the confidence coefficient is given by $100(1 - \alpha)$.) Thus, as the confidence coefficient increases (or, equivalently, as the significance level decreases), it will be more difficult to detect a true departure from the null hypothesis.

Each hypothesis testing method has a corresponding test statistic that possesses a particular null distribution (i.e., when the null hypothesis is assumed to be true). The distribution of the particular test statistic under the null hypothesis sometimes depends on the *df*, which is a function of characteristics of the sample of data such as the sample size, the number of categories a nominal or ordinal variable assumes, etc. It is necessary to know both the significance level and the *df* in order to obtain the critical value, which is then compared to the value of the test statistic calculated using the sample data in order to decide whether or not to reject the null hypothesis.

Much of the remainder of this book will be devoted to discussing different statistical methods for analyzing biomarker data. Many of these methods will involve hypothesis testing, utilizing specific formulas to compute the test statistic and degrees of freedom (if applicable). The hypothesis testing framework described above puts the "burden of proof" on the alternative hypothesis. By default, the null hypothesis is not rejected unless the sample of data provides compelling evidence to the contrary. For example, when $\alpha = 0.05$, there must be a probability of 0.05 or less that we would obtain a sample result (as summarized by the test statistic) as extreme as the one we observed, assuming that our null hypothesis is true. So when the null hypothesis is not rejected, it is not logical to conclude that the null hypothesis is true. This is the foundation and key underlying concept of all of statistical hypothesis testing.

The preceding discussion concerning hypothesis testing and CI estimation assumes the ideal scenario where no selection bias is present, meaning that a representative sample from the *target population* has been obtained. The target population is the population about which statistical inference is being made. For example, the inference from the Faupel-Badger et al. (2006) study that raloxifene increases serum estradiol levels is valid only for premenopausal women who have a high risk of developing breast cancer. Faupel-Badger et al. (2006) identified this as their target population by defining specific *inclusion criteria,* which are the characteristics a subject must possess in order to be allowed to enroll in the study. To be eligible for their study, a potential study subject had to be a female between 23 and 47 years of age who was experiencing regular menses and meeting at least one of the three well-defined clinical criteria for being considered at high risk for developing breast cancer. Once the target population has been defined, the researchers should do everything possible to ensure that a representative sample from that population is obtained. Thus, recruiting study subjects by soliciting volunteers or obtaining some other type of convenient nonrepresentative sample would compromise the validity and generalizability of conclusions drawn from the study results. However, under some circumstances, convenience sampling is the only viable method available for obtaining the study data. See Section 2.2 for a discussion of principles of good study design.

3.7 COMPARING MEANS ACROSS GROUPS

There are occasions when a researcher might want to compare the mean level of a biomarker between two groups (e.g., cases and controls) or among more than two groups (e.g., cancer patients treated with three different chemotherapy regimens). The *equal variance t-test* is the most commonly used statistical method to compare the means of two groups in terms of a continuous DV while *analysis of variance* (ANOVA) is commonly used to compare means across three or more groups. It should be noted that the *t*-test and ANOVA are only appropriate when two assumptions are met: (1) the data in all groups being compared are sampled from a normally distributed population and (2) all groups being compared have the same population variance (Sheskin 2007, pp. 427, 868). Methods for diagnosing violations of these assumptions and alternative statistical methods to use when assumptions are violated are discussed in Chapter 4.

3.7.1 Two Group Comparisons

The question of whether or not two groups differ in terms of the mean level of some biomarker can be formulated as the following null and alternative hypotheses:

$$H_0 : \mu_1 = \mu_2 \text{ vs. } H_a : \mu_1 \neq \mu_2, \tag{3.10}$$

where μ_1 and μ_2 denote the population mean biomarker levels in the two groups.

The equal variance *t*-test (sometimes called Student's *t*-test) is used to test the hypotheses in (3.10) by comparing the means of two independent samples assumed to arise from normal distributions with equal variances. The test statistic for comparing the means of two groups is given by

$$t_0 = \frac{\bar{x}_1 - \bar{x}_2}{s_p \sqrt{\frac{1}{n_1} + \frac{1}{n_2}}}, \tag{3.11}$$

where n_1 and n_2 are the number of observations in the two groups, and s_p is the "pooled" sample standard deviation:

$$s_p = \sqrt{\frac{(n_1 - 1)s_1^2 + (n_2 - 1)s_2^2}{n_1 + n_2 - 2}}.$$

(In this formula, s_1^2 and s_2^2 denote the sample variances for groups 1 and 2, respectively.) Once the value of t_0 in (3.11) has been calculated using the sample data, it is compared with the appropriate critical value; namely, the upper $\alpha/2$-percentage point from a *t*-distribution with $n_1 + n_2 - 2$ degrees of freedom: $t^* = t_{\alpha/2, n_1+n_2-2}$. If the absolute value of t_0 is greater than or equal to t^*, the null hypothesis in (3.10) is rejected. Equivalently, the two-tailed *p*-value can be calculated using a Student's *t*-distribution with $n_1 + n_2 - 2$ *df* and compared with the standard significance level of 0.05.

Example 3.6 Comparison of Two Means

To illustrate the equal variance *t*-test, consider the Na–K ATPase data given in Example 3.1. For the 11 bipolar patients on placebo, $\bar{x}_1 = 0.562$ and, for the 10 patients on lithium, $\bar{x}_2 = 0.790$. For the patients on placebo, $s_1 = 0.252$ and, for the patients on lithium, $s_2 = 0.257$. The "pooled" standard deviation is calculated to be 0.254 and the equal variance *t*-test statistic in (3.11) is given by $t_0 = -2.051$, with 19 *df*. The critical value is given by the upper 0.025-percentage point of a *t*-distribution with 19 *df*: $t_{0.025,\,19} = 2.093$. Since $|-2.051| < 2.093$, the decision is to fail to reject $H_0 : \mu_1 = \mu_2$. Equivalently, using a *t*-distribution with 19 *df*, the test statistic $t_0 = 2.051$ yields a two-tailed *p*-value of 0.054, which also indicates that the null hypothesis should not be rejected since it is greater than 0.05.

The following SAS code can be used to perform the equal variance *t*-test for the data in Example 3.1:

```
proc ttest data=ATPase;
class group;
var NaK_ATPase;
title 't-test comparing bipolar patients on lithium and placebo';
run;
```

Homogeneity, or more accurately, *homoscedasticity*, the equality of population variances in the two groups being compared, is an assumption underlying the equal variance *t*-test and the performance of the *t*-test can be adversely affected when this assumption is not met (Moser et al., 1989). See Section 4.3.2.1 for a discussion of how to deal with apparent violations of the equal variance assumption when comparing the means of two groups.

3.7.2 Multiple-Group Comparisons

The comparison of biomarker levels among more than two groups is sometimes of interest in research studies involving biomarkers. For example, as part of a study examining the relationship between umbilical cord coiling length and maternal diabetes, Lemoine et al. (2013) compared the umbilical cord coiling lengths among ethnic groups (Caucasian, African American, Hispanic, Asian, etc.). The umbilical cord coiling length was calculated as the distance (in cm) between two pairs of coils on a longitudinal section of the cord obtained via ultrasound.

ANOVA is the most commonly used statistical method for this task. Specifically, one-way ANOVA can be used to compare the means of three or more groups, assuming that the biomarker levels in each group are normally distributed and have equal population variances across groups (Sheskin 2007, p. 868). Under these assumptions, ANOVA can be used to test

$$H_0 : \mu_1 = \mu_2 = \cdots = \mu_k \text{ vs. } H_a\text{: at least two means are different,} \quad (3.12)$$

where k is the number of groups being compared. The F-test statistic for this hypothesis is equal to the "mean square between groups" (MSB) divided by the "mean square within groups" (MSW). Thus, $F_0 = \text{MSB/MSW}$, where MSB is given by

$$\text{MSB} = \frac{\sum_{i=1}^{k} n_i(\overline{y}_i - \overline{\overline{y}})^2}{k-1}, \tag{3.13}$$

and MSW is given by

$$\text{MSW} = \frac{\sum_{i=1}^{k} \sum_{j=1}^{n_i} (y_{ij} - \overline{y}_i)^2}{n-k}. \tag{3.14}$$

In these formulas, y_{ij} = the biomarker level of the jth subject in the ith group, $\overline{y}_i$ = the mean biomarker level within the ith group, $\overline{\overline{y}}$ = the "grand mean" of the biomarker levels for all n subjects, k = the number of groups being compared, and n_i = the sample size in group i; $i = 1, 2, \ldots, k$ and $j = 1, 2, \ldots, n_i$.

Note that MSB is an overall measure of how much the group means vary from the grand mean, and MSW is an overall measure of how much the biomarker levels in each group differ from their respective group means. (MSW can also be thought of as a measure of the total error in the ANOVA model, and is sometimes referred to as the "mean square for error" [MSE]). The divisors for each of the mean squares represent the "degrees of freedom" associated with that mean square. A detailed discussion of how degrees of freedom are determined for ANOVA models is beyond the scope of this text; see Kutner et al. (2004, pp. 1359–1361) or another applied linear models textbook for a general approach.

The ANOVA test statistic, given by $F_0 = \text{MSB/MSW}$, is a measure of the relative magnitude of the variability between groups to that within groups. If the variability between groups is sufficiently large relative to the variability within groups, we reject the null hypothesis that all groups have the same population mean. Specifically, the null hypothesis H_0 in (3.12) is rejected if the F-statistic is greater than the appropriate critical value from the F distribution; namely, the upper α-percentage point of the F distribution with $k-1$ and $n-k$ degrees of freedom for the numerator and denominator, respectively.

Example 3.7 One-Way ANOVA

Consider the study by Lemoine et al. (2013) that compared umbilical cord coiling lengths among Caucasians, African Americans, and other ethnicities. The umbilical cord coiling length was calculated as the distance between two pairs of coils on a longitudinal section of the cord, obtained via ultrasound.

Table 3.4 contains a subsample of $n_1 = n_2 = n_3 = 20$ observations of umbilical cord coiling lengths from the three largest ethnic groups in the study (Caucasian, African American, Hispanic). For the data in Table 3.4, $\overline{y}_1 = 3.67$, $\overline{y}_2 = 2.35$, $\overline{y}_3 = 3.05$, $\overline{\overline{y}} = 3.02$, $k = 3$, $n_1 = 20$, $n_2 = 20$, and $n_3 = 20$. Thus, MSB = 8.73 and MSW = 2.32;

TABLE 3.4 Umbilical Cord Coiling Lengths for Caucasian, African American, and Hispanic Subjects

Ethnic Group	Umbilical Cord Coiling Length (cm)									
Caucasian	1.88	1.94	2.46	3.23	1.72	1.12	2.27	0.95	1.74	2.96
	1.60	2.32	5.43	1.94	1.64	1.52	2.06	1.97	5.36	2.83
African American	2.63	4.94	2.36	4.72	2.22	4.50	2.92	4.40	1.52	4.38
	4.44	6.01	4.47	2.25	4.67	2.21	4.83	1.28	4.86	3.75
Hispanic	2.16	1.78	3.07	5.89	2.87	3.95	1.71	1.75	5.36	1.96
	4.03	1.98	2.88	1.27	6.31	1.63	1.53	1.22	7.91	1.64

Source: Data courtesy of Dr. Joseph M. Miller, Jr.

hence, $F_0 = \text{MSB}/\text{MSW} = 3.77$ with 2 and 57 *df*. The ANOVA reveals a significant difference across ethnic groups ($p = 0.029$). Table 3.5 illustrates how an "ANOVA table" is used to summarize the various sources of error for a one-way ANOVA design.

If we fail to reject the null hypothesis in (3.12), we conclude that there are no significant differences among the mean biomarker levels of the k groups. But when the null hypothesis H_0 in (3.12) is rejected, we are usually not satisfied to end the analysis with the conclusion that at least one pair of group means are not equal. It is usually of interest to determine which pairs of group means are significantly different from each other; this is generally referred to as *post hoc analysis* or *pairwise comparisons*.

There are a number of methods that can be used for *post hoc* analysis. One might naïvely propose to use either the t-test to compare each pair of groups in terms of their mean biomarker level. The problem with this approach is that for each individual pairwise comparison, the probability of making a Type I error is equal to the significance level, α. Thus, the *experiment-wise Type I error rate*, defined to be the probability of making at least one Type I error out of all possible pairwise comparisons, will be larger (usually, much larger) than the original α. One commonly used strategy to avoid this so called "alpha inflation" is to use a *Bonferroni adjustment*. The Bonferroni-adjusted α-level (α') for each pairwise comparison is given by

$$\alpha' = \alpha / c, \tag{3.15}$$

where $c = k(k-1)/2$ is the total number of possible pairwise comparisons among the k group means. The test statistic for the equal variance t-test is then computed for each

TABLE 3.5 Analysis of Variance (ANOVA) Table for Example 3.7

Source	SS	*df*	MS	*F*	*P*-value
Ethnicity	17.47	2	8.73	3.77	0.029
Error	132.13	57	2.32	–	–
Total	149.59	59	–	–	–

pairwise comparison, but the critical value from the t-distribution corresponding to α' is used instead of the critical value corresponding to α to determine the statistical significance of each of the $k(k-1)/2$ pairwise comparisons. Sometimes, we are also interested in constructing Bonferroni-adjusted confidence limits; this would be obtained by using the same formula as for an unadjusted CI, but replacing the $\alpha/2$-percentage point with the $\alpha'/2$ value.

A useful feature of using the Bonferroni adjustment is that it is rather easy to obtain Bonferroni-adjusted p-values for each pairwise comparison once the t-test statistics have been calculated. For each test statistic, one finds the usual two-tailed p-value using the appropriate t-distribution, and then multiplies by the number of possible pairwise comparisons. If this Bonferroni-adjusted p-value is less than the desired experiment-wise error rate (usually 0.05), the population means being compared are declared to be significantly different. (Note that if this Bonferroni p-value is calculated to be greater than 1.0, it is truncated at 1.0.)

The *least significant differences* (LSD) method is another approach for *post hoc* analysis. To apply the LSD method, for each pairwise comparison of groups, one computes a modified form of the equal variance t-statistic in (3.11) by substituting the MSW from the ANOVA in place of the pooled variance estimate, s_{p}^2. Then one compares this test statistic to the appropriate critical value; namely, the upper α-percentage point from a Student's t-distribution with $n-k$ degrees of freedom.

Tukey's *Honest Significant Difference* (HSD) test (also called the *Tukey–Kramer (TK) method*) is one of the most commonly used procedures for performing *post hoc* analysis. For example, Bernstein et al. (1999) used Tukey's method to perform all pairwise comparisons of the mean level of their apoptotic index across three groups: (a) "normal" subjects; that is; those with no previous history of polyps or cancer; (b) patients with a history of colorectal cancer; and (c) patients with colorectal adenomas.

The HSD method is very similar to the LSD method. As with the LSD, for each pairwise comparison of groups, one computes a modified form of the equal variance t-statistic in (3.11) by substituting the MSW from the ANOVA in place of the pooled variance estimate s_{p}^2. Instead of comparing this test statistic to a critical value from the Student's t-distribution with $n-k$ degrees of freedom, one uses a critical value from the *Studentized range* distribution. In particular, the modified test statistic used in the HSD method is compared with $\frac{\mathrm{SR}_{\alpha,k,n-k}}{\sqrt{2}}$, where $\mathrm{SR}_{\alpha,g,\upsilon}$ = upper α-percentage point of the distribution of the Studentized range of g normal variates with an estimate of the variance based on υ degrees of freedom. Tables of this distribution are widely available (e.g., http://cse.niaes.affrc.go.jp/miwa/probcalc/s-range/ or Zar 2010, pp. 717–732), and the TK method is easily applied using SAS or another standard statistical software package.

Example 3.8 Tukey–Kramer Method

As stated previously, for the data in Table 3.4, $\bar{y}_1 = 3.67$, $\bar{y}_2 = 2.35$, and $\bar{y}_3 = 3.05$. In addition, from the ANOVA results in Table 3.5, we know that MSE = 2.32. From the tables in Zar (2010) or other sources, we find that the appropriate critical value of the Studentized range distribution is $SR_{0.05,3,57} = 3.40311$; thus, $SR_{0.05,3,57}/\sqrt{2} = 3.40311/\sqrt{2} = 2.406$. So, for example, to compare the mean umbilical cord coiling length for Caucasians versus African Americans, we use the following test statistic:

$$TK_0 = \frac{\bar{x}_1 - \bar{x}_2}{s_p\sqrt{\frac{1}{n_1} + \frac{1}{n_2}}} = \frac{3.67 - 2.35}{\sqrt{2.32\left(\frac{1}{20} + \frac{1}{20}\right)}} = 2.742. \quad (3.16)$$

Since $2.742 > 2.406$, we conclude that there is a significant pairwise difference in mean umbilical cord coiling length between Caucasians and African Americans according to the TK method. A similar calculation to that in (3.16) for the pairwise comparisons of Caucasians versus Hispanics and African Americans versus Hispanics indicates that neither of these pairwise comparisons is statistically significant using the TK method. The LSMEANS statement in either the GLM or MIXED procedures can be used to perform TK pairwise comparisons; a convenient feature of using this approach is that SAS will produce TK-adjusted p-values for the pairwise comparisons, which are then compared with the desired significance level (almost always 0.05 in biomarker studies). For the data in Table 3.4, the TK p-values for the Caucasian versus African American, Caucasian versus Hispanic, and African American versus Hispanic pairwise comparisons are 0.022, 0.323, and 0.404, respectively. Only the Caucasian versus African American pairwise comparison is significant.

When all of the groups being compared in terms of their mean biomarker level have the same population variance, Tukey's method is preferred (Dunnett, 1980a); however, if the variances are not equal, there are other methods that perform better (Dunnett, 1980b). See Section 4.3.2.3 for a discussion of these alternative methods.

SAS can be used to perform all of the tests described here for comparing the means of more than two groups. We recommend Littell et al. (2002) for detailed instructions about how to use SAS to perform ANOVA and other analyses related to linear statistical models.

The SAS code used to perform the ANOVA tests and pairwise comparison methods on the data in Table 3.4 is provided below:

```
data Caucasian;
input coil @@;
ethnicity = 'Caucasian';
datalines;
1.88  1.94  2.46  3.23  1.72  1.12  2.27  0.95  1.74  2.96
1.60  2.32  5.43  1.94  1.64  1.52  2.06  1.97  5.36  2.83
;
run;
```

```
data AA;
input coil @@;
ethnicity = 'AA';
datalines;
2.63  4.94  2.36  4.72  2.22  4.50  2.92  4.40  1.52  4.38
4.44  6.01  4.47  2.25  4.67  2.21  4.83  1.28  4.86  3.75
;
run;

data Hispanic;
input coil @@;
ethnicity = 'Hispanic';
datalines;
2.16  1.78  3.07  5.89  2.87  3.95  1.71  1.75  5.36  1.96
4.03  1.98  2.88  1.27  6.31  1.63  1.53  1.22  7.91  1.64
;
run;

data all;
set Hispanic AA Caucasian;
run;

proc glm data=all;
class ethnicity;
model coil = ethnicity ;
means ethnicity / bon tukey lsd  ;
lsmeans ethnicity  /  pdiff;
title 'Comparison of coil lengths among ethnic groups';
run;
```

3.8 CORRELATION ANALYSIS

Correlation analysis is used to assess the association between two variables. When both variables are normally distributed, Pearson's correlation coefficient (PCC) is the appropriate measure of association. When at least one of the variables is not normally distributed, a nonparametric alternative, Spearman's correlation coefficient (SCC) or Kendall's concordance coefficient (KCC), should be used to measure the association. The SCC and the KCC can also be used to measure the association between ordinal variables. See Section 4.5.1 for a discussion of alternatives to the PCC. SAS code that can be used to perform all of the correlation analyses discussed in this textbook can be found following Example 4.20 and on the companion website.

Pearson's correlation, denoted by ρ in the population, measures the degree of linear association between two continuous variables. PCC can assume values ranging from 1 to -1 (inclusive), with a PCC of 1 (-1) indicating a perfect increasing (decreasing) linear relationship between the two variables and a PCC of 0 indicating no linear relationship. For two continuous random variables X and Y, the PCC is estimated by the sample correlation, r, which is equal to the sample covariance divided by the square root of the product of the sample variances:

$$r = \frac{\widehat{\mathrm{cov}(X, Y)}}{\sqrt{\widehat{\mathrm{var}(X)}\widehat{\mathrm{var}(Y)}}} \tag{3.17}$$

$$\widehat{\mathrm{cov}(X, Y)} = \sum_{i=1}^{n} (x_i - \overline{x})(y_i - \overline{y})/(n - 1),$$

$$\widehat{\mathrm{var}(X)} = \sum_{i=1}^{n} (x_i - \overline{x})^2/(n - 1),$$

and

$$\widehat{\mathrm{var}(Y)} = \sum_{i=1}^{n} (y_i - \overline{y})^2/(n - 1).$$

An equivalent formula, which is particularly useful if the standard deviations of the x- and y-values have already been calculated is (Helsel 2012, p. 218)

$$r = \frac{1}{n-1} \sum_{i=1}^{n} \left(\frac{x_i - \overline{x}}{s_x} \right) \left(\frac{y_i - \overline{y}}{s_y} \right).$$

In terms of hypothesis testing for the PCC, there is an exact test of $H_0 : \rho = 0$ based on the t-distribution. The test statistic is given by

$$t_0 = \frac{r\sqrt{n-2}}{\sqrt{1-r^2}}, \tag{3.18}$$

which is compared with the upper $\alpha/2$-percentage point from a t-distribution with $n - 2$ degrees of freedom. The problem with using this approach to perform statistical inference for the PCC is that the test statistic in (3.18) can be used only to test the null value $\rho_0 = 0$. This means that there is no corresponding CI procedure that will yield a conclusion identical to that obtained when (3.18) is used as the test statistic. Instead, the *Fisher z-transformation* can be used to transform the sample correlation r to a new random variable that is approximately normally distributed. This transformed random variable can then be used to derive a test statistic for testing $H_0 : \rho = \rho_0$, where ρ_0 is any hypothesized value (zero, negative, or positive) of the PCC. This transformed random variable can also be used to derive an approximate CI for the true value of the PCC. The use of the Fisher z-transform is discussed in Section 4.5.2.

An example of hypothesis testing for the PCC can be found in Murphy et al. (2004). In their comparison of urinary biomarkers of tobacco and carcinogen exposure in smokers, the authors found a significant positive correlation between %NNAL glucuronidation and %cotinine glucuronidation in their sample of n = 47 smokers ($r = 0.310$, $p = 0.034$).

The p-value given in Murphy et al. is for the test of the null hypothesis H_0: $\rho = 0$. Testing this hypothesis is equivalent to testing the null hypothesis that the slope is 0 in the simple linear regression (SLR) of Y on X (see Section 3.9.1). It should be noted that concluding that a PCC is significantly different from 0 does not necessarily indicate that there is a clinically relevant association between the two variables. This issue is discussed in more detail in Section 4.5.3.

3.9 REGRESSION ANALYSIS

3.9.1 Simple Linear Regression

In standard statistical notation, the "slope-intercept" form of the equation of a straight line is represented as $Y = \beta_0 + \beta_1 X$, where X and Y represent the values of Cartesian coordinates corresponding to points on the line, β_1 represents the slope of the line, and β_0 denotes the y-intercept of the line (i.e., the point where the line crosses the vertical, or y-axis). But the relationship between two random variables will generally not be perfectly linear. In other words, most, if not all, of the plotted pairs (x, y) from a bivariate sample of data will not fall exactly in a straight line. An error (or disturbance) term is used to quantify each observation's vertical distance from the true linear relationship that relates Y to X.

Using the notation previously defined for the true slope and y-intercept of the regression line, the SLR model takes the form

$$Y = \beta_0 + \beta_1 X + \varepsilon, \tag{3.19}$$

where ε is a normally distributed error term with a mean of 0 and a variance of σ^2. The *least squares regression line* is the straight line that minimizes the sum of squared errors (also called *residuals*) in a sample of bivariate data $\{(x_i, y_i); i = 1, 2, \ldots, n\}$. The quantity to be minimized is given by $\sum_{i=1}^{n} e_i^2 = \sum_{i=1}^{n} (y_i - \hat{y}_i)^2$,where, for the ith individual, $e_i = y_i - \hat{y}_i$ denotes the residual; y_i denotes the observed value of Y; $\hat{y}_i$ denotes the predicted value of Y, $\hat{y}_i = \hat{\beta}_0 + \hat{\beta}_1 x_i$; and x_i denotes the observed value of X; $i = 1, 2, \ldots, n$. The body of statistical techniques used to fit and evaluate the best fitting line to a collection of (x, y) data pairs is called *SLR analysis*.

The slope of the regression line describes the linear relationship between two variables, X and Y. The estimated slope, denoted by $\hat{\beta}_1$, can be interpreted as the estimated change in the mean of Y corresponding to a one unit increase in X. When

$\beta_1 > 0$, Y tends to increase as X increases; when $\beta_1 < 0$, Y tends to decrease as X increases; and when $\beta_1 = 0$, there is no linear relationship between X and Y.

For a bivariate sample of data pairs $\{(x_i, y_i); i = 1, 2, \ldots, n\}$, the estimated slope and intercept of the line in Equation (3.19) are given by

$$\hat{\beta}_1 = \frac{\sum_{i=1}^{n} (x_i - \bar{x})(y_i - \bar{y})}{\sum_{i=1}^{n} (x_i - \bar{x})^2} \tag{3.20}$$

and

$$\hat{\beta}_0 = \bar{y} - \hat{\beta}_1 \bar{x},$$

respectively. The estimated standard errors of the estimated regression parameters are given by

$$\widehat{\text{SE}}(\hat{\beta}_1) = \sqrt{\frac{\text{MSE}}{\sum_{i=1}^{n} (x_i - \bar{x})^2}}$$

and

$$\widehat{\text{SE}}(\hat{\beta}_0) = \sqrt{\text{MSE}\left[\frac{1}{n} + \frac{\bar{x}^2}{\sum_{i=1}^{n} (x_i - \bar{x})^2}\right]},$$

where $\text{MSE} = \sum_{i=1}^{n} (y_i - \hat{y}_i)^2/(n-2)$ denotes the "mean squared error" of the regression model.

Assuming that the sample of Y values $\{y_i; i = 1, 2, \ldots, n\}$ are normally distributed, the null hypotheses H_0: $\beta_1 = 0$ and H_0: $\beta_0 = 0$ can be tested by first calculating the test statistics:

$$t_{01} = \frac{\hat{\beta}_1}{\widehat{\text{SE}}(\hat{\beta}_1)} \tag{3.21}$$

and

$$t_{00} = \frac{\hat{\beta}_0}{\widehat{\text{SE}}(\hat{\beta}_0)}$$

and then comparing the absolute value of t_{00} and t_{01} with the Student's t-distribution with $n - 2$ degrees of freedom.

The statistics in (3.21) can be employed to derive $100(1 - \alpha)\%$ CIs for β_1 and β_0

$$\hat{\beta}_1 \pm t^* \widehat{\text{SE}}(\hat{\beta}_1), \qquad (3.22)$$
$$\hat{\beta}_0 \pm t^* \widehat{\text{SE}}(\hat{\beta}_0),$$

where $t^* = t_{\alpha/2,\, n-2}$ is the upper $\alpha/2$-percentage point of the Student's t-distribution with $n - 2$ *df*.

As an example of the use of SLR in a biomarker study, Södergren et al. (2010) examined the association between age (the IV) and various endothelial biomarker levels (the DVs) in Swedish patients diagnosed with early rheumatoid arthritis. For the biomarker sL-selectin, the fitted SLR equation yielded an estimated slope of −14.4, which can be interpreted to mean that the blood level of sL-selectin in an early rheumatoid arthritis patient is expected to decrease by 14.4 ng/mL for each additional year of age. The test of H_0: $\beta_1 = 0$ indicated that this is a highly significant change ($p < 0.001$).

SLR can be performed using the REG procedure in SAS. An example of SAS code that can be used to fit an SLR model is provided following Example 3.9.

Example 3.9 Simple Linear Regression

As part of a study investigating the role of anemia in pediatric heart disease, Goldberg et al. (2014) compared the serum hemoglobin concentrations (g/dL) of male and female heart disease patients less than 23 years of age. For purposes of this example, we consider the regression of Y = "serum hemoglobin concentration" on X = "age" using the subsample of the original dataset provided in Table 3.6 ($n = 30$). Applying the formulas in Equation (3.20), we obtain the fitted regression line $\hat{Y} = \hat{\beta}_0 + \hat{\beta}_1 X = 10.301 + 0.108X$. Thus, as age increases, there is an estimated mean increase of 0.108 g/dL in serum hemoglobin concentration for each additional year of age. The formulas in (3.20) also yield $\widehat{\text{SE}}(\hat{\beta}_1) = 0.051$ and $\widehat{\text{SE}}(\hat{\beta}_0) = 0.632$. Applying the formulas in (3.21), we obtain the test statistics $t_{01} = 2.14$ for the test of H_0: $\beta_1 = 0$ and $t_{00} = 16.29$ for the test of H_0: $\beta_0 = 0$. Using a t-distribution with $df = 28$, we obtain $p = 0.0411$ for the test of H_0: $\beta_1 = 0$ and, for the test of H_0: $\beta_0 = 0$, we obtain $p < 0.0001$. Thus, the null hypotheses H_0: $\beta_1 = 0$ and H_0: $\beta_0 = 0$ are both rejected. For β_1, this indicates that there is a "significant linear relationship" between serum hemoglobin concentration and age. For β_0, rejection of the null hypothesis indicates that the true y-intercept is not 0, but this is of little practical significance since it merely implies that the serum hemoglobin concentration at birth (i.e., when age is 0 years) is significantly different from 0. In terms of 95% CIs for the true values of the regression parameters, Equation (3.22) yields (0.005–0.212) for β_1 and (9.006–11.596) for β_0. The value of R^2, obtained from Equation (3.24), indicates that only 14.1% of the variation in serum hemoglobin concentration is explained by age alone.

The following SAS code can be used to perform the SLR of serum hemoglobin on age for these data.

```
data heart;
input Subject Hemoglobin Gender $ Age;
1  11.1  male  5.1
...

proc reg data=heart;
model Hemoglobin = age / clb;
run;
```

3.9.2 Multiple Regression

Multiple linear regression (MLR) is an extension of SLR that can accommodate more than one IV, enabling one to examine the effect of each IV on the DV, after adjusting for the effects of the other IVs on the DV. The estimated slope ($\hat{\beta}_k$) for the kth IV can be interpreted as the estimated change in the mean of Y for a one unit increase in X_k after adjusting for the contributions of the other IVs in the MLR model.

For p IVs, the MLR model takes the form

$$Y = \beta_0 + \beta_1 X_1 + \beta_2 X_2 + \cdots + \beta_p X_p + \varepsilon, \tag{3.23}$$

where, for $k = 1, 2, \ldots, p$, X_k represents the kth IV (assumed to be measured without error), β_k represents the coefficient for X_k, and ε is a normally distributed error term with mean 0 and variance σ^2. As with SLR, we use MLR to obtain estimates of the parameters (β_0, $\beta_1, \ldots, \beta_p$), denoted by ($\hat{\beta}_0$, $\hat{\beta}_1 \ldots \hat{\beta}_p$). This is accomplished by using the method of least squares, which minimizes the sum of squared errors $\sum_{i=1}^{n} (y_i - \hat{y}_i)^2$, where y_i denotes the observed value of Y for the ith individual; $\hat{y}_i$ denotes the predicted value of Y for the ith individual, $\hat{y}_i = \hat{\beta}_0 + \sum_{k=1}^{p} \hat{\beta}_k x_{ik}$; and x_{ik}denotes the observed value of the kth IV X_k for the ith individual, $i = 1, 2, \ldots, n$; $k = 1, 2, \ldots, p$.

In Section 3.9.1, SLR was described as a statistical method for modeling the relationship between a single continuous IV and a continuous DV. MLR can accommodate categorical as well as continuous IVs. For a dichotomous IV X_k, an *indicator variable* (sometimes called a "dummy variable") is created so that one of the two categories of the original variable is assigned a value of 0 and the other category is assigned a value of 1. For a nominal variable with more than two categories, one of the categories is designated as the reference group and a separate indicator variable is created for each of the remaining categories, with the indicator variable taking a value of 1 for observations that are in the corresponding category; otherwise the indicator variable is set to 0. No indicator variable is created for the reference category.

For example, suppose that the analyst wishes to incorporate the ethnic origin of the study subjects into an MLR model. In the study data, the nominal variable ethnicity has three levels: Caucasian, African-American, and Hispanic. One way to convert this nominal variable into dummy variables would be to define the reference category to be Hispanic, and create two dummy variables: X_1, which has the value 1 if the study subject is Caucasian, and 0 otherwise; and X_2, which has the value 1 if the study subject is African-American, and 0 otherwise. Hispanic study subjects would then be identified by $X_1 = X_2 = 0$. In this way, all three ethnic origin categories would be included in the MLR model.

Using this variable coding scheme for nominal IVs preserves the interpretation of the estimated regression coefficient $\hat{\beta}_k$ for a dichotomous IV as the estimated increase in the mean of Y corresponding to a one unit increase in the value of X_k (i.e., being in the category corresponding to the indicator variable having a value of 1 as opposed to the reference category having the value of 0), after adjusting for the other IVs in the model.

Ordinal IVs with k ordered values can also be converted into $k - 1$ dummy variables as described above. However, we have generally found it to be more useful not to perform this recoding, but to instead retain the original values of the ordinal IV and treat it as if it were a continuous variable in the MLR analysis.

On occasion, it may be of interest to examine the *interaction* between a quantitative IV and a categorical IV, or between two categorical IVs in an MLR model. The presence of an interaction term in an MLR model implies that the relationship between one of the IVs and the DV depends on the value of the other IV included in the interaction term. For example, Shlipak et al. (2003) used MLR to investigate inflammatory and procoagulant biomarker levels in 5888 elderly subjects by including the IVs age, race, gender, education, renal insufficiency, cardiovascular disease status, diabetes, hypertension, blood pressure, cholesterol, triglycerides, smoking, alcohol consumption, physical activity, and body mass index. They found a significant interaction between the IVs race and renal insufficiency when modeling Factor VII level (one of the biomarkers) as the DV. White study participants with renal insufficiency had Factor VII levels 11% higher than white study participants without renal insufficiency on average, whereas black study participants with renal insufficiency had Factor VII levels an average of 15% higher than black study participants without renal insufficiency.

A quantity that is often used to measure how well a SLR or multiple regression model fits a set of data is the *coefficient of determination* (R^2), which is equal to the proportion of the variation in the DV that is explained by the regression model. It is calculated as the ratio of the regression sum of squares (SSR) to the total sum of squares (SST):

$$R^2 = \frac{\text{SSR}}{\text{SST}} = \frac{\sum_{i=1}^{n} (\hat{y}_i - \bar{y})^2}{\sum_{i=1}^{n} (y_i - \bar{y})^2}. \tag{3.24}$$

Generally, any value of $R^2 \geq 0.75$ indicates that the regression model provides an adequate fit to the data.

The *overall F test* can be used to test the null hypothesis that the coefficients of all IVs in the regression model are 0 versus the alternative hypothesis that at least one of the coefficients is not 0; in other words, to test

$$H_0 : \beta_1 = \beta_2 = \cdots = \beta_p = 0 \text{ vs. } H_a : \text{at least one } \beta_k \text{ is not } 0 \qquad (3.25)$$

The test statistic for the hypothesis in (3.25) is equal to the mean square for regression (MSR) divided by the mean square for error (MSE):

$$F_0 = \frac{\text{MSR}}{\text{MSE}} = \frac{\sum_{i=1}^{n} (\hat{y}_i - \bar{y})^2 / p}{\sum_{i=1}^{n} (y_i - \hat{y}_i)^2 / (n - p - 1)}, \qquad (3.26)$$

which is compared to the appropriate critical value; in this case, the upper α-percentage point of the F distribution with numerator and denominator degrees of freedom equal to p and $n - p - 1$, respectively. Rejecting the null hypothesis in (3.25) implies that the regression model (which accounts for the effects of all of the IVs on the DV) contributes significantly to the prediction of the DV.

Deciding which variables to include in a multiple regression model is challenging. Adding an IV to an MLR model is guaranteed to increase the value of R^2, regardless of its predictive ability. Thus, the increase in R^2 should not be used as the sole criterion for deciding which variable(s) to add to an MLR model because *overfitting* can occur due to inclusion of irrelevant predictors, thereby causing the model to perform poorly when applied to a new set of data that is external to the sample used to fit the model. On the other hand, failure to include important IVs will result in a lower percentage of the variation in the DV being explained by the model, thereby decreasing predictive ability of the MLR model. (Both types of model-building errors fall into the general category of *model misspecification*, which is one of the major pitfalls in regression analysis.)

Numerous statistical criteria (adjusted R^2, Mallow's C_p, Akaike information criterion, Bayesian information criterion, etc.) have been proposed for helping to develop a parsimonious MLR model by balancing quality of model fit versus the number of IVs retained in the model. Automated variable selection methods are also available; these typically involve examining the effect of adding (forward selection) or removing (backward elimination) one IV at a time until some stopping rule is satisfied. An in-depth discussion of variable selection in MLR is beyond the scope of this text, but we caution the data analyst against blindly applying any statistical procedure for variable selection. Instead, clinical relevance and interpretability, as well as statistical significance, should always be considered in light of the purpose of the regression model (e.g., is the MLR model being built only for the identification of IVs significantly associated with the DV, or is it to be used to predict or estimate the response of an individual for which Y cannot be observed?). George Box's (1987) elucidation that "all models are wrong but some are useful" reminds the analyst of the subjectivity inherent to the process of building a regression model. Thus, examination of numerous regression models constructed from the same data set can be informative. All possible subsets and best subsets regression are alternatives to automated variable selection procedures that should always be considered when attempting to build a parsimonious MLR model. Any comprehensive textbook on regression analysis should provide a complete discussion of these issues and other aspects of regression modeling (e.g., Kutner et al. 2004; Montgomery et al. 2012).

In an application of MLR modeling to biomarker data, Södergren et al. (2010) examined the usefulness of various endothelial biomarkers in patients with early rheumatoid arthritis. They repeatedly applied SLR analysis to select candidates for inclusion in their MLR model: "Simple linear regression (variables with $P < 0.05$) together with clinical assumptions, determined which covariates were included in the MLR models." They found a significant positive association between sL-selectin level and endothelial-dependent flow-mediated dilation (a measure of arteriosclerosis) in a SLR model, again in a multiple regression model adjusting for rheumatoid arthritis disease activity score, and yet again in a third MLR model further adjusting for systolic blood pressure and smoking status. While such an approach may indeed result in a clinically useful and parsimonious MLR model, we recommend that one use a more systematic approach to variable selection (e.g., see Kutner et al. 2004, pp. 343–376).

After formulating a "final" MLR model, the analyst should undertake a rigorous examination of regression diagnostics, which includes assessing *multicollinearity* (the effects of intercorrelation among the IVs in the regression model), examining influence statistics to detect possible outliers, and inspecting residual plots to identify patterns that indicate possible violations of the assumptions underlying the MLR model (i.e., linearity, normality, homogeneity, independence of the error terms). (Similar diagnostics are available for examining the quality of SLR models as well.) We strongly encourage our readers to consult textbooks devoted to regression analysis (e.g., Kutner et al. 2004; Montgomery et al. 2012) for a thorough coverage of these topics and other intricacies of regression analysis. We recommend Freund and Littell (2000) for detailed instructions on using SAS for linear regression.

3.9.3 Analysis of Covariance

ANOVA and linear regression are both special cases of what is called the *general linear model*. As illustrated in the examples taken from the studies by Södergren et al. (2010) and Shlipak et al. (2003) (Sections 3.9.1 and 3.9.2, respectively), the IVs in a multiple regression model can be a combination of categorical and continuous predictors. Analysis of covariance (ANCOVA) is another special case of the general linear model; it can be thought of as a mixture of ANOVA (usually with only two groups) and SLR. ANCOVA can be used to determine if the population mean of a continuous DV is equal across groups defined by a single categorical IV, after adjusting for the effect of a continuous covariate that is not of primary interest. The one-way ANCOVA model can be expressed as

$$Y = \beta_0 + \beta_1 X + \beta_2 Z + \varepsilon, \tag{3.27}$$

where Y denotes the continuous DV, X denotes the continuous covariate, Z represents the categorical IV defining the groups to be compared in terms of the mean of Y, and ε denotes the error term that is assumed to be normally distributed with mean 0 and variance σ^2. Note that Z will be defined in terms of a dummy variable if Z is dichotomous, but, as discussed above, more than one dummy variable will be needed if Z has more than two levels. In traditional ANCOVA, it is assumed that there is no interaction between the categorical variable and the continuous covariate. This *homogeneity of regression* assumption implies that the slope of the regression line between Y and X is the same for each level of Z. This assumption can be tested by fitting the model given by

$$Y = \beta_0 + \beta_1 X + \beta_2 Z + \beta_{12} XZ + \varepsilon. \tag{3.28}$$

If the coefficient of the interaction term (β_{12}) is significantly different from 0, the traditional ANCOVA model in Equation (3.27) is not valid. However, a valid statistical analysis can still be performed using multiple regression. (See Kutner et al. 2004, pp. 917–940, for a thorough discussion of ANCOVA.)

In an application of ANCOVA to biomarker data, Tsai et al. (2010) compared the metabolic syndrome-related biomarker levels of 37 medicated schizophrenic patients to that of 30 healthy controls. Applying the equal variance t-test, one does not find a statistically significant difference ($t = 0.76$, $df = 65$, $p = 0.448$) between the mean fasting serum insulin levels of medicated schizophrenic patients (8.4 mU/L $\pm$ 6.4) and that of healthy controls (7.4 mU/L $\pm$ 3.6). However, when Tsai et al. used ANCOVA to adjust for age, the medicated schizophrenic patients had significantly higher mean fasting serum insulin levels than healthy controls ($F = 4.69$; $df = 1, 65$; $p = 0.034$). It is important to note that Tsai et al. did not present the *adjusted* means from their ANCOVA; for example, the estimated mean fasting serum insulin levels, after adjusting for the effect of age. It is considered good statistical practice to report the adjusted means in addition to the unadjusted means any time ANCOVA is used.

Example 3.10 ANCOVA

As part of a study investigating the role of anemia in pediatric heart disease, Goldberg et al. (2014) compared the serum hemoglobin concentrations (g/dL) of male and female heart disease patients less than 23 years of age. The subsample of the original dataset provided in Table 3.6 will be analyzed for the purpose of illustration. Since age is known to influence hemoglobin levels (see Example 3.9), it makes sense to adjust for the effect of age when comparing the serum hemoglobin concentration of males and females. This could be accomplished via ANCOVA, but first the homogeneity of regression assumption should be tested by including the gender × age interaction term in the initial regression model. The SAS code below is used to create a numeric "sex" variable and then create a gender × age interaction term ("gender_age") as the product of "sex" and "age":

```
data heart;
input Subject   Hemoglobin  Gender $  Age;
if gender = "male" then sex = 1;
else if gender = "female" then sex = 0;
gender_age = sex*age;
datalines;
1  11.1  male  5.1
...
```

Next, the SAS code below is used to test the homogeneity of regression assumption:

```
proc reg data=heart;
model Hemoglobin = sex age gender_age;
run;
```

The resulting SAS output indicates that the null hypothesis that there is an interaction between age and gender cannot be rejected at the 5% significance level ($t = 1.71$, $df = 26$, $p = 0.0993$). Thus, the interaction term can be removed before proceeding to fit the ANCOVA model (which includes the gender and age main effects) using the SAS code below. (Note that this code includes the INFLUENCE, VIF, and COLLIN options within the REG procedure which can be used to obtain information about influential observations and assess problems related to multicollinearity as part of the examination of regression diagnostics. See Freund and Littell (2000) for details about using SAS to perform regression diagnostics.)

```
proc reg data=heart;
model Hemoglobin = sex age / influence vif collin;
run;
```

The resulting output from the REG procedure indicates that, after adjusting for the effect of age, the mean serum hemoglobin level for males is estimated to be 2.15 g/dL higher than for females, which represents a statistically significant difference ($t = 3.25$, $df = 27$, $p = 0.0031$). The output also indicates that, after adjusting for the effect of gender, the serum hemoglobin level increases by an estimated mean of 0.115 g/dL for each additional year of age, which is a statistically significant increase ($t = 26.4$, $df = 27$, $p = 0.0137$). Although the ANCOVA model explains a statistically significant proportion of the variation in serum hemoglobin ($F = 8.36$, $df_1 = 2$, $df_2 = 27$, $p = 0.0015$), the R^2 value indicates that only 38.2% of the variation in serum hemoglobin is explained by this model. Thus, if the analyst wishes to build a regression model to accurately predict a heart disease patient's serum hemoglobin level, more candidate IVs should be considered for possible inclusion in the model to improve predictive accuracy.

As indicated in our general discussion of ANCOVA, it is generally considered to be good statistical practice to report the adjusted means, as well as the unadjusted means, any time ANCOVA is used. In the present case, there is very little difference between the unadjusted and adjusted means for the two genders. For males, the unadjusted mean is 10.28 g/dL, whereas the mean adjusted for age is 10.23 g/dL. For females, the unadjusted mean is 12.34 g/dL, whereas the mean adjusted for age is 12.38 g/dL. However, adjusting for age does give a slightly lower p-value for the gender comparison: $p = 0.0042$ without the adjustment and $p = 0.0031$ with the adjustment. In addition to the REG procedure, the GLM procedure can also be used to perform ANCOVA, and can produce the adjusted (using the LSMEANS statement) and unadjusted means (using the MEANS statement), as well as the tests of the age and gender effects. The following SAS code can be used to carry out these analyses for the data in Table 3.6:

```
proc  glm data=heart;
      class gender;
      model Hemoglobin = gender age ;
      means gender;
      lsmeans gender / stderr pdiff;
      title1 'ANCOVA';
      title2 'Adjusted Means';
 run;
```

3.10 ANALYZING CROSS-CLASSIFIED DATA

3.10.1 Testing for Independence

In elementary probability, two events A and B are considered to be *independent* if the occurrence of event A does not affect the probability of the occurrence of event B and vice versa. For example, suppose an experiment consists of tossing a balanced coin and rolling a fair die. It is reasonable to assume that the outcome of the roll of the die does not depend in any way on the outcome of the toss of the coin, so it is reasonable to assume that getting Heads on the coin (Event A) and getting a 6 on the die (Event B) are independent.

If A and B are independent events, then according to the Law of Probability for Independent Events (also known as the "multiplication rule"), the probability that both events will occur simultaneously is equal to the product of the probabilities of the individual events:

$$P(A \text{ and } B) = P(A) \times P(B). \tag{3.29}$$

The χ^2 (chi-squared) test is commonly used to test the null hypothesis of independence between two nominal variables, both of which could be dichotomous. (See Section 4.9.4.2 for discussion of an alternative method.) The χ^2 test uses the multiplication rule to compute the expected frequency of all possible combinations of

TABLE 3.6 Gender, Age, and Serum Hemoglobin Concentrations of 30 Heart Disease Patients Less Than 23 Years of Age

Subject	Hemoglobin (g/dL)	Gender	Age (years)
1	11.1	Male	5.1
2	10.5	Female	19.9
3	12.2	Male	15.8
4	12.8	Male	21.6
5	10.8	Male	7.0
6	9.4	Male	1.0
7	11.9	Male	3.5
8	10.8	Male	14.3
9	13.0	Female	3.7
10	14.2	Male	3.9
11	6.7	Female	1.6
12	8.4	Female	1.6
13	10.2	Male	0.5
14	15.6	Male	15.1
15	9.3	Female	0.4
16	10.2	Female	22.2
17	10.4	Male	0.7
18	12.1	Female	11.6
19	15.2	Male	17.4
20	13.1	Male	16.0
21	8.1	Female	12.4
22	8.4	Female	17.5
23	11.0	Female	16.2
24	11.0	Female	0.3
25	11.0	Female	1.6
26	11.2	Male	4.3
27	11.4	Female	18.0
28	12.1	Male	8.5
29	12.8	Female	18.3
30	16.5	Male	19.3

Source: Data courtesy of Dr. Jack Price.

the categories of the two nominal variables under the assumption that the null hypothesis of independence is true, and then compares these "expected" frequencies to the frequencies actually observed in the sample data. Both the expected and observed frequencies are calculated from a sample of cross-classified data consisting of n observations. The "canonical form" of a 2×2 table for assessing the independence of two nominal variables with two categories each is given in Table 3.7.

Consider two nominal variables X and Y having I and J distinct categories, respectively. A two-way *contingency table* with I rows and J columns can be used to represent all possible combinations of each category of X (the "row variable") with each category of Y (the "column variable"). (Each of these combinations is referred

TABLE 3.7 Canonical Form of a 2 × 2 Table for Assessing Independence of Two Nominal Variables with Two Categories Each.

	Level of Variable 2		
Level of Variable 1	1	2	Total
1	n_{11}	n_{12}	$n_{1\bullet}$
2	n_{21}	n_{22}	$n_{2\bullet}$
Total	$n_{\bullet 1}$	$n_{\bullet 2}$	n

to as a *cell*.) The *observed frequency* for each of the IJ cells is obtained by counting the number of subjects in the sample that fall into that cell, and the *relative frequency* for each cell is then found by dividing the observed frequency by the total sample size, n. Relative frequencies for each row and column in the $I \times J$ table are calculated in a similar manner.

Using the "multiplication rule" for independent events given in (3.29), the product of the relative frequencies for row i and column j is used to estimate the expected proportion of all n observations that would fall into cell (i, j) under the null hypothesis that the row variable X and the column variable Y are independent. This proportion is then multiplied by n in order to obtain the expected frequency (i.e., expected cell count) for cell (i, j) under the null hypothesis. For each of the IJ cells in the contingency table, the difference between the observed and the expected frequency is squared and this squared value is then divided by the expected cell count in that cell. These quantities are then summed across all cells to obtain the χ^2 test statistic:

$$\chi_0^2 = \sum_{i=1}^{I} \sum_{j=1}^{J} \frac{(n_{ij} - \hat{\mu}_{ij})}{\hat{\mu}_{ij}}, \qquad (3.30)$$

where the expected count in cell (i, j) is given by

$$\hat{\mu}_{ij} = n \left(\frac{n_{i\bullet}}{n} \right) \left(\frac{n_{\bullet j}}{n} \right) = \frac{n_{i\bullet} n_{\bullet j}}{n}.$$

In these formulas, $n_{i\bullet}$ is the total number of observations in the ith row, $n_{\bullet j}$ is the total number of observations in the jth column, and n_{ij} is the number of observations in cell (i, j).

The most common type of contingency table found in biomarker studies is the 2×2 (i.e., two rows and two columns), as in Table 3.7. For a 2×2 table, there is a shortcut computational formula for the χ^2 test statistic in (3.30):

$$\chi_0^2 = \frac{n \left(n_{11} n_{22} - n_{12} n_{21} \right)^2}{n_{1\bullet} n_{2\bullet} n_{\bullet 1} n_{\bullet 2}}. \qquad (3.31)$$

Once computed, the χ^2 test statistic in (3.30) is compared with the appropriate critical value; namely, the upper α-percentage point from a χ^2distribution with $(I-1)(J-1)$ degrees of freedom. If the test statistic is greater than this critical value, we reject the null hypothesis of independence and conclude that there is a significant association between X and Y. A general discussion of how to determine degrees of freedom for cross-classified data is beyond the scope of this textbook. An excellent description of this at a very basic level can be found in Agresti (2007, p. 37).

The FREQ procedure in SAS can be used the perform the χ^2 test for an $I \times J$ contingency table of any dimension, as well as the alternatives to the traditional χ^2 test that are described in Section 4.9.

Example 3.11 The χ^2 Test

As an example of the application of the χ^2 test to biomarker data, consider the study by Ayadi et al. (2010). Based on immunohistochemical staining results (positive or negative) using surgical tissue specimens obtained from 57 patients diagnosed with ovarian carcinoma (see Table 3.8), they wished to determine if expression of the estrogen receptor (ER) is independent of the expression of the progesterone receptor (PR). The χ^2 test indicates that PR and ER expression are *not* independent ($\chi^2 = 24.1$, $df = 1, p < 0.001$).

The SAS code to perform the χ^2 test for an association between PR and ER expression is provided below:

```
data Ayadi;
input PR $ ER $ count;
datalines;
+ + 33
+ - 5
- + 4
- - 15
;
run;
```

TABLE 3.8 Association between ER and PR Expression in 57 Ovarian Cancer Patients[a]

	ER		
PR	Positive	Negative	Total
Positive	33 (24.7)	5 (13.3)	38
Negative	4 (12.3)	15 (6.7)	19
Total	37	20	57

Source: Adapted from Table 3 of Ayadi et al. (2010, p. 122). Public Domain.
[a]Observed cell counts are given in the body of the table, with expected frequencies in parenthesis.

```
proc freq data=Ayadi;
tables PR*ER / chisq ;
weight count;
title1 'ER and PR Expression in Ovarian Cancer Patients';
title2 'Chi-square Test for Independence';
run;
```

3.10.2 Comparison of Proportions

A frequent objective of biomedical research involving biomarkers is to evaluate the effects of exposure to a possible risk factor for a certain disease. For example, does exposure to environmental (second-hand) cigarette smoke increase one's risk of lung cancer? An intuitive way to evaluate such a risk factor is to compare the estimated probability of disease for those exposed to the risk factor under study versus the estimated probability of disease for those not exposed to the risk factor (commonly referred to as the "unexposed"). Assuming that one has a representative sample from the target population of interest, the true probabilities of disease for the exposed (π_1) and unexposed (π_2) individuals can be estimated by the proportion of exposed study participants with disease (p_1) and the proportion of unexposed study participants with disease (p_2), respectively. An approximate $100(1-\alpha)\%$ CI for the true difference between the proportions (i.e., $\pi_1 - \pi_2$), also known as the *risk difference* or the *attributable risk* (see Section 4.9.1.3) is given by the familiar Wald interval:

$$(p_1 - p_2) \pm z_{\alpha/2}\hat{\sigma}_{\mathrm{d}}, \tag{3.32}$$

where the estimated standard error of the difference in proportions is given by

$$\hat{\sigma}_{\mathrm{d}} = \sqrt{\frac{p_1(1-p_1)}{n_1} + \frac{p_2(1-p_2)}{n_2}}.$$

If this CI does not include 0, the null hypothesis $H_0 : \pi_1 = \pi_2$ is rejected.

In biomedical research (and in most applications involving biomarkers), it is more common for researchers to compare the probability of disease for those exposed versus those not exposed by examining the ratio of the probabilities instead of the difference, i.e., π_1/π_2 rather than $\pi_1 - \pi_2$. (For a related discussion, see Agresti 2007, pp. 27–28.) This ratio of proportions is called the *relative risk* (RR) and is estimated in the sample by

$$\widehat{\mathrm{RR}} = p_1/p_2. \tag{3.33}$$

(The RR is also referred to as the *risk ratio*.) Because the sampling distribution of $\widehat{\mathrm{RR}}$ tends to be highly skewed, the natural logarithm is used to transform $\widehat{\mathrm{RR}}$ to a random variable that more closely resembles the normal distribution. The log-transformed

$\widehat{RR}$ is then used to derive an approximate CI for the true RR. Thus, an approximate $100(1-\alpha)\%$ CI for the true RR is given by

$$\exp\left[\ln(p_1/p_2) \pm z_{\alpha/2}\sqrt{\frac{1-p_1}{n_1p_1}+\frac{1-p_2}{n_2p_2}}\right], \tag{3.34}$$

where n_1 and n_2 represent the number of exposed and unexposed subjects, respectively, and "exp" denoted the exponentiation operator e^X.

If the CI in (3.34) includes the "null value" of 1, we conclude that there is no association between the risk factor and the disease. On the other hand, if both endpoints of the CI are greater than 1, we conclude that exposure to the risk factor significantly increases the risk of disease. If both endpoints of the CI are less than 1, the interpretation is that exposure significantly reduces the risk of disease. An approximate test of the null hypothesis H_0 : RR = 1 can be performed by calculating the following test statistic and then referring it to the standard normal:

$$z_0 = \frac{\ln(p_1/p_2)}{\sqrt{\frac{1-p_1}{n_1p_1}+\frac{1-p_2}{n_2p_2}}}. \tag{3.35}$$

An example of the use of the RR in a study involving biomarkers can be found in Rabinovitch et al. (2011). The authors investigated the association between urinary leukotriene E4 levels and risk of severe exacerbations in asthmatic children exposed to second-hand tobacco smoke (SHS). As part of their study, they examined the risk for asthmatic children exposed to second-hand smoke to have an emergency department (ED) or urgent care (UC) visit. They found that, "Three (12.5%) of 24 non–SHS-exposed children and 9 (45%) of 20 SHS-exposed children required an ED or UC visit during the study period. Exposure to SHS was significantly ($P = 0.02$) associated with an ED or UC visit (RR, 3.6; 95% CI, 1.1–11.5)."

The RR is not an appropriate measure of the association between exposure and disease if the study participants cannot be considered to be a representative sample of exposed and unexposed subjects; for example, as in a case–control study (Section 2.2.3). For further discussion of this and related issues, see Sections 2.3.1 and 4.9.1, where we provide guidance on choosing the most appropriate measure of association in a research study.

The most commonly used alternative to the risk ratio for measuring association is the *odds ratio* (OR), which is an appropriate measure of association under a wide variety of research scenarios. The OR is equal to the ratio of the odds of disease for the exposed study participants, divided by the odds of disease for the unexposed. (If π represents the probability that an event will occur, the *odds* that the event will occur is defined to be $\pi\ /\ (1-\pi)$.) Thus, using the proportions of disease among the

TABLE 3.9 Canonical 2 × 2 Table for Assessing the E-D Association

	Disease		
Exposure	Present (D+)	Absent (D−)	Total
Present (E+)	a	b	$a+b$
Absent (E−)	c	d	$c+d$
Total	$a+c$	$b+d$	n

exposed and unexposed in the sample, an estimate of the true OR can be calculated as follows:

$$\widehat{\text{OR}} = \frac{p_1/(1-p_1)}{p_2/(1-p_2)}. \tag{3.36}$$

The canonical 2 × 2 table for examining the exposure–disease (E–D) association using the "a, b, c, d" notation is given in Table 3.9. As with the sampling distribution of $\widehat{\text{RR}}$, the sampling distribution of $\widehat{\text{OR}}$ tends to be highly skewed, so the natural logarithm is used to transform $\widehat{\text{OR}}$ to a random variable that is approximately normally distributed. This log-transformed $\widehat{\text{OR}}$ is then used to derive an approximate CI for the true OR. An approximate $100(1-\alpha)\%$ CI for the true OR is given by

$$\exp\left[\ln(\widehat{\text{OR}}) \pm z_{\alpha/2}\sqrt{\frac{1}{a}+\frac{1}{b}+\frac{1}{c}+\frac{1}{d}}\right], \tag{3.37}$$

where the numbers of exposed subjects with disease, exposed subjects without disease, unexposed subjects with disease, and unexposed subjects without disease are represented by a, b, c, and d, respectively. Note that, using this notation, $\widehat{\text{OR}} = ad/bc$. An approximate test of the null hypothesis H_0 : OR = 1 can be performed by calculating the following test statistic and comparing it with the standard normal distribution:

$$z_0 = \frac{\ln(\widehat{\text{OR}})}{\sqrt{\frac{1}{a}+\frac{1}{b}+\frac{1}{c}+\frac{1}{d}}}. \tag{3.38}$$

The FREQ procedure in SAS can be used to perform these analyses for the OR, as well as the alternative methods that are described in Section 4.9.

Example 3.12 The Odds Ratio

Hobbs et al. (2005) examined the association of low plasma methionine level (<24.17 μmol/L) in pregnant women with the presence of congenital heart defects in

TABLE 3.10 Frequency of Low and Normal Plasma Methionine Levels and Births with and without Congenital Heart Defects in 313 Pregnant Women

	Disease		
Exposure	Congenital Heart Defect	No Heart Defect	Total
Low methionine level	103	27	130
Normal methionine level	120	63	183
Total	223	90	313

Source: Adapted from Table 4 of Hobbs et al. (2005, p. 151) with permission from the American Society for Nutrition.

their offspring. Of the 223 mothers whose infants had a congenital heart defect (the cases), 103 (46.2%) had a low plasma methionine level; of the 90 mothers whose infants did not have a heart defect (the controls), 27 (30.0%) had a low methionine level, yielding an estimated OR of $\widehat{\text{OR}} = 2.00$, with a 95% CI for the true OR of (1.19, 3.38). This indicates a significant *increase* in the odds of congenital heart defects for pregnant women with plasma methionine below 24.17 μmol/L since both endpoints of the CI are greater than 1. The data from this study are displayed in the usual "*a*, *b*, *c*, *d*" format in Table 3.10.

The SAS code used to analyze the contingency table shown in Table 3.10 is provided below. We highly recommend the book by Stokes et al. (2012) as a very useful reference for understanding how to use SAS (especially the FREQ procedure) to analyze categorical data effectively.

```
data Hobbs;
input methionine $ heart $ count;
datalines;
low defect 103
low normal 27
normal defect 120
normal normal 63
;
run;

proc freq data=Hobbs;
tables  methionine*heart / relrisk;
weight count;
title1 'Methionine Levels and Heart Defect Status';
title2 'Odds Ratio';
run;
```

PROBLEMS

3.1. Data on the systolic pulmonary artery pressure (SPAP) (mm Hg) and right atrial emptying rate (RAER) (counts per second assessed using radionuclide labeled red blood cells) of 26 hypothetical chronic obstructive pulmonary disease (COPD) patients are shown in the following table.

A. Compute the following descriptive statistics on for the SPAP and RAER sample data in the table: sample median, mode, $\bar{x}$, s^2, s, CV, $p_{0.25}$, $p_{0.75}$, $\widehat{SEM}$, 95% CI on μ.

B. Compute the PCC to assess the linear association between SPAP and RAER using the data in the table. Is there a statistically significant association between right atrial emptying rate and systolic pulmonary artery pressure? What proportion of the variation in systolic pulmonary artery pressure is explained by right atrial emptying rate?

C. Use simple linear regression to compute the predicted change in systolic pulmonary artery pressure for every count per second increase in right atrial emptying rate.

D. Generate a scatter plot to display the relationship between right atrial emptying rate (x-axis) and systolic pulmonary artery pressure (y-axis).

The Systolic Pulmonary Artery Pressure and Right Atrial Emptying Rate of 26 Hypothetical Chronic Obstructive Pulmonary Disease (COPD) Patients

Subject	Systolic Pulmonary Artery Pressure (mm Hg)	Right Atrial Emptying Rate (counts per second)
1	64.1	34.1
2	61.9	17.0
3	81.8	26.0
4	44.3	35.8
5	34.5	71.1
6	32.9	63.0
7	20.8	60.6
8	41.4	59.6
9	45.0	43.3
10	75.5	30.8
11	61.0	19.3
12	59.6	13.2
13	49.9	39.8
14	58.9	51.4
15	32.8	63.2
16	31.0	59.7
17	24.2	68.3

(*continued*)

Subject	Systolic Pulmonary Artery Pressure (mm Hg)	Right Atrial Emptying Rate (counts per second)
18	29.5	66.1
19	19.3	65.1
20	21.6	70.2
21	27.2	68.5
22	24.5	83.2
23	13.9	73.8
24	30.3	27.3
25	38.1	92.0
26	39.5	41.0

3.2. Ross et al. (1992) conducted a nested case–control study (for each hepatocellular carcinoma case, "5 or 10 controls were randomly selected from cohort members without liver cancer") to examine the presence of detectable urinary aflatoxins in subjects with and without hepatocellular carcinoma. Of the 22 study participants with hepatocellular carcinoma, 13 had detectable urinary aflatoxins. Of the 140 participants without hepatocellular carcinoma, 53 had detectable urinary aflatoxins. Construct a 2×2 table from this information and assess the association between presence of aflatoxin in the urine and hepatocellular carcinoma status.

3.3. Lund et al. (2001) conducted a retrospective cohort study to compare the risk of hyperlipidemia in schizophrenic patients taking Clozapine versus other antipsychotic drugs by examining medical and pharmacy claims from the Iowa Medicaid program. (Although hyperlipidemia was dichotomized as "yes" or "no" for this example, there are a number of subcategories of hyperlipidemia that are characterized by an excess of serum lipids such as cholesterol, cholesterol esters, phospholipids, and triglycerides.) Use the data in the following table to determine if there is a difference in risk of hyperlipidemia in schizophrenic patients taking Clozapine compared to other antipsychotic drugs. Compute the estimated proportion and 95% CI on the true proportion of schizophrenic patients with hyperlipidemia separately for those taking Clozapine and other antipsychotic drugs.

Type of antipsychotic drug and hyperlipidemia status of 2891 schizophrenic patients

		Hyperlipidemia?	
		Yes	No
Drug	Clozapine	26	492
	Other Antipsychotic	93	2280

3.4. Suppose a study of the utility of α-methylacyl coenzyme A racemase (AMACR) as a tissue biomarker for prostate cancer yielded the results in the following table.

A. Compute descriptive statistics (n, $\bar{x}$, and s) and the 95% confidence interval on the mean AMACR expression level for each of the three tissue types.

B. Use box plots to display the AMACR expression levels for each tissue type.

C. Use ANOVA to compare the mean AMACR expression level for each of the three tissue types. If necessary, use the Tukey–Kramer (TK) method for *post hoc* analysis.

AMACR expression level (Cy5/Cy3 ratio) in prostate samples from three types of tissue.

Benign	Hyperplastic	Malignant
1.4	0.9	3.7
1.0	1.8	5.3
1.0	0.6	1.2
0.7	2.1	5.1
1.4	2.1	5.4
1.3	0.6	2.2
1.3	1.4	3.4
1.3	1.7	3.5
1.6	1.8	6.2
1.0	2.3	3.2
0.7	1.5	6.4
1.0	1.1	4.2
1.1	1.8	1.5
0.6	0.8	
0.8	1.2	
0.5	0.8	
1.2		
0.9		
1.4		
0.9		
1.1		
0.8		
1.4		

3.5. Hartung et al. (2005) used an Oregon Medicaid claims database to conduct a case–control study with a 6:1 case:control matching ratio to investigate the association between Thiazolidinedione therapy and heart failure. Controls were matched with cases on age and gender. Of the 288 heart failure subjects, 59 had received Thiazolidinedione therapy. Of the 1652 study subjects who had not experienced heart failure, 216 had received Thiazolidinedione therapy. Construct a 2×2 table from this information and assess the association between Thiazolidinedione therapy and heart failure.

4

FREQUENTLY ENCOUNTERED CHALLENGES IN ANALYZING BIOMARKER DATA AND HOW TO DEAL WITH THEM

4.1 INTRODUCTION

The proper analysis of biomarker data often requires that the analyst employ statistical methods that are not usually covered in introductory statistics courses or textbooks. In this chapter, we illustrate some of the challenges faced in dealing with biomarker data using examples from the biomarker literature and our own experience. For each of these challenges, we provide descriptions and illustrations of those statistical methods that we have found to be most useful in dealing with these challenges. It is often the case that biomarker data require "non-standard" analyses because of the presence of non-normality, heterogeneity, dependence, clustering, censoring, etc. Sample sizes in biomarker studies can be rather small, so that large-sample approximations to the null distributions of test statistics are no longer valid. For these reasons, we have recommended that exact methods be used whenever possible, and have emphasized the use of distribution-free and robust methods when available. In many instances, we have used published studies from the scientific literature to illustrate improper or inadequate applications of "standard" statistical analyses when dealing with biomarker data. While it may seem that we have been overly critical of the authors of these studies, our intent has been simply to demonstrate that many of the published analyses of biomarker data analyses have not made full use of the vast array of statistical tools that are readily available for these analyses. We readily acknowledge that the statistical analyses that appear in print usually represent the best that could be done at the time of publication due to unavoidable limitations in terms of time, personnel, or resources, and that more thorough (or even different)

Analysis of Biomarker Data: A Practical Guide, First Edition. Stephen W. Looney and Joseph L. Hagan.

analyses could have been performed under different circumstances. Our primary goal in writing this chapter is to provide our readers with statistical tools that they can use to conduct proper analyses of biomarker data in their future research endeavors. We hope that we have been able to "fill the gap" in terms of tools that some analysts may not have been aware of or had access to because of lack of software, etc.

To the greatest extent possible, we have based our recommendations in this Chapter and elsewhere in this book on the published advice of recognized authorities in the field. In addition, we have drawn on our combined experience of over 45 years of analyzing data from many different fields of scientific research. We emphasize statistical methods and procedures that can be implemented using widely available statistical software, and we provide software code (primarily SAS) that can be used to carry out the recommended analyses. However, since statistics is a dynamic field, many of the recommendations contained in this chapter may soon prove to be obsolete because of new developments in the discipline and/or new advances in statistical software.

4.2 NON-NORMALLY DISTRIBUTED DATA

4.2.1 The Effects of Non-Normality

Many commonly used statistical procedures are based on the assumption that the variables being examined in the data analysis follow a particular statistical distribution. Of course, the most common underlying distributional assumption is the normal. For example, Student's t-test, the most commonly used method to compare the mean biomarker level between two groups, is based on the assumption that the biomarker data follow a normal distribution. (See Section 3.7.1.) A bivariate normal distribution, in which both X and Y have a normal distribution, is assumed for the two variables being examined in a correlation analysis using Pearson's correlation coefficient (PCC, see Section 3.8). The serious adverse effects that violations of underlying distributional assumption(s) can have on the performance of a statistical procedure are well known (Algina et al. 1994; Wilcox 1987, pp. 103–104, 130). Hence, attempting to verify the assumption that the data are normally distributed prior to undertaking a data analysis is a worthwhile endeavor. However, it is an unfortunate fact that many analysts working with biomarker data ignore the underlying distributional assumptions and/or make no attempt to check these assumptions before proceeding with an analysis of biomarker data. Statements such as "due to the skewed nature of the data, nonparametric statistical methods were used" sometimes appear in the Methods or Results section of a published analysis of biomarker data, but there is typically no indication that any formal test of the underlying distributional assumption was ever performed. For example, Atawodi et al. (1998), when describing their examination of hemoglobin adducts as biomarkers of exposure to tobacco smoke, state that "because the distribution of HPB-Hb adduct levels was not normal, we used the nonparametric Kruskal-Wallis test ..." (p. 819). However, they offer no justification for why they concluded that the adduct levels were not normally distributed.

Apart from verifying the assumption of normality as a prelude to applying a statistical test based on this assumption, it may also be of interest to verify that a sample of biomarker values are normally distributed so that previously established standards or tests based on the normal distribution may be applied. For example, in MacRae et al. (2003), the authors examined the feasibility of using the Beckman Coulter Access Analyzer to obtain maternal serum values for three commonly used biomarkers for assigning patient-specific risk for Down's syndrome at mid-trimester. MacRae et al. used probability plots (Section 4.2.2.1) and the Shapiro–Wilk (S-W) test (Section 4.2.2.3) to determine if serum concentrations of serum α-fetoprotein, unconjugated estriol, and human chorionic gonadotropin obtained using the Beckman Coulter analyzer were normally distributed after applying a $\log_{10}$ transformation. It was necessary to establish normality of these biomarkers so that patient-specific risks could be calculated using published Gaussian (i.e., normal) distribution parameters for the biomarkers that were estimated using data from previously available immunoassays.

4.2.2 Testing Distributional Assumptions

Many authors have proposed methods for determining whether or not a particular distributional assumption is reasonable for a set of observed data. (The general term describing these methods is *goodness-of-fit* tests.) In fact, several books have been written dealing with this topic (e.g., D'Agostino and Stephens 1986; Huber-Carol et al. 2002), and many articles have been published comparing the performance of various commonly used methods for testing particular distributional assumptions. Most of these articles deal with goodness-of-fit tests for the normal distribution (e.g., Shapiro et al. 1968; Pearson et al. 1977; Henderson 2006). We focus our attention on two areas related to testing the assumption of normality for a set of biomarker data: (1) graphical methods, which are the most commonly used approach, and (2) formal goodness-of-fit tests for the normal distribution that have been shown to have good statistical properties. For a more thorough treatment, see Thode (2002). It is important to note that tests of the normality assumption can also be used to test whether a set of data follow the lognormal distribution; that is, after applying the (natural) logarithmic transformation to the original measurements, do the transformed measurements follow a normal distribution? A similar approach can be used to determine whether *any* transformation results in data that more closely resemble the normal distribution (see Section 4.2.3.1).

4.2.2.1 Graphical Methods for Assessing Normality Several authors have proposed graphical methods for verifying the assumption of normality (D'Agostino 1986), and these methods continue to be an area of active methodological research (Aldor-Noiman et al. 2013). These methods include quantile–quantile (Q–Q) plots and probability–probability (P–P) plots (Wilk and Gnanadesikan 1968), both of which are special cases of probability plots (Gerson 1975). All of these plots, as well as many others, can be constructed using the UNIVARIATE procedure in SAS.

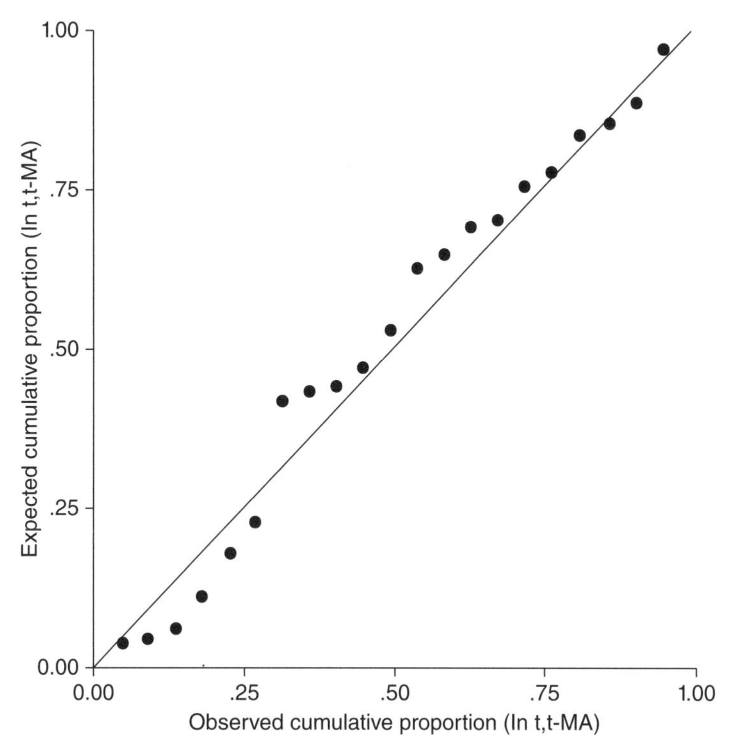

FIGURE 4.1 Normal probability plot of urinary *trans, trans* muconic acid (*t,t*-MA) log concentrations. Reprinted from Figure 2 of Lagorio et al. (1998) with permission from Oxford University Press.

Probability Plots Probability plots are commonly used to assess the normality of biomarker data; for example, Lagorio et al. (1998) used one in their evaluation of *trans, trans* muconic acid (*t,t*-MA) as a biomarker for low-level exposure to benzene. They used the plot to determine if the log-transformed urinary concentrations of *t,t*-MA obtained in their study followed a normal distribution (Figure 4.1). From a visual examination of their plot, they concluded that the normality assumption was justified.

While it is true that a probability plot is a valuable tool for assessing the normality assumption, we feel that it would have been preferable for Lagorio et al. to augment their plot with a formal statistical test based on the plot in order to confirm their subjective conclusion that the log concentration of *t,t*-MA did, in fact, follow a normal distribution. Such a test, the correlation coefficient (CC) test for normality, was proposed by Looney and Gulledge (1985a). In their assessment of the normality of the log concentrations of their biomarker, Lagorio et al. used the S-W test (Section 4.2.2.3) in conjunction with their probability plots. However, this test does not directly address the linearity of the probability plot. We recommend that any time normal probability plots are used to assess normality, they be accompanied by the CC test for normality.

Correlation Coefficient Test for Normality We wish to test the following hypotheses:

H_0: The sample observations are from a normal distribution (mean and variance unspecified).

$$\text{vs.} \tag{4.1}$$

H_a: The sample observations are not from a normal distribution.

To construct a normal probability plot, suppose that the sample of biomarker data is composed of n independent observations $\{x_1, x_2, \ldots x_n\}$. Let $\{x_{[1]}, x_{[2]}, \cdots, x_{[n]}\}$ denote the *order statistics* of the sample; in other words, the n observations after they have been arranged in order from smallest to largest. Suppose that the true distribution of the sample observations can be described by the normal cumulative distribution function (cdf) $\Phi[(x-\mu)/\sigma]$, where μ and σ are the unknown mean and standard deviation of the normal distribution, respectively. In other words,

$$\Phi[(x-\mu)/\sigma] = \int_{-\infty}^{(x-\mu)/\sigma} \frac{1}{\sqrt{2\pi}} e^{-z^2/2} dz, \tag{4.2}$$

where the integrand is the probability density function of the standard normal distribution. (Note that $\Phi[(x-\mu)/\sigma]$ in (4.2) corresponds to the area under the standard normal curve to the left of $z = (x-\mu)/\sigma$.) To construct a normal probability plot, the sample order statistic $x_{[i]}$ is plotted against $z_i = \Phi^{-1}(p_i)$, where p_i is an estimate of $\Phi[(x_{[i]} - \mu)/\sigma]$. In other words, z_i is the estimated $100\,p_i$th percentile of the standard normal distribution. (For example, if $p_i = .5$, then z_i = 50th percentile = 0.) The estimate p_i is called the "plotting position." If the hypothesized normal distribution is correct for the true distribution of $\{x_1, x_2, \ldots x_n\}$, then the resulting probability plot of z_i vs. $x_{[i]}$ will be approximately linear, with slope σ and y-intercept μ. The choice of a plotting position for a normal probability plot is not straightforward and various choices have been recommended over the years (Looney and Gulledge 1984). Simulation results by Looney and Gulledge (1984, 1985a, b) suggest that a reasonable choice is the Blom plotting position given by

$$p_i = (i - 0.375)/(n + 0.25). \tag{4.3}$$

This is the default plotting position used by the UNIVARIATE procedure in SAS to construct a normal probability plot. The use of this plotting position to construct a normal probability plot is illustrated in Example 4.1.

Once the plotting position has been selected and the probability plot constructed, it would be useful to have an objective criterion for interpreting the plot. If the hypothesized normal distribution is the correct one, then the normal probability plot will be approximately linear. Since the PCC between z_i and $x_{[i]}$ will be equal to one if the plot is exactly linear, Looney and Gulledge (1985a) proposed that one use it to measure the linearity of the probability plot, and developed a goodness-of-fit test for the normal distribution based on this CC, denoted by r_{cc}. This is the

TABLE 4.1 Empirical Percentage Points for the Correlation Coefficient Test for Normality

	Level of Significance (α)				
n	0.10	0.05	0.025	0.01	0.005
5	0.903	0.880	0.865	0.826	0.807
6	0.910	0.888	0.866	0.838	0.820
7	0.918	0.898	0.877	0.850	0.828
8	0.924	0.906	0.887	0.861	0.840
9	0.930	0.912	0.894	0.871	0.854
10	0.934	0.918	0.901	0.879	0.862
12	0.942	0.928	0.912	0.892	0.876
14	0.948	0.935	0.923	0.905	0.890
16	0.953	0.941	0.929	0.913	0.899
18	0.957	0.946	0.935	0.920	0.908
20	0.960	0.951	0.940	0.926	0.916
22	0.963	0.954	0.945	0.933	0.923
24	0.965	0.957	0.949	0.937	0.927
26	0.967	0.960	0.952	0.941	0.932
28	0.969	0.962	0.955	0.944	0.936
30	0.971	0.964	0.957	0.947	0.939
40	0.977	0.972	0.966	0.959	0.953
50	0.981	0.977	0.972	0.966	0.961
60	0.984	0.980	0.976	0.971	0.967
70	0.986	0.983	0.979	0.975	0.971
80	0.987	0.985	0.982	0.978	0.975
90	0.988	0.986	0.984	0.980	0.977
100	0.989	0.987	0.985	0.982	0.979

Source: Adapted from Table 2 of Looney and Gulledge (1985a, p. 78), Public Domain.

CC test for normality mentioned earlier. Simulation results indicate that this test has good statistical power for detecting a wide variety of non-normal distributions under the null hypothesis that the data follow a normal distribution (Looney and Gulledge 1985a).

Since the order statistics $\{x_{[1]}, x_{[2]}, \ldots, x_{[n]}\}$ used to construct the normal probability plot are highly correlated and heteroscedastic, the usual distributional results for the PCC do not apply, and the Fisher z-transform (Section 4.5.2) cannot be used to calculate p-values for r_{cc}. Instead, Looney and Gulledge used simulation to generate empirical percentage points for the null distribution of r_{cc}. An abbreviated table of these percentage points is provided in Table 4.1. We now illustrate the use of this test for the semaphorin concentrations given in Table 3.2.

Example 4.1 Probability Plot and Correlation Coefficient Test

Probability plots for the semaphorin concentrations given in Table 3.2 are provided for the original (untransformed) data in Figure 4.2, and for the log-transformed

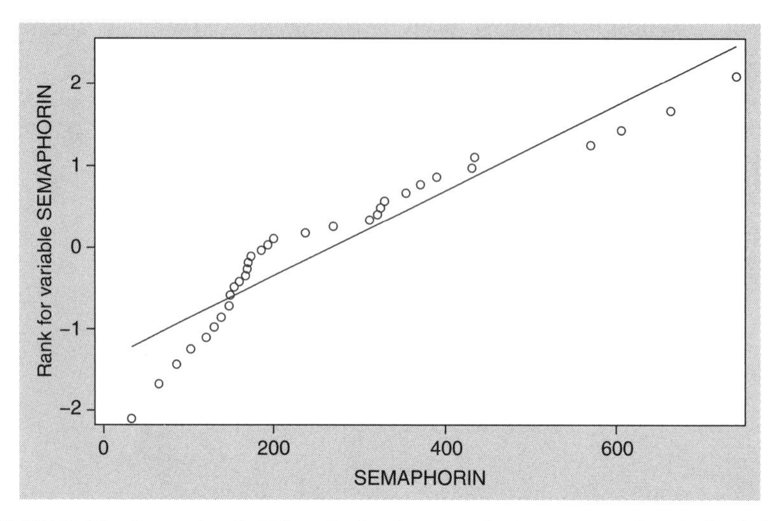

FIGURE 4.2 Normal probability plot for the semaphorin concentrations in Table 3.2.

data in Figure 4.3, respectively. There is a definite nonlinear pattern in the plot in Figure 4.2; thus, it appears that the original data are not normally distributed. On the other hand, the pattern in the probability plot in Figure 4.3 does appear to be roughly linear, suggesting that the log-transformed semaphorin data do in fact follow a normal distribution. The CC test for the original data yields r_{cc} = 0.938, with a p-value of 0.005; whereas, for the log-transformed data, r_{cc} = 0.982, with a p-value of 0.290. (Both p-values were obtained using linear interpolation in Table 4.1.) These hypothesis testing results confirm our subjective interpretations of the probability plots.

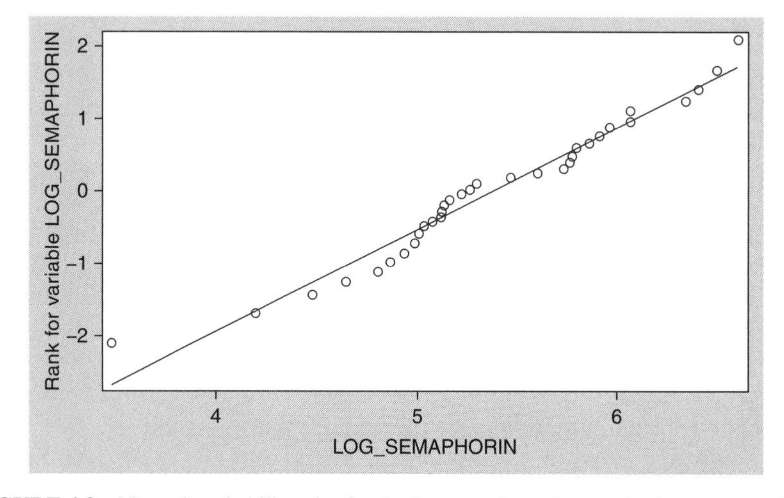

FIGURE 4.3 Normal probability plot for the log-transformed semaphorin concentrations.

The following SAS code can be used to generate the probability plot in Figure 4.2 and to calculate the test statistic r_{cc} for the CC test for normality for the untransformed semaphorin data. It is also provided on the companion website.

```
data SEMA;
input semaphorin @@;
datalines;
310.0 185.0 237.0 166.5 328.5 319.5
739.5 149.3 168.0 159.8 153.0 322.9
430.5 353.0 130.0 88.0  32.0  121.5
662.5 199.5 388.5 139.0 146.0 269.0
433.0 570.0 173.0 66.0  104.0 170.0
146.0 605.0 370.0 194.0
;
run;

proc rank data = SEMA normal = blom out = plot_pos;
     var semaphorin;
     ranks quantile;
     run;

ods listing close;
ods html;
proc sgscatter data = plot_pos;
     plot quantile * semaphorin / reg;
     title1 'Normal Probability Plot';
     run;
ods html close;
ods listing;

proc corr data = plot_pos nosimple noprob;
     var quantile;
     with semaphorin;
     title2 'Correlation Coefficient Test Statistic';
     run;
```

Normal Density Plots A graphical method that is not as widely used as the probability plot but can nevertheless provide very useful insight into possible departures from the normality assumption is the *normal density plot* (Jones and Daly 1995; Hazelton 2003). This plot is easier to interpret than the normal probability plot because it is based on a direct comparison of a particular plot of the sample data vs. an overlay of the familiar bell-shaped curve that represents the normal distribution. Normal density plots can be constructed using STATA statistical software (StataCorp LP, College Station, TX, 2009), and STATA code that can be used to construct the plot for the data in Table 3.2 is provided following Example 4.2.

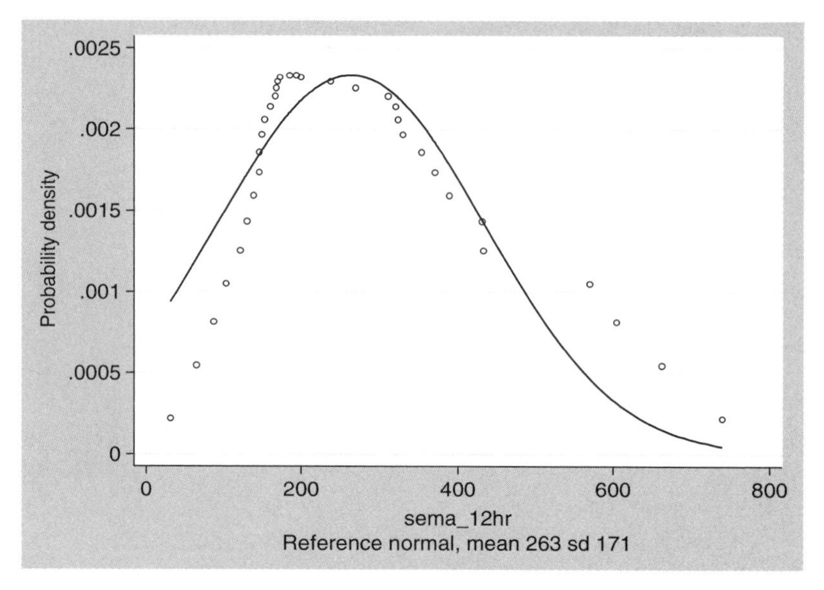

FIGURE 4.4 Normal density plot for the semaphorin concentrations in Table 3.2.

Example 4.2 Normal Density Plot

Normal density plots for the semaphorin concentrations given in Table 3.2 are provided for the original data in Figure 4.4, and for the log-transformed data in Figure 4.5, respectively. Based on Figure 4.4, it appears that the data are not normally distributed and positively skewed, whereas Figure 4.5 seems to indicate that the log

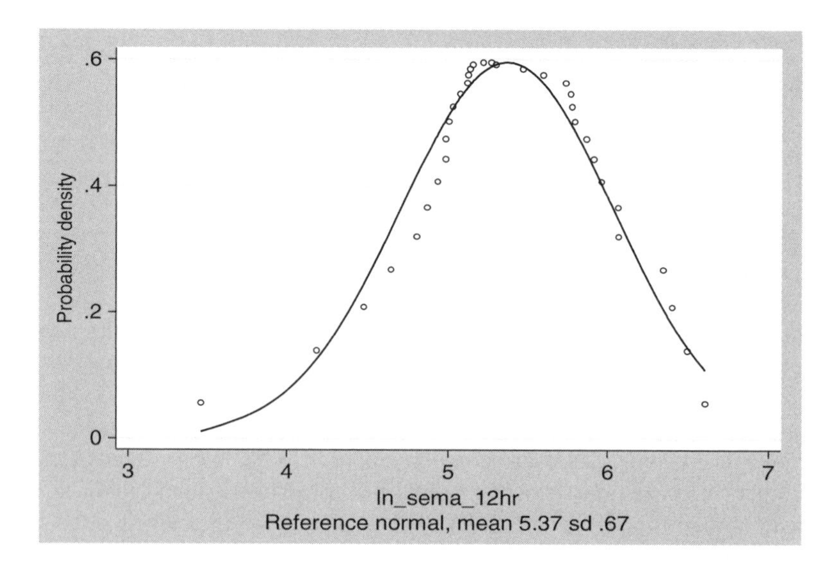

FIGURE 4.5 Normal density plot for the log-transformed semaphorin concentrations.

transformation worked; that is, the log-transformed semaphorin data do follow a normal distribution. These conclusions are consistent with our conclusions based on the probability plots and CC test results given in Example 4.1.

The following STATA statement was used to generate the normal density plot for the semaphorin concentrations given in Table 3.2.

```
dpplot sema_12hr, param(263 171)
```

Note that the data are stored in the STATA data set named "sema_12hr," and the mean and variance of the semaphorin concentrations are given in the "param" statement. The following STATA statement was used to generate the normal density plot for the log-transformed semaphorin concentrations given in Table 3.3.

```
dpplot ln_sema_12hr, param(5.37 0.67)
```

The log-transformed data are stored in the STATA data set named "ln_sema_12hr," and the mean and variance of the transformed semaphorin concentrations are given in the "param" statement.

4.2.2.2 Measures of Skewness and Kurtosis In addition to graphical displays that can be used to help us get a sense of whether or not the assumption of normality is reasonable for a sample of biomarker data, we have also found it useful to calculate numerical summaries that give us an idea of how much the sample data deviate from the normal distribution. Several such summaries have been proposed over the years, but the most commonly used numerical measures are the *coefficient of skewness*, denoted by $\sqrt{b_1}$, and the *coefficient of kurtosis*, denoted by b_2. The population version of the skewness coefficient, $\sqrt{\beta_1}$, is a measure of how far the true distribution of the data deviates from symmetry. If the true distribution is symmetric about the mean, $\sqrt{\beta_1} = 0$. If the distribution is positively skewed (i.e., skewed right), $\sqrt{\beta_1} > 0$, and, if the distribution is negatively skewed (i.e., skewed left), $\sqrt{\beta_1} < 0$. These concepts of symmetry and skewness were illustrated in Section 3.4.

In a similar vein, the sample skewness coefficient, $\sqrt{b_1}$, can also be thought of as a measure of how symmetric the sample data are; for data that are perfectly symmetric about the sample mean, $\sqrt{b_1} = 0$. For data that are positively skewed, $\sqrt{b_1} > 0$, and, for data that are negatively skewed, $\sqrt{b_1} < 0$. The sample skewness coefficient is calculated using the following formula:

$$\sqrt{b_1} = \frac{\sqrt{n}\sum_{i=1}^{n}(x_i - \bar{x})^3}{\left(\sum_{i=1}^{n}(x_i - \bar{x})^2\right)^{3/2}}. \tag{4.4}$$

Note that the sum of squared deviations in the denominator is the numerator of the sample variance.

The population version of the kurtosis coefficient, β_2, is a measure of how heavy the "tails" of the distribution are. The kurtosis of a distribution is interpreted by comparing the value of β_2 with the value of kurtosis for the normal distribution, which is equal to 3. Distributions with kurtosis equal to 3 are known as *mesokurtic*. Distributions with greater kurtosis than the normal are known as *leptokurtic*, $\beta_2 > 3$. Distributions with smaller kurtosis than the normal are known as *platykurtic*, $\beta_2 < 3$. If $\beta_2 > 3$, it is more likely that one would observe an extreme value from the distribution (e.g., three standard deviations from the mean) than it would be to observe such an extreme value from the normal distribution. Similarly, if $\beta_2 < 3$, it is less likely that one would observe an extreme value than if the data were normally distributed. For a given sample of data, we calculate the sample measure of kurtosis, b_2, and compare it with the value 3. The measure of kurtosis that is reported by many statistical software packages, including SAS, is $g_2 = b_2 - 3$. Thus, if $g_2 < 0$, we say that the sample data have *negative kurtosis*; if $g_2 > 0$, we say that the sample data have *positive kurtosis*.

The sample kurtosis coefficient is calculated using the following formula:

$$b_2 = \frac{n \sum_{i=1}^{n} (x_i - \bar{x})^4}{\left(\sum_{i=1}^{n} (x_i - \bar{x})^2 \right)^2}. \tag{4.5}$$

As with the sample skewness, the sum of squared deviations in the denominator is the numerator of the sample variance.

Example 4.3 Measures of Skewness and Kurtosis

For the untransformed semaphorin concentrations in Table 3.2, $\sqrt{b_1} = 1.19$ and $g_2 = 0.82$. This confirms our general impression from the normal density plot in Figure 4.4 that the data are positively skewed, with a slight degree of positive kurtosis. After applying the log transformation to the data, we obtain $\sqrt{b_1} = -0.36$, and $g_2 = 0.58$. This confirms our general impression from the normal density plot in Figure 4.5 that the log-transformed data are closer to being symmetric, with a slightly smaller degree of positive kurtosis. These general impressions are confirmed by the results of the CC test of normality for these data (Example 4.1).

The skewness coefficient, $\sqrt{b_1}$, and the measure of kurtosis, g_2, are provided as part of the standard output of the UNIVARIATE procedure in SAS. Thus, the following SAS code can be used to calculate the measures of skewness and kurtosis for the data in Table 3.2.

```
proc univariate data = SEMA;
var semaphorin;
title 'Measures of Skewness and Kurtosis';
run;
```

Note that SAS code for creating the SAS data set `SEMA` was provided with Example 3.1.

Authors of studies involving biomarker data often make statements such as "The biomarker data were highly skewed, so a log transformation was applied" or "Because of the extreme skewness in the data, nonparametric statistical tests were used" (Atawodi et al. 1998; Strachan et al. 1990). We feel that it is important to provide justification for such statements by, for example, providing the value of the sample skewness coefficient for the biomarker data under consideration. As stated by Zar (2010, p. 90) in the context of general biostatistical data analysis, "In practice, researchers seldom calculate these symmetry and kurtosis measures." While we agree with this statement, we nevertheless feel that it is important to routinely provide such numerical measures (along with the mean and standard deviation) when summarizing biomarker data. One benefit of doing so is to provide the reader with an indication of the type of departure from the normality assumption, if normality appears to be violated. The robustness of standard statistical procedures (t-test, Pearson correlation, regression analysis) to violations of the normality assumption typically depends on the nature and the extent of the deviation of the data from normality (Wilcox 2012, pp. 1–5). In addition to their use as descriptive measures, the skewness and kurtosis coefficients can also be used to perform formal tests of the normality assumption. D'Agostino et al. (1990) describe these tests and provide an SAS macro that can be used to perform them.

4.2.2.3 Formal Hypothesis Tests of the Normality Assumption Based on our experience, graphical examination of biomarker data is usually extremely valuable in assessing a distributional assumption. However, as with any graphical display of data, interpretation of a probability plot or normal density plot is inherently subjective. Therefore, one should never base the assessment of a distributional assumption entirely on the interpretation of a graphical display. In their evaluation of the use of a bile acid-induced apoptosis assay as a measure of colon cancer risk, Bernstein et al. (1999) stated that their apoptotic index (AI) "had a Gaussian distribution, as assessed by a box plot, Q–Q plot, and histogram" (p. 2354). Since each of these methods is a graphical technique, different data analysts could interpret these plots differently. (At least one of these graphical displays should have been included in the article, so that the reader could interpret it for themselves.)

It is our strong belief that any time a graphical method is used to assess a distributional assumption, this assessment should be augmented with a formal statistical test of the assumption, which may itself be based on results obtained from the graphical display. As we have already discussed (Section 4.2.2.1), the test statistic for the CC test for normality can be calculated directly from the plotting positions used to construct a normal probability plot. If one prefers the normal density plot to the probability plot, a formal test of the distributional assumption based on this plot is also available (Jones and Daly 1995; Hazelton 2003).

Shapiro–Wilk Test While graphical evaluation can be very useful when examining the appropriateness of the normality assumption for a set of biomarker data, one may wish to proceed directly to a formal goodness-of-fit test and avoid the complications inherent in the subjective evaluation of graphical displays. The formal hypothesis test that we recommend for general use is the S-W test (Shapiro and Wilk, 1965). Simulation studies have shown that the S-W test has good statistical power against a wide variety of non-normal distributions, and generally outperforms competing goodness-of-fit tests (see Shapiro et al. 1968). While the S-W test is not based directly on a graphical method for assessing normality, we have found it to be a valuable adjunct to such methods, and it was used for this purpose by Lagorio et al. (1998) in the study examining the usefulness of (*t,t*-MA) as a biomarker for exposure to benzene. Other authors have also used the S-W test to test the normality assumption when analyzing biomarker data, including Buckley et al. (1995) and MacRae et al. (2003). As described below, the S-W test is a lower-tailed test (i.e., small values of the test statistic indicate rejection of the normality assumption), with $p < 0.05$ indicating that the assumption of normality should be rejected. In their examination of a urinary biomarker for benzo[*a*]pyrene, Buckley et al. (1995, p. 261) incorrectly interpreted the S-W p-value on several occasions, concluding that a p-value of 0.013 was not significant for the test of the normality assumption, whereas a p-value of 0.07 was significant.

Suppose that a sample of biomarker data is composed of n independent observations $\{x_1, x_2, \dots x_n\}$. As in our discussion of probability plots, let $\{x_{[1]}, x_{[2]}, \dots, x_{[n]}\}$ denote the order statistics of the sample. The S-W test statistic is given by

$$W_0 = \frac{\left[\sum_{i=1}^{n} a_i x_{[i]}\right]^2}{\sum_{i=1}^{n} (x_i - \bar{x})^2}, \tag{4.6}$$

where the a_is are constants that depend on n (see Royston 1982). As with the CC test for normality, the hypotheses to be tested (Equation 4.1) are:

H_0: The sample observations are from a normal distribution (mean and variance unspecified).

vs.

H_a: The sample observations are not from a normal distribution.

Even though the S-W test is not based directly on a graphical method for assessing normality (unlike the CC test for normality discussed in Section 4.2.2.1), it does have a strong connection with probability plots. Shapiro and Wilk based their test statistic on the ratio of two estimators of the true population variance σ^2: the square of the generalized least squares estimate of the slope of the regression line fitted to the probability plot and the sample variance calculated from the x_is. If the hypothesized normal distribution is the appropriate model, these estimates of σ^2 will be close to each other, and their ratio will be close to one. Departures from normality would be indicated by values significantly less than one. Note that, unlike the CC test for normality, the S-W test does not directly address the nonlinearity of the probability plot.

As mentioned previously, the null hypothesis H_0 in (4.1) is rejected for small values of W_0. The distribution of W is strongly negatively skewed when the data follow a normal distribution; however, W can be transformed to approximate normality when

$7 \leq n \leq 2000$ (Royston 1982, 1989, 1992). For $3 \leq n \leq 6$, the methods described by Wilk and Shapiro (1968) should be used to find the exact lower-tailed p-value. (Note that this implies that the S-W test can be applied for samples as small as $n = 3$.) The statistical performance of the S-W test is greatly affected by the presence of tied observations in the sample data, so it is particularly important to adjust for ties when applying the S-W test (Royston 1989). Many statistical packages are capable of performing the adjusted-for-ties version of the S-W test; however, some packages ignore this adjustment. The implementation of the S-W test in SAS (via the UNIVARIATE procedure) incorporates the adjustment for ties.

Example 4.4 Shapiro–Wilk Test for Normality

To illustrate the application of the S-W test, once again consider the semaphorin data in Table 3.2. Based on the normal probability plot in Figure 4.2, the normal density plot in Figure 4.4, and the sample skewness and kurtosis for these data ($\sqrt{b_1} = 1.19$, $g_2 = 0.82$), we concluded that there appeared to be a violation of the normality assumption. This is confirmed by the results of the S-W test for these data, after adjusting for the effect of ties: $W_0 = 0.88$, $p = 0.001$. After applying the log transformation to these data, we concluded that the assumption of normality was reasonable for the transformed data, based on the normal probability plot in Figure 4.3, the normal density plot in Figure 4.5 and the sample skewness and kurtosis for the transformed data, ($\sqrt{b_1} = -0.36$, $g_2 = 0.58$). These subjective impressions are confirmed by the results of the S-W test for the transformed data, after adjusting for the effect of ties: $W_0 = 0.97$, $p = 0.390$.

The UNIVARIATE procedure in SAS can be used to perform the S-W test, adjusted for ties, by specifying the `normal` option in the PROC UNIVARIATE statement. Thus, the following SAS code can be used to calculate the S-W test for the semaphorin data in Table 3.2.

```
proc univariate normal data = SEMA;
     var semaphorin;
     title 'Shapiro-Wilk Test Adjusted for Ties';
     run;
```

SAS code for creating the SAS data set `SEMA` was provided with Example 3.1.

Note that the p-values for the S-W test are very similar to those obtained using the CC test for normality when applied to the original and log-transformed data ($p = 0.005$ and $p = 0.298$, respectively). The lower p-value for the S-W test for the untransformed data is consistent with the fact that the S-W test has been shown to be the most powerful goodness-of-fit test for normality under most conditions (see Shapiro et al. 1968). However, if one desires a statistical test result that is directly tied to a normal probability plot, we recommend that the CC test for normality be used instead. It compares favorably with the S-W test in terms of power against most non-normal distributions (Looney and Gulledge 1985a, b).

4.2.3 Remedial Measures for Violation of a Distributional Assumption

Once it has been determined that the distributional assumption underlying a statistical procedure (most commonly, normality) is violated for a particular set of data, at least three approaches have been recommended: (a) attempt to find a transformation to apply to the observations that will result in a new set of data for which the required distributional assumption appears to be valid, (b) use an alternative statistical procedure that is "robust" to a violation of the distributional assumption, or (c) use a "distribution-free" method that does not depend on the assumption that the data follow any particular statistical distribution. (It may also be the case that the detected departure from the assumed distribution is not important enough to adversely affect the results of the proposed statistical analysis. For a discussion of this point, see Wilcox (1987, pp. 103–104, 130).)

Robust statistical methods are beyond the scope of this textbook, although we briefly discuss them in Section 4.2.3.2. For a thorough treatment of robust statistical analysis, see Huber (1996) and Wilcox (2012). In particular, Wilcox provides a multitude of R programs that can be used to perform various robust estimation and hypothesis testing procedures.

Distribution-free (also called *nonparametric*) alternatives to statistical methods that are based on the normality assumption (often referred to as "normal-theory methods") are discussed in various places throughout this chapter. For example, Section 4.2.3.3 covers distribution-free methods for comparing two groups, and Section 4.5.1. covers distribution-free measures of association. In the following section, we discuss approaches that can be used to identify an appropriate transformation when the sample of biomarker data appears to violate a distributional assumption.

4.2.3.1 Choosing a Transformation The logarithmic transformation, performed by applying $\log_e$, the "natural" logarithm, or "log base e" to each observation in the data set, is commonly used in the analysis of biomarker data (see Atawodi et al. 1998; MacRae et al. 2003; Strachan et al. 1990). While it is true that log transformations have the potential to render right-skewed data much more symmetrical when compared to the original untransformed data, there is no guarantee that a log transformation will achieve its intended purpose. Note, however, that the log transformation does appear to have achieved its intended purpose for the semaphorin biomarker data in Table 3.2, as discussed in Examples 4.1–4.4.

In studies involving biomarker data, authors typically provide no rationale for using a log transformation; they sometimes justify applying the logarithm to the observed data prior to analysis by saying something similar to "the log transformation is commonly used when analyzing data of this type." At the very least, before proceeding with the any statistical analysis, the log-transformed data should be tested for normality as described in Section 4.2.2. If the results of the goodness-of-fit testing indicate that the log-transformed data are not normally distributed, then there are many other possible data transformations that are available. Several authors have identified particular "families" of possible data transformations, including the Box–Cox family (Box and Cox 1964), the Tukey "ladder of powers" (Tukey 1977, pp. 88–93), the

Johnson S_u family (Johnson 1949), and the Pearson family (Stuart and Ord, 1987, pp. 210–220). The Box–Cox approach to finding a transformation is particularly appealing because there is a formal statistical test that one can use to determine if the chosen transformation is "statistically significant" (see "Technical Details for the Box–Cox" below). However, identifying the appropriate Box–Cox transformation to use for a particular set of data can be computationally difficult (Atkinson, 1973). SAS code that can be used to select the appropriate Box–Cox transformation parameter for any set of data is provided following Example 4.5 and on the companion website. The TRANSREG procedure in SAS can also be used to find an appropriate transformation for X or Y or both when performing regression analysis.

The Tukey "ladder of powers" is also appealing as a method of identifying the appropriate transformation in that it requires one to consider only a small number of possible transformations in order to achieve normality. The so-called "variance stabilizing" (VS) transformations, which may also yield a transformed variable that is approximately normally distributed, are available for certain non-normal distributions; for example, proportions can be transformed to approximate normality using $Arcsin\sqrt{p}$, the VS transformation for the binomial, and count data can be transformed using $\sqrt{X}$, the VS transformation for the Poisson distribution (Snedecor and Cochran 1980, pp. 287–292). Regardless of the method that is used to select a transformation, the transformed data should be tested for normality in order to verify that the correct transformation has been selected (see Section 4.2.2). Once it has been verified that the transformation has achieved its intended purpose, one can proceed to the next stage of the statistical analysis. For an example in which this approach was applied to biomarker data, see MacRae et al. (2003).

*Box–Cox Method** The idea behind the Box–Cox approach is that maximum likelihood estimation (MLE) is used to estimate the value of the unknown parameter λ such that $y^{(\lambda)}$ is normally distributed, where $y^{(\lambda)}$ is defined by

$$y^{(\lambda)} = \left\{ \begin{array}{ll} \dfrac{y^{\lambda} - 1}{\lambda}, & \lambda \neq 0 \\ \log y, & \lambda = 0 \end{array} \right\}. \tag{4.7}$$

(Note that adding a constant to y or multiplying y by a constant, as is done in the definition of $y^{(\lambda)}$ in (4.7) when $\lambda \neq 0$, will have no effect on the values of the skewness and kurtosis coefficients for the transformed data, nor will these operations affect the CC test or the S-W test results. This property is referred to as "location and scale invariance.")

Using MLE, the optimal value of the transformation parameter, denoted by λ^*, is obtained by maximizing the log-likelihood function, given by

$$\ell(\lambda) = -\frac{n}{2}\log\left[\frac{1}{n}\sum_{i=1}^{n}\left(y_i^{(\lambda)} - \overline{y^{(\lambda)}}\right)^2\right] + (\lambda - 1)\sum_{i=1}^{n}\log y_i, \tag{4.8}$$

TABLE 4.2 The Tukey Ladder of Powers for Identifying a Transformation

Power (p)	Transformation	Name	Comments
3	Y^3	Cube	Infrequently used power
2	Y^2	Square	Largest commonly used power
1	Y	Original data	No transformation
$\frac{1}{2}$	$\sqrt{Y}$	Square root	Commonly used power
"0"	log Y or $\log_{10}(Y)$	Logarithm	Commonly used power
$-\frac{1}{2}$	$-1/\sqrt{Y}$	Reciprocal root	Commonly used power
-1	$-1/Y$	Reciprocal	Commonly used power
-2	$-1/Y^2$	Reciprocal square	Smallest commonly used power
-3	$-1/Y^3$	Reciprocal cube	Infrequently used power

Source: Adapted from Berenson et al. (1983, Table 11.4, pp. 319–320). Reprinted with permission of Pearson Education, Inc., Upper Saddle River, NJ.

where

$$\overline{y^{(\lambda)}} = \frac{1}{n}\sum_{i=1}^{n} y_i^{(\lambda)}.$$

Once the MLE λ^* has been obtained, one can determine if the chosen transformation is "statistically significant" by performing the likelihood ratio test of the null hypothesis $H_0 : \lambda = 1$.

Tukey Ladder of Powers Tukey (1977) introduced the idea of a "ladder of powers" for transformations, which can be used as a guide in selecting the appropriate transformation once a violation of the normality assumption has been detected. The basic idea is to identify the value of p such that the "power transformation" Y^p accomplishes the desired result; namely, that the transformed data are approximately normally distributed. This approach is exemplified in Table 4.2 (see Berenson et al. 1983).

An implication of using the ladder of powers is that exponents greater than 2 or less than -2 are rarely, if ever, used, and that only the powers in the interval $(-2, 2)$ that are listed in Table 4.2 should be considered. Of course, this differs from the Box–Cox approach, in which a much greater selection of powers is considered. In the SAS code for the Box–Cox method by Dimakos (1997) that is provided following Example 4.5, for example, all of the powers from -2 to $+2$ in increments of 0.1 are considered as possible transformations. The SAS code by Coleman (2004) that is available on the companion website is much more precise, and provides an estimate of the transformation parameter to five decimal places.

Example 4.5 Finding a Transformation

Table 4.3 contains a summary of the results after applying each of the transformations in the ladder of powers to the original semaphorin data in Table 3.2. Note that, as the value of the transformation parameter moves toward 0 (i.e., the log transformation), the skewness, kurtosis-3, and S-W test results steadily improve. The $\sqrt[5]{X}$

TABLE 4.3 Normality Test Results for Transformed Semaphorin Data

Transformed Variable	Skewness	Kurtosis-3	Shapiro-Wilk p-Value
X^2	2.08	4.01	<0.001
X	**1.19**	**0.82**	**0.001**
$\sqrt{X}$	0.56	−0.15	0.155
$\sqrt[5]{X}$	0.06	−0.05	0.560
log X	**−0.36**	**0.58**	**0.390**
$-1/\sqrt{X}$	1.79	5.50	<0.001
$-1/X$	3.41	14.89	<0.001
$-1/X^2$	5.25	29.04	<0.001

(or, equivalently, $X^{0.2}$) transformation is included in Table 4.3 only because this is the value of the transformation parameter produced by the Box–Cox estimation routine, as implemented in SAS. As confirmed by the results in Table 4.3, this transformation yields the best diagnostic results for the transformed data, with sample values of skewness and kurtosis-3 almost equal to zero, and a S-W p-value that is larger than that for any other transformation. (Note that the SAS code by Coleman (2004) that is available on the companion website produces a value of 0.16786 for the transformation parameter. This yields even better results $\sqrt{b_1} = -0.004$, $g_2 = 0.011$, and S-W p-value = 0.568.) However, according to the Tukey ladder of powers, a transformation parameter of $p = 0.2$ is rarely used in practice. The log transformation is much more commonly used, especially with biomarker data, and the results for log X are almost as good as those for $\sqrt[5]{X}$ (Table 4.3). Thus, in practice, the semaphorin data would be transformed by taking the natural logarithm, rather than the fifth root. (Note that $\log_{10}$ could also be used to transform the data, and would yield exactly the same skewness and kurtosis values and S-W p-value since $\log_e$ logarithms can be obtained from $\log_{10}$ logarithms simply by multiplying by $\log_e 10$.)

The SAS code given below (Dimakos 1997) and provided on the companion website can be used to search for the Box–Cox parameter among all powers from −2 to +2 in increments of 0.1. Other selections for the possible powers to consider can be specified using the `min=` , `max=`, and `step=` input parameters in the call to the `bctrans` SAS macro. One also needs to specify the total number of λ values to be considered (in this example, 31) using the `r=` input parameter.

```
%macro bctrans(data=,out=,var=,r=, min= ,max=, step=) ;


proc iml;
use &data;
read all var {&var} into x;
n=nrow(x); one=j(n,1,1); mat=j(&r,2,0);
lnx=log(x); sumlog=sum(lnx);
start;
i=0;
min1 = &min;
```

```
max1 = &max;
step1 = &step;
r1 = &r;
do lam=&min to &max by &step;
i =i+1;
lambda = round (lam, .01 );
x2=x##lambda;
x3 = x##lambda - one;
x4 = ((x##lambda) - one)/lambda;
mean2 = x4[:];
if lambda= 0 then xl=log(x); else xl= ((x##lambda) -
one)/lambda;
mean=xl[:];
d=xl- mean;
ss=ssq(d)/n;
l = -.5*n*log(ss)+((lambda- 1)*sumlog);
mat[i,1] = lambda;
mat[i,2] = l;
end;
finish;
run;

print "Lambdas and their l(lambda) values",
mat[format=8.3];
create lambdas from mat;
append from mat;
quit;

data lambdas;
set lambdas;
rename col1=lambda col2 = l;
run;

proc plot data=lambdas nolegend;
plot l*lambda;
title 'lambda vs. l(lambda) values';
run;
quit;

proc sort data=lambdas;
by descending l;
run;

data &out;
set lambdas;
```

```
if _n_>1 then delete;
run;

proc print data=&out;
title 'Highest lambda and l(lambda) value';
run;

proc iml;
use &data;
read all var {&var} into old;
use &out;
read all var {lambda l} into power;
if power=0 then new=log(old);
else new=old##power[1];
create final from new;
append from new;
quit;

data final;
set final;
rename col1=&var;
run;

%mend bctrans;

%bctrans(data=sema,out=boxcox,var=semaphorin,r=31,min=
-2,max=1,step=.1)
```

SAS code reproduced here with permission of the author.

The following SAS code can be used to calculate the measures of skewness and kurtosis and perform the S-W test for the transformed data obtained by the applying the ladder of powers approach to the semaphorin data. This SAS code also performs these calculations for the data after the selected Box–Cox transformation ($\lambda = 0.2$) has been applied.

```
data sema_trans;
     set sema;
     sema_minus_2 = semaphorin ** (-2);
     sema_recip = 1/semaphorin;
     sema_recip_root = 1/sqrt(semaphorin);
     sema_log = log(semaphorin);
     sema_sqrt = sqrt(semaphorin);
     sema_sqr = semaphorin ** 2;
     sema_point2bc = (semaphorin ** (.2) - 1) / (.2);
```

```
proc univariate normal data = sema_trans;
     var sema_minus_2 sema_recip sema_recip_root sema_log
         sema_sqrt sema_sqr;
     title1 'Normality Assessment for Transformed Variables';
     title2 'Ladder of Powers';
     run;

proc univariate normal data = sema_trans;
     var sema_point2bc;
     title1 'Normality Assessment for Transformed Variable';
     title2 'Box-Cox Transformation';
run;
```

SAS code for creating the SAS data set SEMA was provided with Example 3.1.

4.2.3.2 Using a Robust Statistical Procedure Loosely speaking, the term "robust" is used in statistics to refer to a statistical method that is not adversely affected in any meaningful way by violations of the assumptions underlying it (Scheffé 1959, p. 361; Dodge 2003, pp. 353–354). For example, the *t*-test is thought by many to perform quite well in terms of Type I error rate and power, regardless of whether or not the underlying assumptions of normality and homogeneity of variances are satisfied. However, it is known that this is not the case, especially when n is relatively small (Wilcox 1987, pp. 103–104; Wilcox 2012, pp. 9–10). The "robustness" of any statistical procedure generally depends on the sample size, and the performance of most statistical procedures in the presence of violations of assumptions improves as n increases. However, there are exceptions; for example, if n is too large, goodness-of-fit tests such as S-W are likely to reject the null hypothesis, even if the departure from normality is of no consequence. Generally speaking, tests for comparing means (*t*-test, ANOVA) are reasonably robust against violations of the normality assumption, whereas tests for comparing variances (the *F*-test, Bartlett's test) are much less robust against this violation (Milliken and Johnson 1984, pp. 16–28).

The term "robust" is also used in a more formal sense in statistics to refer to a very specialized class of statistical methods that are designed specifically to minimize the adverse effects that the presence of outliers and/or violations of the underlying distributional assumption might have (e.g., "robust regression" techniques such as least absolute regression and least median of squares regression). Robust alternatives (e.g., M-estimates, adaptive estimates) have been proposed for many estimation and hypothesis testing situations (Huber 1996; Wilcox 2012), but very few of them are available in commonly used statistical packages. Note, however, that Wilcox (2012) has recently provided a multitude of R programs that can be used to perform various robust estimation and hypothesis testing procedures. We encourage readers who are interested in learning more about robust methods to consult this comprehensive text.

TABLE 4.4 Nonparametric Alternatives for Some Commonly Used Tests That Are Based on the Assumption of Normality

Normal-Theory Test	Distribution-Free Alternative Method	Section
Paired t-test	Wilcoxon signed ranks test	4.4.2.2
	Sign test	4.4.2.3
Two-sample t-test	Mann–Whitney–Wilcoxon test	4.2.3.3
	Median test	4.2.3.3
F-test for equality of variances	Conover test	4.2.3.3
ANOVA	Kruskal–Wallis test	4.2.3.3
	k-sample median test	4.2.3.3
Bonferroni pairwise comparisons	Dunn's method	4.2.3.3
Pearson correlation	Spearman correlation	4.5.1.1
	Kendall's tau	4.5.1.2

4.2.3.3 Distribution-Free Alternatives It is well known that both the t-test and ANOVA are generally robust against violations of the normality assumption; however, if certain types of departures from normality are present, this can seriously affect the performance of these methods in terms of Type I error rate and statistical power (Algina et al. 1994). If one applies the methods for testing the underlying assumption of normality described in Section 4.2.2 and finds a significant departure from normality in any of the groups being compared, then we recommend that they consider using the appropriate distribution-free alternative indicated in Table 4.4 instead of the normal-theory-based test. (Note that distribution-free statistical procedures are also referred to as *nonparametric methods*. See Conover (1999) for a thorough discussion of these techniques.)

Mann–Whitney–Wilcoxon Test Several published analyses of biomarker data have used the Mann–Whitney–Wilcoxon (M-W-W) test when comparing two groups in terms of a continuous variable that appears to be non-normally distributed (Granella et al. 1996; Qiao et al. 1997). For example, in Granella et al. (1996), the authors compared 9 subjects with the lowest level of exposure to cigarettes (<5 cigarettes smoked per day) vs. the 8 subjects with the highest level (11 or more cigarettes per day) in terms of mutagenic activity and found a statistically significant difference using the M-W-W test ($p < 0.001$). This procedure is very similar to the equal-variance t-test, except that instead of comparing the mean biomarker levels of two groups, one compares the mean ranks of the biomarker levels in the two groups.

The M-W-W test is designed to test the following hypotheses:

H_0: The two populations have identical distributions

$$\text{vs.} \tag{4.9}$$

H_a: One of the populations tends to yield larger observations than the other.

Sometimes the alternative hypothesis is stated as follows (see Conover 1999, p. 290):

H_a: The populations do not have identical means.

Suppose that the data consist of n independent observations $\{x_1, x_2, \ldots x_n\}$ in Group 1 and m independent observations $\{y_1, y_2, \ldots y_m\}$ in Group 2. To perform the M-W-W test, first arrange the combined sample of $N = n + m$ observations from the two groups from smallest to largest and assign a rank of 1 to the smallest observation and a rank of N to the largest observation. If two or more of the sample values are tied at a particular value, then assign the *mid-rank* to each of the tied observations. The mid-rank is obtained by averaging the ranks of all of the observations that are tied at a particular value. This process is illustrated in Example 4.6.

Denote the ranks (including any mid-ranks) of the n Group 1 observations by $\{R(x_1), R(x_2), \ldots R(x_n)\}$. Define S to be sum of the ranks of the observations in Group 1, $S = \sum_{i=1}^{n} R(x_i)$, and T to be the sum of the squared ranks: $T = \sum_{i=1}^{n} [R(x_i)]^2$. Then the test statistic for the M-W-W test is given by

$$z_0 = \frac{S - n(N+1)/2}{\left[\frac{nm}{N(N-1)}T - \frac{nm(N+1)^2}{4(N-1)}\right]^{1/2}}. \tag{4.10}$$

The value of this test statistic can then be compared against the standard normal to obtain an approximate p-value. If there are no ties in the x-values and $N < 20$, tables of the exact distribution of S are also available (Conover 1999, Table A7). The exact distribution of S can be produced by StatXact and by the NPAR1WAY procedure in SAS, provided that the sample sizes in the two groups are not too large.

Example 4.6 Mann–Whitney–Wilcoxon Test

Consider the hypothetical data in Table 4.5 comparing the levels of a biomarker between two groups of subjects; one possessing Genotype MM (n = 19) and one possessing Genotype MN (m = 23). A histogram of the biomarker levels in each group indicates an apparent violation of the normality assumption in both groups, with the data for Genotype MM demonstrating negative skewness, and the data for Genotype MN demonstrating positive skewness (Figure 4.6). In fact, the skewness coefficients bear this out: $\sqrt{b_1} = -1.39$ for Genotype MM and $\sqrt{b_1} = 1.33$ for Genotype MN. Statistical evidence of departure from the normality assumption in both groups is provided by the S-W test: $p = 0.014$ for Genotype MM and $p = 0.001$ for Genotype MN. Thus, it would not be appropriate to use the two-sample t-test to

TABLE 4.5 Hypothetical Biomarker Levels for Two Genotypes

Genotype	Biomarker Level
MM	44, 50, 42, 44, 48, 38, 42, 50, 47, 49, 49, 40, 44, 48, 41, 34, 41, 30, 22
MN	48, 31, 31, 36, 29, 31, 39, 69, 34, 31, 34, 26, 35, 58, 37, 41, 36, 32, 57, 64, 28, 28, 43

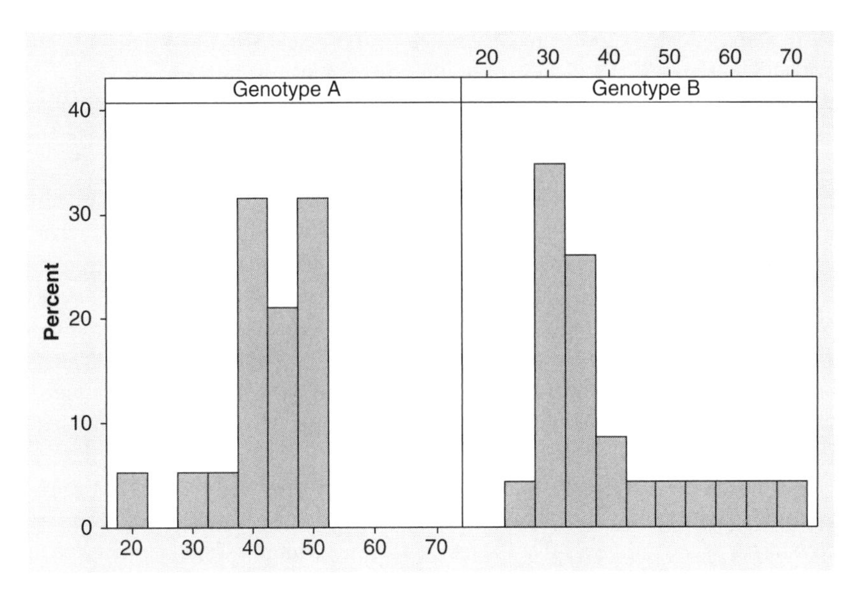

FIGURE 4.6 Histograms of hypothetical biomarker data by Genotype.

compare the two groups in terms of mean biomarker level, and one should consider using the M-W-W test instead.

To illustrate the M-W-W test, consider Table 4.6, in which ranks and mid-ranks have been assigned to the data in Table 4.5. As an example of the calculation of mid-ranks, consider the four samples that are tied at a biomarker level of 31 in the combined data for Genotypes MM and MN. After ordering the 42 total observations in the combined sample from smallest to largest, we see that the value 31 falls into positions 7, 8, 9, and 10 in the ranked data (Table 4.6). Thus, the mid-rank assigned to the value 31 is given by$(7 + 8 + 9 + 10)/4 = 8.5$, as can be seen in the fourth row of Table 4.6.

For the data in Table 4.5, $n = 19$, $m = 23$, $N = 42$. Using the ranks and mid-ranks in Table 4.6, and applying the formula in (4.10), we obtain $S = 487$, $T = 15734.25$, $z_0 = 1.986$, $p = 0.0470$. The exact p-value is also 0.0470. Thus, we can conclude that

TABLE 4.6 Ranks and Mid-Ranks for Combined Sample of Hypothetical Biomarker Levels for Two Genotypes

Sorted Biomarker Data	22[a], 26, 28, 28, 29, 30[a], 31, 31, 31, 31, 32, 34[a], 34, 34, 35, 36, 36, 37, 38[a], 39, 40[a], 41[a], 41[a], 41, 42[a], 42[a], 43, 44[a], 44[a], 44[a], 47[a], 48[a], 48[a], 48, 49[a], 49[a], 50[a], 50[a], 57, 58, 64, 69
Ranks and Mid-ranks	1.0, 2.0, 3.5, 3.5, 5.0, 6.0, 8.5, 8.5, 8.5, 8.5, 11.0, 13.0, 13.0, 13.0, 15.0, 16.5, 16.5, 18.0, 19.0, 20.0, 21.0, 23.0, 23.0, 23.0, 25.5, 25.5, 27.0, 29.0, 29.0, 29.0, 31.0, 33.0, 33.0, 33.0, 35.5, 35.5, 37.5, 37.5, 39.0, 40.0, 41.0, 42.0

[a]Indicates that the observation came from those subjects with Genotype MM.

there is a statistically significant difference in the distribution of biomarker levels between Genotypes MM and MN, although the evidence is not very strong.

An interesting feature of the M-W-W test statistic is that it can be shown to be equivalent to the test statistic obtained when the equal-variance t-test statistic (3.11) is calculated using the ranks of the x-values $\{R(x_1), R(x_2), \ldots R(x_n)\}$ (Conover and Iman 1981). The t-distribution with $n + m - 2$ degrees of freedom can then be used to calculate an approximate p-value and simulation studies have shown that the t-approximation to the M-W-W test is more accurate than the z-approximation under many conditions (Iman 1976). For the data in Table 4.5, the t-approximation to the M-W-W test yields an approximate p-value of 0.0552, whereas the normal approximation yields an approximate p-value of 0.0466 and the exact p-value is 0.0470. Thus, the t-approximation to the null distribution of the M-W-W test statistic is much less accurate than the z-approximation for these data. That is why we recommend that the exact method be used whenever possible.

StatXact and the NPAR1WAY procedure in SAS can be used to perform the M-W-W test, and calculate the exact p-value (with mid-P adjustment), as long as n and m are not too large. We recommend that the exact p-value (with mid-P adjustment) be used whenever possible. If the software fails to calculate the exact p-value because m and n are too large, then we recommend that the z-approximation be used. SAS includes a continuity correction for the z-approximation to the p-value for the M-W-W test; however, Conover (1999, pp. 274–275) recommends that the continuity correction not be used when ties are present. The output from the NPAR1WAY procedure when the `wilcoxon` option is specified also includes the results for the application of the Kruskal–Wallis (K-W) test with χ^2 approximation. Since the K-W test is equivalent to the M-W-W test when there are only two groups, the z-approximate p-value for the M-W-W test is the same as the χ^2-approximate p-value for the K-W test. The z-test statistic for the M-W-W test in (4.10) can be obtained by taking the positive square root of the χ^2 test statistic for the K-W test.

The SAS code provided below and on the companion website can be used to perform the M-W-W test for the data in Table 4.5. Even though the sample sizes are not that large (n = 19 for Genotype MM and m = 23 for Genotype MN), these data exceed the capabilities of SAS to perform the exact test. However, StatXact is able to carry out the exact analysis.

```
data MM;
input biomarker @@;
genotype = 'MM' ;
datalines;
44 50 42 44 48 38 42 50 47 49 49 40 44 48 41 34 41 30 22
;

data MN;
input biomarker @@;
genotype = 'MN';
```

```
datalines;
48  31  31  36  29  31  39  69  34  31  34  26  35  58  37  41
36  32  57  64  28  28  43
;

data Table4_5 ;
set MM MN ;
run;

proc npar1way data = Table4_5 wilcoxon;
class genotype;
var biomarker ;
*exact wilcoxon;
run;
```

It is interesting to note that neither the equal-variance t-test (t = 1.02, df = 40, p = 0.3157), nor the unequal-variance t-test (t = 1.06, df = 36.96, p = 0.2946), yielded a statistically significant difference in mean biomarker level between those subjects having Genotype MM and those having Genotype MN. This illustrates the fact that, despite the mistaken impression held by many statistical practitioners, distribution-free tests such as the M-W-W are not always inferior to normal-theory methods such as the t-test in terms of power. While it is true that the t-test is slightly more powerful than the M-W-W when the data do, in fact, come from a normal distribution, this is not necessarily the case if the data are from a non-normal distribution. If the data in both groups are normally distributed, then the asymptotic relative efficiency (ARE) of the M-W-W relative to the t-test is 95.5%; roughly speaking, this means that if N = 100 is required to achieve the desired power (usually 80% using a significance level of 0.05) for the M-W-W test, then N = 96 would be required for the t-test (Siegel and Castellan 1988, pp. 21–22). However, if the data come from a uniform distribution, the ARE of the M-W-W relative to the t-test is 100%; if the data come from a double exponential distribution, this ARE is 150%. (Roughly speaking, the latter result means that if N = 100 is required for the M-W-W test, then N = 150 would be required for the t-test.) Regardless of the true parent population, the ARE of the M-W-W to the t-test is never less than 86.4% (Conover 1999, p. 284). Since the power advantage of the t-test over the M-W-W is relatively small when the data do arise from a normal distribution, some would argue that one should always use the M-W-W test for the two-sample problem, especially since there is no infallible method for determining if the data in the two groups are truly normally distributed.

A key aspect of applying the M-W-W test that is often overlooked is that this method is intended to detect what are called "shift alternatives"; that is, the alternative hypothesis is that the two populations being compared have identical shapes, but one is a "shifted" version of the other. This implies that the populations being compared have equal variability. Typically, no consideration is given to this variability issue when the M-W-W test is applied in practice. We recommend that one test the assumption of equal variability in the two populations prior to applying the M-W-W test; the method we recommend is the Conover test (Conover 1999, pp. 300–303), which has been shown to be generally superior to other tests of homogeneity (Conover et al. 1981). If the Conover test detects a difference in variability between the two populations being compared, then the median test can be used instead. (Each of these tests is described below.) The median test does not depend on the assumption that the two populations being compared have identical shapes.

Another common misconception that is related to this idea of detecting a shift alternative is that the M-W-W can be used to test for equality of medians between two populations. In fact, this is not the case; however, the median test can be used for this purpose.

The Conover Test The Conover test is used to test the assumption of equal variability in two populations. The null and alternative hypotheses are thus given by

$$\begin{aligned} &H_0\text{: } X \text{ and } Y \text{ are identically distributed, except for possibly different means.} \\ &\qquad\qquad\qquad\text{vs.} \\ &H_a\text{: } \mathrm{Var}(X) \neq \mathrm{Var}(Y). \end{aligned} \tag{4.11}$$

To perform the Conover test, suppose that the data consist of n independent observations $\{x_1, x_2, \ldots x_n\}$ in Group 1 and m independent observations $\{y_1, y_2, \ldots y_m\}$ in Group 2. The first step in performing the Conover test is to convert each x- and y-value to its absolute deviation from the sample mean in each group: $u_i = |x_i - \bar{x}|$, $i = 1, 2, \ldots, n$; $v_j = |y_j - \bar{y}|$, $j = 1, 2, \ldots, m$. Now, arrange the combined sample of $N = n + m$ absolute deviations from smallest to largest and assign a rank of 1 to the smallest absolute deviation and a rank of N to the largest. If two or more of the absolute deviations are tied at a particular value, then assign the mid-rank to each of the tied deviations, as was done when computing the mid-ranks of the raw data in the calculation of the M-W-W test statistic in Example 4.6.

Denote the ranks (including any mid-ranks) of the n deviations in Group 1 by $\{R(u_1), R(u_2), \ldots R(u_n)\}$ and by $\{R(v_1), R(v_2), \ldots R(v_n)\}$ in Group 2. If there are no ties of u-values with v-values, then the sum of the squared ranks of the u-values can be used as the test statistic:

$$S = \sum_{i=1}^{n} R^2(u_i).$$

Tables of percentage points of the exact distribution of S for $n \leq 10$ and $m \leq 10$ can be found in Conover (1999). If there are ties between the u- and v-values, then the following test statistic should be used:

$$z_0 = \frac{S - n\overline{R^2}}{\left[\frac{nm}{N(N-1)} \sum_{i=1}^{N} R_i^4 - \frac{nm}{N-1}\left(\overline{R^2}\right)^2\right]^{1/2}}, \tag{4.12}$$

where $\overline{R^2}$ is the average squared rank in the combined sample:

$$\overline{R^2} = \left\{ \sum_{i=1}^{n} [R^2(u_i)] + \sum_{i=1}^{m} [R^2(v_i)] \right\} / N,$$

and $\sum_{i=1}^{N} R_i^4$ is the sum of the fourth power of the ranks:

$$\sum_{i=1}^{N} R_i^4 = \left\{ \sum_{i=1}^{n} [R^4(u_i)] + \sum_{i=1}^{m} [R^4(v_i)] \right\}.$$

An approximate p-value for the test statistic z_0 in (4.12) can be obtained using the standard normal distribution. Extensive simulations (Conover et al. 1981) demonstrated that the Conover test is generally preferable to other methods for comparing two populations in terms of variability. The approximate and exact versions of the two-group Conover test are available in StatXact and in the NPAR1WAY procedure in SAS.

Example 4.7 Conover Test

For the data in Table 4.5, $S = 7876.5$ and $z_0 = -2.11$, with an approximate p-value of 0.035. Note that the exact p-value is 0.0330. Thus, there is an indication that the variability in biomarker level differs significantly between those having Genotype MM and those having Genotype MN.

The following SAS code can be used to perform the approximate version of the Conover test for the data in Table 4.5. Even though the sample sizes are not that large (n = 19 for Genotype MM and m = 23 for Genotype MN), these data exceed the capabilities of SAS to perform the exact test. However, StatXact is able to perform the exact analysis.

```
proc npar1way data= Table4_5 conover;
class genotype;
var biomarker ;
*exact conover;
run;
```

SAS code for creating the SAS data set `Table4_5` was provided with Example 4.6.

The results for the Conover test for the data in Table 4.5 suggest that the M-W-W test is not appropriate for comparing the two genotypes in terms of biomarker level. The inappropriateness of the M-W-W test for these data is also indicated by fact that the distributions of the biomarker levels in the two groups appear to differ in shape, with biomarker levels being skewed left for Genotype MM and skewed right for Genotype MN (Figure 4.6). Given these results, our recommendation would be

TABLE 4.7 Observed Frequencies for Performing the Median Test

	Group 1	Group 2	Total
Number of values > M	n_{11}	n_{12}	$n_{1\bullet}$
Number of values ≤ M	n_{21}	n_{22}	$n_{2\bullet}$
Total	n	m	N

to use the median test instead of the M-W-W test to compare those having Genotype MM with those having Genotype MN.

Two-Sample Median Test The median test is nothing more than a very specialized application of the general chi-square test for independence that was covered in Section 3.10.1. It is applicable when one wishes to test the hypothesis that the medians in two or more populations are equal. We will first consider the case in which one wishes to compare two population medians; that is, one wishes to test the following hypotheses:

$$H_0 : M_1 = M_2 \text{ vs. } H_a : M_1 \neq M_2, \tag{4.13}$$

where M_1 is the median in Population 1 and M_2 is the median in Population 2.

As in our discussion of the M-W-W and Conover tests, suppose that the data consist of n independent observations $\{x_1, x_2, \ldots x_n\}$ in Group 1 and m independent observations $\{y_1, y_2, \ldots y_m\}$ in Group 2, and that the two samples of data are independent of each other. The first step in applying the median test is to find the median of the combined sample of $N = n + m$ data values; this value, called the *grand median*, is denoted by M. The next step is to count the number of data values above and below the grand median in each group, and put the results in a 2×2 table, as illustrated in Table 4.7.

Under the null hypothesis $H_0 : M_1 = M_2$, the magnitude of the observation (i.e., either greater than or less than or equal to M) is independent of whether it belongs to Group 1 or Group 2. So, we can test H_0 by using the chi-square procedure described in Section 3.10.1 to test the null hypothesis that the row classification in Table 4.7 is independent of the column classification. Using the computational formula in Equation (3.31) and changing notation slightly, we obtain the following test statistic:

$$\chi_0^2 = \frac{N\left(n_{11}n_{22} - n_{12}n_{21}\right)^2}{nmn_{1\bullet}n_{2\bullet}}. \tag{4.14}$$

An approximate p-value for the median test can be calculated by comparing the test statistic in (4.14) against the chi-squared distribution with one degree of freedom. The exact version of the χ^2 test, which is equivalent to Fisher's exact test (Section 4.9.4.2) for a 2×2 table (Davis 1986), can be used to perform an exact test

TABLE 4.8 Observed Frequencies for Performing the Median Test for Hypothetical Biomarker Data

	Group 1	Group 2	Total
Number of values $> M$	14	7	21
Number of values $\leq M$	5	16	21
Total	19	23	42

of the null hypothesis H_0 in (4.13). There is also a k-sample version of the median test that can be used to compare the medians of any number of populations. This test is described below.

Example 4.8 Two-Sample Median Test

For the hypothetical biomarker data in Table 4.5, the sample medians are $m_1 = 44$, $m_2 = 35$, and the grand median is $M = 40.5$. The 2×2 table for performing the median test for these data is given in Table 4.8.

Based on these results, $\chi_0^2 = 7.78$, $df = 1$, and the approximate p-value = 0.0053. The exact p-value is 0.0122 and the mid-P value (Section 4.9.4.1) is $2[0.0061 - \frac{1}{2}(0.0053)] = 0.0069$. Thus, there is strong evidence that the population medians in the two groups are not equal and that we should reject the null hypothesis H_0: $M_1 = M_2$ in favor of the alternative H_a: $M_1 \neq M_2$. Note that the median test, which is widely thought to be much less powerful than the t-test and the M-W-W test, actually yields a much stronger degree of evidence against the null hypothesis (as measured by the p-value) than either of these tests ($p = 0.0470$ for M-W-W and $p = 0.3157$ for the t-test).

StatXact can be used to perform both the exact and approximate versions of the median test. The median test is available in the NPAR1WAY procedure in SAS; however, the results for the approximate test based on chi-square do not agree with the results obtained using StatXact. (Note that the exact results do agree with StatXact.) This is apparently due to a discrepancy between the "median" scores used by SAS when performing the median test and the chi-square formulation of the test as we have described it here. However, the FREQ procedure in SAS can be used to perform the median test and obtain approximate and exact p-values that correspond to those using StatXact. Therefore, we recommend using the FREQ procedure to perform the median test. The following SAS code can be used to perform the median test for the data in Table 4.5. It makes use of the cross-classified data in Table 4.8. We also provide SAS code utilizing the NPAR1WAY procedure that can be used to perform the exact version of the median test for the data in Table 4.5.

```
data two_group;
input gt_median group count @@;
cards;
```

```
1 1 14  1 2 7
2 1  5  2 2 16
;

proc freq data = two_group order = data; weight count;
     tables gt_median * group;
     exact chisq;
     title 'Median Test';
     run;

proc npar1way data = Table4_5 median;
     class genotype;
     var biomarker;
     exact median;
     title1 'Median Test';
     title2 'Use Exact Output Only';
     run;
```

Note that SAS code for creating the SAS data set `Table4_5` was provided with Example 4.6.

While it is true that the t-test is more powerful than both the M-W-W test and the median test when the data do, in fact, come from a normal distribution; this is not necessarily the case if the data are from a non-normal distribution. If the data in both groups come from a normal population, the ARE of the median test relative to the t-test is only 63.7%; roughly speaking, this means that if $n = 100$ is required to achieve the desired power (usually 80% at a significance level of 0.05) for the median test, then $n = 64$ would be required for the t-test. If the data come from a uniform distribution, the ARE of the median test relative to the t-test is only 33.3%; however, if the data come from a double exponential distribution, this ARE is 200%. In other words, for data that arise from a double exponential distribution, if $n = 100$ is required to achieve the desired power for the median test, then $n = 200$ would be required for the t-test. When comparing the median test to the M-W-W test, the AREs are 66.7%, 33.3%, and 133.3% for the normal, uniform, and double exponential distributions, respectively (Conover 1999, p. 285). Thus, depending on the true distribution of the data, the median test can actually be the most powerful of the three. What this means from a practical point of view is that the analyst should proceed very carefully if the sample data appear to violate the normality assumption; if so, then distribution-free methods such as the M-W-W and sign test should be considered.

Kruskal–Wallis Test The K-W test, which is equivalent to the M-W-W procedure when comparing two groups, has been used with biomarker data (Amorim et al. 1997; Atawodi et al. 1998). As with the M-W-W procedure, a key aspect of applying the K-W test that is often overlooked is that it is intended to detect "shift alternatives"; in other words, the k populations being compared have identical shapes, but at least one is a "shifted" version of at least one of the others. The null and alternative hypotheses are thus given by

H_0: All k populations have identical distributions.

$$\text{vs.} \tag{4.15}$$

H_a: At least one of the populations tends to yield larger observations than at least one of the others.

Sometimes, the alternative hypothesis is stated as

H_a: Not all of the k populations have the same mean (Conover 1999).

Stating the hypotheses as in (4.15) implies that the populations being compared have equal variability. Typically, no consideration is given to this issue when applying the K-W test to biomarker data. We recommend that one test the assumption of equal variability in the k populations using the k-sample Conover test, which is described below. This test is available in the NPAR1WAY procedure in SAS.

*Technical Details for the Kruskal–Wallis Test** We wish to compare k different populations, using a random sample of size n_i from Population i, $i = 1, 2, \ldots, k$. It is assumed that these random samples are independent of each other. Denote the sample of data from the ith population by $\{x_{i1}, x_{i2}, \ldots x_{in_i}\}$. Now arrange the combined sample of $N = n_1 + n_2 + \cdots + n_k$ observations from smallest to largest and assign a rank of 1 to the smallest observation and a rank of N to the largest. If two or more of the sample values are tied at a particular value, then assign the mid-rank to each of the tied observations, as illustrated for the M-W-W test in Example 4.6.

Denote the ranks (including any mid-ranks) of the n_i observations in Group i by $\{R(x_{i1}), R(x_{i2}), \ldots R(x_{ini})\}$. Define R_i to be the sum of the ranks assigned to the observations in Group i, $R_i = \sum_{j=1}^{n_i} R(x_{ij})$, $i = 1, 2, \ldots, k$. Then the test statistic for the K-W test is given by

$$\chi_0^2 = \frac{1}{S^2}\left[\sum_{i=1}^{k}\frac{R_i^2}{n_i} - \frac{N(N+1)^2}{4}\right], \tag{4.16}$$

where

$$S^2 = \frac{1}{N-1}\left[\sum_{i=1}^{k}\sum_{j=1}^{n_i} R(x_{ij})^2 - \frac{N(N+1)^2}{4}\right].$$

The value of this test statistic is then compared against the chi-squared distribution with $k - 1$ degrees of freedom to obtain an approximate p-value.

Example 4.9 Kruskal–Wallis Test

Consider the hypothetical data in Table 4.9 comparing the levels of a biomarker between three groups of subjects; those possessing Genotype MM (n = 20), those having Genotype MN (n = 23), and those with Genotype NN (n = 15). Histograms of

TABLE 4.9 Hypothetical Biomarker Levels for Three Genotypes

Genotype	Biomarker Level
MM	44, 50, 42, 41, 44, 48, 38, 42, 50, 47, 49, 49, 40, 44, 48, 41, 34, 41, 30, 22
MN	48, 31, 31, 36, 29, 31, 39, 69, 34, 31, 34, 26, 35, 58, 37, 41, 36, 32, 57, 64, 28, 28, 43
NN	35, 29, 47, 32, 36, 37, 4, 36, 34, 39, 38, 37, 52, 45, 41

the biomarker levels indicate an apparent violation of the normality assumption in all the three groups, with the data for those with Genotype MM demonstrating negative skewness, the data for Genotype MN demonstrating positive skewness, and the data for Genotype NN indicating the presence of an apparent outlier (Figure 4.7). The shape of the histogram for Genotype NN suggests that if we removed the outlying data value, the data would appear to be symmetric. For purposes of this example, we will assume that there is no valid scientific reason to remove this biomarker reading, and we will retain it in all further analyses of these data.

The sample skewness coefficients all indicate a high degree of departure from the normality assumption: $\sqrt{b_1} = -1.39$ for Genotype MM, $\sqrt{b_1} = 1.33$ for Genotype MN, and $\sqrt{b_1} = -1.87$ for Genotype NN. Statistical evidence of departure from the normality assumption in all the three groups is provided by the S-W test: $p = 0.014$ for MM, $p = 0.001$ for MN, and $p = 0.006$ for NN. Thus, it would not be appropriate to use ANOVA to compare the three groups in terms of biomarker level.

Based on the data in Table 4.9, the value of the K-W test statistic is $\chi_0^2 = 6.27$, $df = 2$, approximate p-value $= 0.0435$. Note that the usual one-way ANOVA

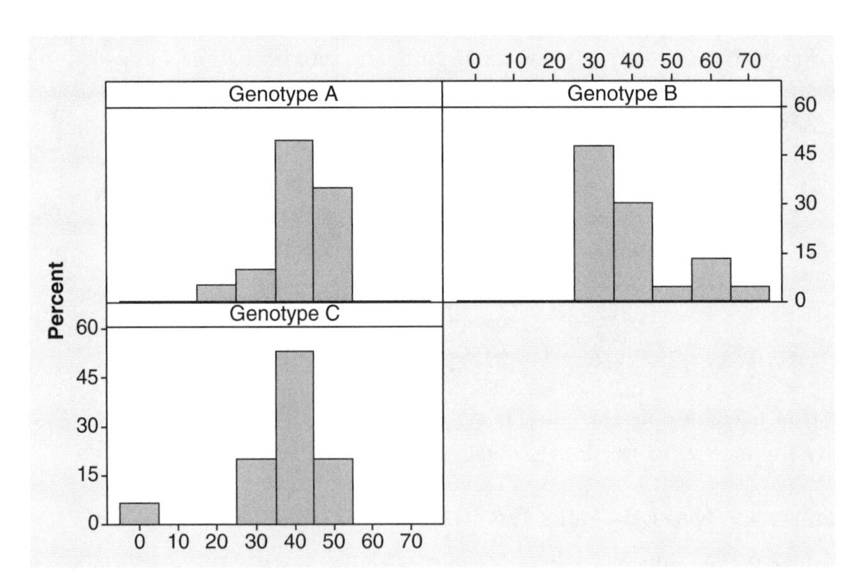

FIGURE 4.7 Histograms for hypothetical biomarker levels for subjects possessing one of the three genotypes.

F-test fails to detect a significant difference among the three genotypes: $F_{2,55} = 1.52$, $p = 0.2270$.

StatXact and the NPAR1WAY procedure in SAS can be used to perform the K-W test using the chi-square approximation, and calculate exact p-values (and mid-P adjustment), as long as none of the n_is are too large. We recommend that the exact p-value with mid-P adjustment be used whenever available. If the software fails to calculate the exact p-value because one or more of the n_is are too large, then we recommend that the χ^2-approximation be used. Even though the sample sizes in Example 4.9 are not that large ($n_1 = 20$ for Genotype MM, $n_2 = 23$ for MN, and $n_3 = 15$ for NN), these data exceed the capabilities of both SAS and StatXact to perform the exact test. Using the simulation option in StatXact yields an estimated exact p-value of 0.0423 with a 99% confidence interval (CI) of (0.0371, 0.0475).

The following SAS code can be used to perform the approximate version of the K-W test for the data in Table 4.9:

```
data MM;
input biomarker @@;
genotype = 'MM' ;
datalines;
44  50  42  41  44  48  38  42  50  47  49  49  40  44  48  41
34  41  30  22
;

data MN;
input biomarker @@;
genotype = 'MN';
datalines;
48  31  31  36  29  31  39  69  34  31  34  26  35  58  37  41
36  32  57  64  28  28  43
;

data NN;
input biomarker @@;
genotype = 'NN';
datalines;
35  29  47  32  36  37  4  36  34  39  38  37  52  45  41
;

data Table4_9 ;
set MM MN NN;
run;

proc npar1way data= Table4_9 wilcoxon;
class genotype;
```

```
var biomarker ;
*exact wilcoxon;
run;
```

An interesting feature of the K-W test statistic in (4.16) is that it can be shown to be equivalent to the F-test statistic for a one-way ANOVA (Section 3.7.2) calculated using the ranks of the x-values $\{R(x_{11}), R(x_{12}), \ldots R(x_{k,n_k})\}$ instead of the original data (Conover and Iman 1981). The F-distribution with k and $n - k$ degrees of freedom can thus be used to calculate an approximate p-value for the K-W test and simulation studies have shown that the F-approximation to the K-W test is more accurate than the χ^2-approximation under many conditions (Iman and Davenport 1976). This approximation is not available in either StatXact and SAS; however, the F-approximation is easily obtained by using the RANK procedure in SAS to calculate the ranks (and mid-ranks, if any) of the original data, and then using the GLM procedure to perform the usual one-way ANOVA F-test on the ranks as if they were the original data. For the data in Table 4.9, the F-approximation to the K-W test yields $F_{2,55} = 3.40$, $p = 0.0406$. (Recall that the approximate p-value based on the chi-square approximation was 0.0435). The following SAS code can be used to carry out the calculations for the F-approximation to the K-W test. Note that SAS code for creating the `k_group` SAS data set was provided following Example 4.9.

```
proc rank data = Table4_9 out = Table4_9_r ;
     var biomarker;
     ranks biomarker_r;

proc npar1way data= Table4_9_r anova;
     class genotype;
     var biomarker_r ;
     title1 'F-test Approximation to Kruskal-Wallis';
     run;
```

It is important to note that the M-W-W and K-W tests, as well as all other distribution-free methods that are based on ranks, are invariant with respect to logarithmic and all other monotonic transformations of the data. In other words, transforming the data using the log or other transformation as discussed in Section 4.2.3.1 will not affect the results of the statistical analysis when one of the methods based on ranks is used. Atawodi et al. (1998) were apparently unaware of this fact when they analyzed both the original and log-transformed data in their study using the K-W test and obtained "virtually identical results" (p. 820).

All of the distribution-free methods discussed in this textbook are available in StatXact and in the NPAR1WAY procedure in SAS. We prefer to use StatXact to perform these methods since it produces exact p-values whenever possible; many commonly used statistical packages are capable only of producing approximate p-values when applying nonparametric methods. (Note that, with each new version of SAS, more and more exact procedures are implemented; therefore, it is important to check the SAS documentation each time a new version is released.) Not using the exact version of the K-W test may explain why Atawodi et al. (1998) found discrepancies when comparing their K-W results.

However, it may be that the total sample size (or one or more of the group sizes) are too large for the software to carry out the exact version of the test. In this case, there should be no harm in using the approximate version of the test since this is precisely when the approximate p-value will be very similar (if not identical) to the exact p-value.

As with the M-W-W test, a key aspect of applying the K-W test (which is equivalent to the M-W-W test when there are only two groups) that is often overlooked is that this method is intended to detect "shift alternatives"; that is, the alternative hypothesis is that the distributions of biomarker levels in the k populations being compared have identical shapes, but at least one is a "shifted" version of at least one of the others. This implies that the populations being compared have equal variability in terms of biomarker level. Typically, no consideration is given to this variability issue when the K-W test is applied in practice. As in our discussion of the M-W-W test, we recommend that one use the k-sample Conover test (described below) to confirm or deny the assumption of equal variability in the k populations prior to applying the K-W test. If the Conover test detects a difference in variability among the k populations being compared, then we recommend that one use the k-sample median test, which is described below, instead of the K-W test. The median test does not depend on the assumption that the k populations have identical shapes.

The Dunn Method of Pairwise Comparisons If we fail to reject the null hypothesis H_0 in (4.15) using the K-W test, we conclude that there is no significant difference among the k groups in terms of biomarker level. But if the null hypothesis is rejected, it is usually of interest to determine which of the populations differ from the others in terms of biomarker level. As in the parametric Analysis of Variance (ANOVA, Section 3.7.2), this is generally referred to as "post hoc analysis" or "pairwise comparisons."

The preferred distribution-free method for pairwise comparisons is the Dunn method (Gibbons and Chakraborti 2003, p. 367), which is performed as follows. Let $\overline{R_i} = \sum_{j=1}^{n_i} R(x_{ij})/n_i$, the mean rank of the n_i observations in Group i, $i = 1, 2, \ldots, k$, and let $N = \sum_{i=1}^{k} n_i$. Then, to compare any two groups, say i and j, where $1 \leq i < j \leq k$, calculate

$$z_{ij} = \frac{\overline{R_i} - \overline{R_j}}{\sqrt{[N(N+1)/12]\,[(1/n_i) + (1/n_j)]}}, \tag{4.17}$$

and compare the value of z_{ij} with the upper α'-percentage point of the standard normal distribution, where α' is the Bonferroni-adjusted α-level for all possible pairwise comparisons among k groups, given by

$$\alpha'=\alpha/c, \tag{4.18}$$

where $c = k(k-1)/2$. (See Section 3.7.2 for a description of the Bonferroni method of pairwise comparisons in the general ANOVA.)

One advantage of using this method is that it is rather easy to obtain Bonferroni-adjusted p-values for each pairwise comparison once the test statistics z_{ij} in (4.17) have been calculated. For each z_{ij}, one finds the two-tailed p-value using the standard normal distribution, and then multiplies by the number of possible pairwise comparisons. This yields:

$$\text{Dunn } p\text{-value} = c[2 \cdot \Pr(Z > |z_{ij}|)] = k(k-1)\Pr(Z > |z_{ij}|). \tag{4.19}$$

If this p-value is less than the desired experiment-wise error rate (usually 0.05), populations i and j are declared to be significantly different. (Note that if the Dunn p-value is calculated to be greater than 1.0, it is truncated at 1.0.) The Dunn method is illustrated in Example 4.10.

Example 4.10 Dunn's Method of Pairwise Comparisons

For the data in Table 4.9, $n_1 = 20$, $n_2 = 23$, $n_3 = 15$, and $N = 58$. From the output from the NPAR1WAY procedure applied to these data, we find the following mean ranks in each group: $\overline{R_1} = 37.125$, $\overline{R_2} = 25.087$, and $\overline{R_3} = 26.100$. Applying (4.17) and (4.19), we find for the comparison of Genotypes MM and MN, $z_{12} = 2.33$, Bonferroni-adjusted Dunn p-value = 0.059; for Genotypes MM and NN, $z_{13} = 1.91$, adjusted p-value = 0.168; and for Genotypes MN and NN, $z_{23} = 0.18$, adjusted p-value = 1.000. Despite the apparent difference among the three groups detected by the K-W test ($p = 0.044$), the Dunn method fails to detect any significant pairwise differences among the three groups. Thus, we are unable to conclude that subjects possessing one of the three Genotypes differ significantly from subjects possessing one of the other Genotypes in terms of biomarker level.

SAS code that can be used to carry out Dunn's method for the data in Table 4.9 is available on the companion website. It was adapted from SAS code downloaded from the following website on August 27, 2013.

http://www.misug.org/uploads/8/1/9/1/8191072/pjuneau_nonparam_comp.zip
See also Juneau (2004).

k-Sample Conover Test The two-sample Conover test described previously can be used to test the assumption of equal variability in two populations. This test can be extended and used to test the assumption of equal variability in k populations. The hypotheses to be tested are

H_0: All k populations are identical, except for possibly different means.

$$\text{vs.} \tag{4.20}$$

H_a: At least two of the population variances are not equal to each other.

To perform the k-sample version of the Conover test, we first convert the sample values in each of the k groups to their absolute deviations from their respective sample mean, just as in the two-sample version of this test. Next, the combined sample of all N absolute deviations from the k groups are ordered from smallest to largest and a rank of 1 is assigned to the smallest deviation, and a rank of N to the largest. Mid-ranks are again used if there are ties among the deviations. Next, calculate the sum of squares of the deviations in each of the k samples, and denote these sums of squared ranks by $S_1, S_2, \ldots, S_k$. The test statistic for testing the hypotheses in (4.20) is then given by

$$\chi_0^2 = \frac{\sum_{j=1}^{k} \frac{S_j^2}{n_j} - N\left(\overline{S}\right)^2}{D^2}, \tag{4.21}$$

where

n_j = the number of sample values in Group j,

$$N = n_1 + n_2 + \cdots + n_k,$$

$$\overline{S} = \sum_{j=1}^{k} S_j/N,$$

and

$$D^2 = \left\{ \sum_{i=1}^{N} R_i^4 - N\left(\overline{S}\right)^2 \right\} /(N-1).$$

An approximate p-value for the test statistic χ_0^2 in (4.21) can be obtained using the χ^2 distribution with $k - 1$ degrees of freedom. Approximate and exact p-values for the k-sample Conover test are available in the NPAR1WAY procedure in SAS. (Note that, at the time of this writing, the k-sample Conover test was not available in the most recent release of StatXact-9.) SAS code for performing the Conover test for the data in Table 4.9 is provided following Example 4.11.

Example 4.11 ***k*-Sample Conover Test**

The histograms in Figure 4.7 for the data in Table 4.9 suggested that the distributions of the biomarker readings for subjects possessing one of the three genotypes are not identical in shape. Applying the Conover test to compare the variability in the three populations almost reaches the usual 0.05 level of statistical significance: $\chi_0^2 = 6.25$,

$df = 2$, approximate p-value $= 0.054$. In fact, those subjects with Genotype MM and those with Genotype MN do differ significantly in terms of variability at the 0.05 level: $\chi_0^2 = 5.11$, $df = 1$, approximate p-value $= 0.024$. Given that there is some evidence that the variability differs among the three groups, we recommend using the k-sample median test to compare the biomarker levels for subjects having one of the three genotypes.

The following SAS code can be used to perform the k-sample Conover test for the data in Table 4.9. SAS code for creating the `Table4_9` SAS data set was provided following Example 4.9.

```
proc npar1way data= Table4_9 conover;
class genotype;
var biomarker ;
*exact conover;
run;
```

k-Sample Median Test Let k denote the number of population medians to be compared. As with the other tests discussed in this section, assume that we have a random sample of size n_i from population i, $i = 1, 2, \ldots, k$. Let M_i denote the median of population i. We wish to test the following hypotheses:

$$H_0 : M_1 = M_2 = \cdots = M_k \text{ vs.} \tag{4.22}$$

$$H_a\text{: at least two of the medians are different.}$$

As in the two-sample median test in the section described previously we first find the grand median of the combined sample of $N = n_1 + n_2 + \cdots + n_k$ data values, which we denote by M. Now, compute O_{1i} = number of observations in the ith sample that are greater than M, and O_{2i} = number of observations in the ith sample that are less than or equal to M for $i = 1, 2, \ldots k$. Next, arrange these results into a $2 \times k$ contingency table as in Table 4.10.

In this table, $O_{1.}$ denotes the total number of data values above the grand median in all samples combined, and $O_{2.}$ denotes the total number of data values less than or equal to the grand median in all samples combined. Thus, $O_{1\bullet} + O_{2\bullet} = N$, the total number of observations.

Under the null hypothesis $H_0 : M_1 = M_2 = \cdots = M_k$, the size of the observation is independent of the population it came from. So, we can test H_0 in (4.22) by using the chi-square procedure described in Section 3.10.1 to test the null hypothesis that the row classification of Table 4.10 is independent of the column classification. Using

TABLE 4.10 Observed Frequencies for Performing the *k*-Sample Median Test

	Group 1	Group 2	...	Group k	Total
Number of values > M	O_{11}	O_{12}	...	O_{1k}	$O_{1.}$
Number of values ≤ M	O_{21}	O_{22}	...	O_{2k}	$O_{2.}$
Total	n_1	n_2		n_k	N

the formula in Equation (3.30), and changing notation to be consistent with Table 4.10, we obtain the following test statistic:

$$\chi_0^2 = \sum_{i=1}^{2}\sum_{j=1}^{k} \frac{\left(O_{ij} - \hat{\mu}_{ij}\right)^2}{\hat{\mu}_{ij}}, \tag{4.23}$$

where the expected count in cell (i, j) is given by

$$\hat{\mu}_{ij} = N\left(\frac{n_i O_{1\bullet}}{N}\right)\left(\frac{n_j O_{2\bullet}}{N}\right). \tag{4.24}$$

After some algebra, (4.23) simplifies to the following formula, which is more amenable to hand calculation:

$$\chi_0^2 = \frac{N^2}{O_{1\bullet}O_{2\bullet}} \sum_{j=1}^{k} \frac{O_{1j}^2}{n_j} - \frac{NO_{1\bullet}}{O_{2\bullet}}. \tag{4.25}$$

An approximate p-value for the k-sample median test can be calculated by using a chi-squared distribution with $k - 1$ degrees of freedom. The exact version of the chi-square test can be used to perform an exact test of the hypotheses in (4.22). This is done by calculating the exact p-value for the test statistic in (4.25), in a manner similar to that described for the Fisher–Freeman–Halton (F-F-H) test statistic (Section 4.9.7.1). The k-sample median test is illustrated in Example 4.12.

Example 4.12 *k*-Sample Median Test

For the hypothetical biomarker data in Table 4.9, the sample medians in the three groups are $m_1 = 43, m_2 = 35$, $m_2 = 37$, respectively, and the grand median is $M = 38.5$. The 2×3 table for performing the median test for these data is given in Table 4.11.

Based on these results, $\chi_0^2 = 11.00$, $df = 2$, approximate p-value = 0.0041, exact p-value = 0.0044, mid-P value = 0.0044 – ½(0.0009) = 0.0040. Thus, there is strong evidence that the median biomarker levels of individuals having one of the three genotypes are not the same; therefore, we should reject the null hypothesis H_0: $M_1 = M_2 = M_3$ in favor of the alternative that at least two of the population medians are different. In fact, using the two-sample median test to compare each pair of genotypes in terms of biomarker level yields p-values of 0.005 for MM vs. MN, 0.007 for MM vs. NN, and 0.299 for MN vs. NN. This yields Bonferroni-adjusted p-values of 0.015, 0.021, and 0.897. Thus, there is a significant difference in median biomarker level between individuals with Genotype MM and those with Genotype MN and between those individuals with Genotype MM and those with Genotype NN. These differences were not detected using ANOVA (one-way ANOVA F-test $p = 0.2270$), nor with the K-W test followed by Dunn pairwise comparisons (Example 4.10). This is another illustration of the fact that the median test, which is mistakenly thought by many practitioners to be much less powerful than ANOVA and

TABLE 4.11 Observed Frequencies for Performing the *k*-Sample Median Test

	Group 1	Group 2	Group 3	Total
Number of values > *38.5*	16	8	5	29
Number of values ≤ *38.5*	4	15	10	29
Total	20	23	15	58

K-W under all conditions, can actually detect differences among groups that these other methods might miss.

StatXact and SAS can both be used to perform the k-sample median test using the chi-square approximation, and calculate exact p-values, as long as none of the n_is are too large. As with other distribution-free methods discussed in this textbook, we recommend that the exact p-value be used whenever possible. If the statistical software fails to calculate the exact p-value because one or more of the n_is are too large, it should be safe to use the p-value based on the chi-square approximation (since the chi-square approximation is valid specifically when n is sufficiently large). The chi-square approximation for the k-sample median test is available in the NPAR1WAY procedure in SAS; however, just as with the two-sample median test, the approximate results obtained using NPAR1WAY do not agree with the results obtained using StatXact. (Note that the exact results obtained using NPAR1WAY do agree with StatXact.) This is apparently due to a discrepancy between the "median" scores used by SAS when performing the k-sample median test and the chi-square formulation of the test as we have described it here. However, the correct version of the k-sample median test with chi-square and exact p-values, can be performed using the FREQ procedure in SAS.

The following SAS code can be used to obtain the correct chi-square approximate p-value for the k-sample median test for the data in Table 4.9. It makes use of the cross-classified data in Table 4.11. We also provide SAS code utilizing the NPAR1WAY procedure to produce the exact version of the k-sample median test for the data in Table 4.9. SAS code for creating the `Table4_9` SAS data set was provided following Example 4.9.

```
data Table4_11;
input gt_median genotype count @@;
cards;
1 1 16  1 2  8  1 3  5
2 1  4  2 2 15  2 3 10
;

proc freq  data = Table4_11; weight count;
     tables gt_median * genotype;
     exact chisq;
     title1 'k-Sample Median Test';
     title2 'Based on Exact Chi-Square Test';
     run;
```

```
proc npar1way data = Table4_9 median;
     class genotype;
     var biomarker ;
     exact median;
     title1 'k-Sample Median Test';
     title2 'Use Exact Output Only';
     run;
```

4.3 HETEROGENEITY OF VARIANCE

4.3.1 The Effects of Heterogeneity

Many commonly used statistical procedures for comparing two or more groups in terms of biomarker level are based on the assumption that the population variances of the biomarker levels in the groups being compared are equal. Examples include Student's t-test and one-way ANOVA. (See Sections 3.7.1 and 3.7.2.) The assumption of equal variances among groups is sometimes referred to as *homoscedasticity* or *homogeneity of variances*. Violations of this assumption are referred to as *heteroscedasticity* or *heterogeneity of variances*. The serious adverse effects that heteroscedasticity can have on the performance of commonly used procedures for comparing two or more population means are well known (Algina et al. 1994; Wilcox 1987, pp. 102, 129). However, it is an unfortunate fact that many analysts working with biomarker data ignore the underlying homoscedasticity assumption and make no attempt to either verify this assumption and/or make use of a procedure that is robust to its violation. In this section, we discuss several approaches that can be used to mitigate any adverse effects that violations of the homoscedasticity assumption can have on the comparison of two or more groups in terms of mean biomarker level.

4.3.2 The Importance of Heterogeneity in the Comparison of Means

4.3.2.1 Comparisons of Two Groups The most commonly used method for comparing two groups in terms of their mean biomarker level is the t-test. The "usual" t-test (sometimes called the "equal-variance t-test" or "pooled variance t-test") that is typically used in biomarker studies depends very strongly on the underlying assumption that the population variances in the two groups being compared are equal (Moser et al. 1989). The approach for dealing with the equal variance issue that is most commonly presented in textbooks is to use the F-test for testing equality of population variances or some other method for comparing variances to verify the homogeneity assumption prior to applying the equal-variance t-test (Markowski and Markowski 1990; Moser and Stevens 1992). If the results of the test of variances indicate that the null hypothesis of equal variances should not be rejected, then one applies the "usual" t-test to compare the means of the two groups. If the test of variances indicates that the hypothesis of equal variances should be rejected, then one applies an alternative approach that does not depend on the underlying homogeneity assumption.

Assuming that the preliminary F-test indicates that the homogeneity assumption does not hold, the most commonly used alternative method is the "unequal-variance t-test" (sometimes referred to as the "Welch test" or "Satterthwaite's approximation"). This test is typically available in any statistical package that can perform the equal-variance t-test (but not Excel). However, based on their simulation results, Markowski and Markowski (1990) concluded that the preliminary F-test is "flawed"; in addition, Moser and Stevens (1992) demonstrated via simulation that performing the preliminary F-test of the homogeneity assumption contributes nothing of value and, in fact, it is safe to use the unequal-variance t-test any time one wishes to compare the means of two normal populations. This is because the unequal-variance t-test performs almost as well as the equal-variance t-test when the variances of the two normal populations being compared are equal, and can substantially outperform the equal-variance t-test when the population variances are unequal. Hence, we recommend the routine use of the unequal-variance t-test any time two normal populations are being compared in terms of mean biomarker level. (This recommendation is valid, of course, only if there is reason to believe that the biomarker levels are normally distributed in both groups. If the methods for assessing the normality assumption described in Section 4.2.2 indicate that the data are not normally distributed in either of the two groups, then a distribution-free alternative to the t-test such as the M-W-W test or the median test (Section 4.2.3.3) should be considered.)

We wish to test the following hypotheses:

$$\begin{aligned} H_0 &: \ \mu_1 = \mu_2 \\ H_a &: \ \mu_1 \neq \mu_2 \end{aligned} \tag{4.26}$$

where μ_1 is the mean in Population 1 and μ_2 is the mean in Population 2. The test statistic for the unequal-variance t-test is given by

$$t_{0u} = \frac{(\bar{x}_1 - \bar{x}_2)}{\sqrt{\frac{s_1^2}{n_1} + \frac{s_2^2}{n_2}}} \tag{4.27}$$

where $\bar{x}_1$, s_1^2, and n_1 denote the mean, variance, and sample size, respectively, for the biomarker levels in Group 1; and $\bar{x}_2$, s_2^2, and n_2 denote the mean, variance, and sample size, respectively, for the biomarker levels in Group 2. To perform the test of the hypotheses in (4.26), compare the value of t_{0u} in (4.27) with the critical value from the Student's t-distribution with the following approximate degrees of freedom:

$$\upsilon = \frac{\left(\frac{1}{n_1} + \frac{u}{n_2}\right)^2}{\frac{1}{n_1^2(n_1-1)} + \frac{u^2}{n_2^2(n_2-1)}}, \tag{4.28}$$

where $u = {}^{s_2^2}/_{s_1^2}$. (Note that υ in (4.28) reduces to $2n - 2$ whenever $u = 1$ and $n_1 = n_2 = n$. Under these conditions, the unequal-variance t-test statistic in (4.27) with degrees of freedom given by (4.28) is equivalent to the equal-variance t-test statistic in Equation (3.11).)

There is no guarantee that the approximate degrees of freedom υ in (4.28) will be an integer. It can be shown that $\min(n_1, n_2) \leq \upsilon \leq n_1 + n_2 - 2$. A conservative approach would be to use the integer closest to but less than υ. However, most standard statistical packages are capable of performing the unequal-variance t-test with *df* given by (4.28) even with fractional degrees of freedom. (Note that Excel is not.) Software is available for calculating critical values and p-values for the t-distribution with fractional degrees of freedom; one such example is StatCalc, which accompanies the textbook by Krishnamoorthy (2006). The TTEST procedure in SAS provides results for both the equal and unequal-variance t-test, in addition to the results of the F-test for comparing the variances of the two groups.

Example 4.13 Unequal-Variance *t*-Test

To illustrate the effects of variance heterogeneity in a two-group comparison of mean biomarker levels, consider the study by Salmi et al. (2002). These investigators examined the potential usefulness of soluble vascular adhesion protein-1 (sVAP-1) as a biomarker for monitoring and predicting the extent of ongoing atherosclerotic processes. Salmi et al. compared the mean sVAP-1 level of diabetic subjects on insulin treatment only ($\bar{x}_1 = 148$, $s_1 = 114$, $n_1 = 7$) with that of diabetic subjects on other treatments ($\bar{x}_2 = 113$, $s_2 = 6$, $n_2 = 41$) using the equal-variance t-test (Section 3.7.1), which indicated that diabetics on insulin treatment only have a significantly higher mean sVAP-1 level ($t_0 = 2.06$, $df = 46$, one-tailed $p = 0.023$). However, the authors ignored the heterogeneity of variance in the two groups they compared: $s_1^2 = 12996$ vs. $s_2^2 = 36$, $F_0 = 361$, $df = (6,40)$, $p < 0.001$. Had they used the unequal-variance t-test, as recommended by Moser and Stevens (1992), they would not have concluded that the mean sVAP-1 levels of the two groups were significantly different: $t_{0u} = 0.81$, $\upsilon = 6.01$, one-tailed $p = 0.224$). Even without performing the formal F-test of homogeneity of variances in the two groups, there can be little doubt that the two population variances are unequal. Thus, we contend that the results based on the unequal-variance t-test provide a more valid comparison of the two groups in terms of mean sVAP-1 level. (Note that we recommend that the unequal-variance t-test be used any time one wishes to compare the mean biomarker levels of two groups using data that appear to be normally distributed, so we would not have considered using the equal-variance t-test on those grounds, regardless of an examination of the sample variances or results of the F-test of homogeneity.)

The following SAS code can be used to perform the equal and unequal-variance t-tests and the F-test of variances for the sVAP-1 data in Salmi et al. (2002). Note that a special data set has to be created in order to input the summary statistics since the raw data were not provided in Salmi et al.

```
DATA salmi;
     INPUT Obs Group $ _TYPE_ _FREQ_ _STAT_ $ sVAP_1;
     DATALINES;
 1 insulin   0  7 N     7.000
 2 insulin   0  7 MIN    .
 3 insulin   0  7 MAX    .
 4 insulin   0  7 MEAN  148
 5 insulin   0  7 STD   114
 6 other_tx  0 41 N     41.000
 7 other_tx  0 41 MIN    .
 8 other_tx  0 41 MAX    .
 9 other_tx  0 41 MEAN  113
10 other_tx  0 41 STD   6
;

proc ttest data = salmi SIDES = U;
   class Group;
   var sVAP_1;
run;
```

4.3.2.2 Comparisons of More Than Two Groups In Section 3.7.2, we described the method most commonly used to compare mean biomarker levels across $k > 2$ groups; namely, the one-way ANOVA F-test. As we pointed out in the preceding section, the most commonly used method for comparing two groups in terms of their mean biomarker, the "equal-variance t-test," depends very strongly on the assumption that the population variances in the two groups being compared are equal. The same is true for the one-way ANOVA F-test. As pointed out by Wilcox (1987, p. 129), several authors have shown that violation of the homoscedasticity assumption can seriously affect the Type I error rate and the power of the ANOVA F-test, even when there are equal sample sizes in the k groups (Brown and Forsythe 1974; Ramsey 1980; Scheffé 1959). In Section 4.3.2.1, we described the unequal-variance t-test (attributed to both Welch (1937) and Satterthwaite (1946)), which does not depend on the assumption of equal variances when comparing the means of two groups. In this section, we describe a generalization of the unequal-variance t-test to the comparison of $k > 2$ means from normal populations proposed by Welch (1951).

Recall from Section 3.7.2, that the test statistic for the usual one-way ANOVA F-test is equal to the "Mean square between groups" (MSB) divided by the "mean square within groups" (MSW). From Equation (3.13), MSB is given by

$$\text{MSB} = \frac{\sum_{i=1}^{k} n_i \left(\bar{y}_i - \bar{\bar{y}}\right)^2}{k-1},$$

where $\bar{y}_i$ = the mean biomarker level within the ith group, $\bar{\bar{y}}$ = the "grand mean" of the biomarker levels for all n subjects combined, k = the number of groups being compared, and n_i = the sample size within group i; $i = 1, 2, \ldots, k$ and $j = 1, 2, \ldots, n_i$. In the Welch test, the squared deviations of the group means from the grand mean appearing in the numerator of MSB are weighted not by the group size, but by the reciprocal of the squared standard error in that group, $w_i = n_i/s_i^2$:

$$\mathrm{MSB}_w = \frac{\sum_{i=1}^{k} w_i \left(\bar{y}_i - \tilde{y}\right)^2}{k-1}. \tag{4.29}$$

Furthermore, the grand mean $\bar{\bar{y}}$ in (3.13) is replaced by

$$\tilde{y} = \frac{\sum_{i=1}^{k} w_i \bar{y}_i}{\sum_{i=1}^{k} w_i}, \tag{4.30}$$

which is the weighted average of the group means. The Welch test statistic is then given by

$$W_0 = \frac{\mathrm{MSB_w}}{1 + (2/3)(k-2)\Lambda}, \tag{4.31}$$

where

$$\Lambda = \frac{3\sum_{i=1}^{k}\left\{\left[1 - \left(w_j \Big/ \sum_{i=1}^{k} w_j\right)\right]^2 \Big/ \left(n_i - 1\right)\right\}}{k-1}. \tag{4.32}$$

When the null hypothesis $H_0 : \mu_1 = \mu_2 = \cdots = \mu_k$ is true, W_0 given in (4.31) is approximately distributed as F with $k - 1$ and $1/\Lambda$ degrees of freedom. Thus, H_0 is rejected if the value of W_0 calculated from the data is greater than the upper α-percentage point of the F-distribution with $k - 1$ and $1/\Lambda$ degrees of freedom for the numerator and denominator, respectively. As in the unequal-variance t-test, there is no guarantee that $1/\Lambda$ will be an integer. Just as with the t-distribution with fractional degrees of freedom, software is available for calculating critical values and p-values for the F-distribution with fractional degrees of freedom; one such example is StatCalc (Krishnamoorthy 2006).

The GLM procedure in SAS can be used to perform the Welch test for comparing more than two means. SAS code for performing this test for the data in Table 3.4 is given following Example 4.14.

Example 4.14 Welch Test for Comparing k > 2 Group Means

Recall Example 3.7, in which we considered the study by Lemoine et al (2013), who compared mean umbilical cord coiling length (the biomarker) among Caucasians,

TABLE 4.12 Descriptive Statistics for Data on Umbilical Cord Coiling Lengths

Group	Sample Mean ($\bar{x}_i$)	Sample Variance (s_i^2)	Sample Size (n_i)
Caucasians	2.35	1.4066	20
African Americans	3.67	1.8349	20
Hispanics	3.05	3.7124	20

African Americans, and other ethnicities (Hispanics, Asians, etc.). The data for this study are given in Table 3.4, and the group means, variances, and sample sizes are provided in Table 4.12.

Based on these summary statistics, homoscedasticity appears to be violated since the sample variance for Hispanics is over twice as large as that for the other two groups. This subjective impression is confirmed by the results of the k-sample Conover test $\chi_0^2 = 9.23$, $df = 2$, approximate p-value $= 0.0099$, which provides strong evidence of a significant departure from the homoscedasticity assumption (Section 4.2.3.3). Applying the Welch test, we obtain $W_0 = 5.32$, $df_1 = 2$, $df_2 = 36.819$, approximate p-value $= 0.009$. For the F-test, we obtain $F_0 = 3.77$, $df_1 = 2$, $df_2 = 57$, p-value $= 0.029$. Both the Welch test and the usual ANOVA F-test indicate that $H_0 : \mu_1 = \mu_2 = \mu_3$ should be rejected; however, the evidence against the null hypothesis (as measured by the p-value) is much stronger for the Welch test.

The following SAS code can be used to perform the Welch test for the data in Table 3.4:

```
proc glm data = all;
    class ethnicity;
    model coil = ethnicity;
    means ethnicity / welch;
    title1 'Welch Test for 1-way ANOVA';
    run;
```

Note that SAS code for creating the SAS data set `all` was provided with Example 3.8 (and can also be found on the companion website.)

4.3.2.3 Multiple Comparisons In the analysis of biomarker data, it is often the case that one wishes to compare the means of three or more groups. For example, in Bernstein et al. (1999), the investigators compared three groups in terms of the mean level of their apoptotic index (AI): (a) "normal" subjects with no history of polyps or cancer; (b) patients with a history of colorectal cancer; and (c) patients with benign colorectal adenomas. Bernstein et al. used the Tukey–Kramer (T-K) method to perform all possible pairwise comparisons among the three group means. The T-K method (Section 3.7.2) is the technique of choice if the population variances of the three groups are equal (Dunnett 1980a); however, if the variances are not equal, the methods known as Dunnett's C, Dunnett's T3, and Games–Howell are preferable (Dunnett 1980b; Maxwell and Delaney 2004, pp. 212–213). These methods (especially Dunnett's T3) are very similar to the unequal-variance t-test that we recommended for general use in Section 4.3.2.1. The T-K, Games–Howell, Dunnett's C, and Dunnett's T3 procedures are all available in the Statistical Package for the Social Sciences (SPSS). The T-K method is available in SAS. The T-K and Dunnett's T3 procedures are available in R.

*Technical Details for Multiple Comparison Methods** Let μ_i and σ_i^2 denote the population mean and population variance, respectively, in group i, $1 \leq i \leq k$, where k denotes the number of groups to be compared. Let $\bar{x}_i$ denote the sample mean and let s_i^2 denote the unbiased estimate of σ_i^2 based on υ_i degrees of freedom in group i. We wish to find a set of $100(1 - \alpha)\%$ joint CI estimates for the $k(k-1)/2$ differences $\mu_i - \mu_j$, $1 \leq i < j \leq k$. Both the Dunnett's C and T3 methods involve constructing joint CI estimates of the form

$$\bar{x}_i - \bar{x}_j \pm c_{ij,\alpha,k}\sqrt{\frac{s_i^2}{n_i} + \frac{s_j^2}{n_j}}, \tag{4.33}$$

where $c_{ij,\alpha,k}$ is a critical value chosen so that the joint confidence coefficient is as close as possible to $1 - \alpha$. For Dunnett's T3 procedure, it is also possible to calculate adjusted p-values for each pairwise comparison of means.

For Dunnett's C procedure,

$$c_{ij,\alpha,k} = \frac{\mathrm{SR}_{\alpha,k,\upsilon_{ij}^*}}{\sqrt{2}}, \tag{4.34}$$

where

$$\mathrm{SR}_{\alpha,k,\upsilon_{ij}^*} = \frac{\dfrac{\mathrm{SR}_{\alpha,k,\upsilon_i} s_i^2}{n_i} + \dfrac{\mathrm{SR}_{\alpha,k,\upsilon_j} s_j^2}{n_j}}{\dfrac{s_i^2}{n_i} + \dfrac{s_j^2}{n_j}}$$

and $\mathrm{SR}_{\alpha,k,\upsilon}$ denotes the upper α-percentage point of the distribution of the Studentized range of k normal variates with an estimate of the variance based on υ degrees of freedom. Tables of the SR distribution are widely available; for example, see http://cse.niaes.affrc.go.jp/miwa/probcalc/s-range/srng_tbl.html#fivepercent (accessed March 3, 2014).

For Dunnett's T3 procedure,

$$c_{ij,\alpha,k} = \text{SMM}_{\alpha,k^*,\hat{\upsilon}_{ij}}, \tag{4.35}$$

where $\text{SMM}_{\alpha,k^*,\hat{\upsilon}_{ij}}$ denotes the upper α-percentage point of the Studentized maximum modulus (SMM) distribution of $k^* = k(k-1)/2$ uncorrelated normal variates with degrees of freedom $\hat{\upsilon}_{ij}$ given by

$$\widehat{\upsilon_{ij}} = \frac{\left(\frac{s_i^2}{n_i} + \frac{s_j^2}{n_j}\right)^2}{\frac{s_i^4}{n_i^2(\upsilon_i)} + \frac{s_j^4}{n_j^2(\upsilon_j)}}. \tag{4.36}$$

Note the similarity of the formula for $\widehat{\upsilon_{ij}}$ in (4.36) to that of the degrees of freedom for the unequal-variance t-test given in (4.28), after making the substitution $u = s_j^2/s_i^2$ in (4.36).

Tables of the percentage points of the SMM distribution for integer degrees of freedom are readily available (e.g., Maxwell and Delaney 2004, pp. A14–A16). As recommended by Dunnett (1980b), percentage points of the SMM distribution for fractional degrees of freedom can be estimated using quadratic interpolation based on the reciprocals of the degrees of freedom corresponding to percentage points in the published tables.

Example 4.15 Dunnett's C and T3 Pairwise Comparison Methods

Again recall Example 3.7, in which we considered the comparison by Lemoine et al. (2013) of umbilical cord coiling lengths among Caucasians, African Americans, and other ethnicities (Hispanics, Asians, etc.). Table 4.12 contains the group means, variances, and sample sizes for these data.

In Section 3.7.2, we illustrated the use of the T-K method to perform all pairwise comparisons among the three groups. The T-K p-values and associated 95% CIs are given in Table 4.13. The only significant difference was between Caucasians and African Americans ($p = 0.022$). Table 4.13 also contains the results for all pairwise comparisons using the Dunnett T3 and Dunnett C methods. Note that the p-value for the Caucasian vs. African American comparison is somewhat smaller for the T3 method than for the T-K method, and that there is very little difference between the Dunnett T3 and Dunnett C results in terms of the CIs. Since there was evidence of unequal variances among the three groups (Conover's test, $\chi_0^2 = 9.23$, $df = 2$, $p = 0.0099$), the Dunnett T3 (or C) results would be preferable.

R code that can be used to perform Dunnett's T3 method for the data in Table 3.4 is provided in the following Table 4.13.

TABLE 4.13 Pairwise Comparisons for Umbilical Cord Coiling Length Data

Method	C vs. AA	C vs. H	AA vs. H
Tukey–Kramer	0.022[a]	0.323	0.404
	(−2.48, −0.16)	(−1.86, 0.46)	(−0.54, 1.78)
Dunnett's T3	0.007	0.436	0.562
	(−2.33, −0.32)	(−1.97, 0.57)	(−0.70, 1.94)
Dunnett's C	—	—	—
	(−2.34, −0.30)	(−1.98, 0.59)	(−0.71, 1.96)
Bonferroni adjusted unequal variance t-tests	0.007	0.532	0.735
	(−2.33, −0.31)	(−1.98, 0.58)	(−0.70, 1.95)

C, Caucasian; AA, African American; H, Hispanic.
[a]The top entry in each cell is the p-value for that pairwise comparison using the indicated method; the bottom entry is the 95% confidence interval for the true difference in means.

```
# install and load the DTK package
install.packages("DTK", dependencies=TRUE)
library(DTK)
# enter each genotype's biomarker data
MM <- c(44, 50, 42, 41, 44, 48, 38, 42, 50, 47, 49, 49, 40, 44, 48, 41, 34, 41, 30, 22)
MN <- c(48, 31, 31, 36, 29, 31, 39, 69, 34, 31, 34, 26, 35, 58, 37, 41, 36, 32, 57, 64, 28, 28, 43)
NN <- c(35, 29, 47, 32, 36, 37, 4, 36, 34, 39, 38, 37, 52, 45, 41)

# combine all three genotype's biomarker data
biomarker <- c(MM, MN, NN)

# create "genotype" factor variable
genotype <- c(rep("MM", length(MM)), rep("MN", length(MN)), rep("NN", length(NN)))
# perform DTK test, output results and generate plot
DTK.result<-DTK.test(x=biomarker,f=genotype,a=0.05)
DTK.result
DTK.plot(DTK.result)
```

The following SPSS syntax can be used to perform the T-K, Dunnett T3, and Dunnett C analyses for the data in Table 3.4. It also performs the Welch version of the one-way ANOVA F-test, which was discussed in Section 4.3.2.2.

```
oneway length by group
/statistics descriptives welch
/missing analysis
/posthoc=tukey t3 c alpha(0.05).
```

As a practical matter, a natural question to ask is whether it is worth the extra trouble to use the Dunnett C or T3 procedures instead of the much more commonly used Tukey-Kramer method. This issue is complicated by (1) the fact that performing a "pre-test" of the homoscedasticity assumption in one-way ANOVA is generally not recommended since any test of the assumption may not have sufficient power to detect heteroscedasticity in situations when the assumption of homoscedasticity should be abandoned, even when the data are normally distributed (Wilcox 1987, p. 143); and (2) the Dunnett C and T3 procedures are not available in SAS. We feel that a reasonable way to proceed is to use the Tukey-Kramer method as long as the group sizes are roughly comparable. If there is wide variation, then we recommend that the Dunnett T3 method be used since it can be performed using the freely available R software. If the analyst has access to SPSS, then the T-K, Dunnett T3, or Dunnett C methods can be applied, as appropriate. (SPSS can also perform the Games–Howell method of pairwise comparisons, which some authors have recommended under certain conditions (Maxwell and Delaney 2004, p. 213)).

Another reasonable approach that could be extremely conservative under some conditions would be to use the unequal-variance t-test with Bonferroni adjustment to perform all pairwise comparisons among the group means. This would be consistent with using the Welch version of the one-way ANOVA F-test to test the null hypothesis $H_0 : \mu_1 = \mu_2 = \cdots = \mu_k$, which is the appropriate test to use in the presence of heteroscedasticity (and very little is lost even when using this method in the presence of homoscedasticity). The results obtained using this approach are provided in Table 4.13. Note that there is essentially no difference between the intervals produced by the unequal-variance t-test using a Bonferroni-adjusted 98.33% confidence coefficient and either the T3 or C CIs. The p-value for Dunnett's T3 and the Bonferroni-adjusted p-value for the comparison of Caucasians vs. African Americans (the only significant pairwise comparison) agree to within three decimal places (p = 0.007 for both).

4.4 DEPENDENT GROUPS

4.4.1 The Consequences of Ignoring Dependence Among Groups

In most comparisons of mean biomarker level between two groups, the biomarker levels in one group can safely be assumed to be independent of the biomarker levels in the other group. That is, there is no reason to believe that knowing the biomarker level of any individual in one group will provide any useful information about the biomarker level of an individual in another group. In a randomized clinical trial (Section 2.2.7), in which study participants are randomly assigned to one treatment group or the other, independence between groups is assured, provided the randomization is properly carried out. Even if the study is not randomized, it may be reasonable to assume that the groups being compared are independent. In Example 3.6, we considered a study in which the investigators wished to compare the mean Na–K ATPase level of 11 bipolar patients on placebo vs. the mean Na–K ATPase level of 10 bipolar patients on lithium. There was no overlap between the 11 patients receiving placebo and the 10 patients being treated with lithium. Thus, we can safely assume that these two groups of patients are independent as far as the comparison of their mean Na–K

ATPase levels are concerned, and we can apply the usual two-sample *t*-test. However, suppose that there was overlap between the two groups; in other words, suppose that some of the patients were studied in both the placebo condition and in the lithium-treated condition. Then, obviously, the two groups cannot be treated as independent. In Section 4.4.2, we consider methods that can be used when *all* of the patients receive both treatments; frequently, this takes the form of a "before and after" design. That is, patients are studied prior to receiving some treatment (i.e., at *baseline*), and then again after receiving the treatment (i.e., at *follow-up*). In Example 4.16, we consider the study by Naylor et al. (1976), in which the investigators examined erythrocyte sodium (ES) concentration as a potential biomarker for the response to lithium treatment in patients with bipolar illness. The ES levels were measured in 10 bipolar patients before and after treatment with lithium. Obviously, since the same patients are being studied under both treatment conditions, it would not be reasonable to assume that the two groups (prior to lithium treatment and following lithium treatment) are independent. We would say that the ES levels for each subject under the two treatment conditions are "paired"; hence, the term "paired *t*-test" is used to describe the most commonly used method for analyzing data from this type of study.

Sometimes the "pairing" of the observations in the two groups is not so obvious. For example, in studies involving identical twins, it is often assumed that the data for one twin is paired with the data for the other twin, and the methods described in Section 4.4.2.1 are used to determine if there are significant twin-related differences. In matched case–control studies (Section 2.2.3), dependence is deliberately introduced by matching each subject with the disease (the *case*) to one or more subjects without the disease (the *controls*) on the basis of attributes that are assumed to be confounders of the true exposure–disease (E-D) association. The most commonly used matching criteria are age, race, and gender, but many other criteria have been used in this type of study. Because the cases and controls are matched and are therefore similar in terms of the matching criteria, any biomarker determinations made on them must now be assumed to be dependent, and the methods of Section 4.4.2 should be used for comparing cases and controls in terms of mean biomarker level. Similarly, if one wishes to compare two "dependent groups" in terms of a proportion, the methods in Section 4.4.3 should be used. Similarly, if the primary focus of the study is to use the odds ratio (OR) to measure the E-D association between some exposure (perhaps based on a dichotomized biomarker) and some disease outcome, the methods described in Section 4.9.4.4 should be used, rather than the standard analyses for ORs (Section 3.10.2).

There can be serious consequences if the dependence between the groups being compared is not taken into account in the statistical analysis. Failure to incorporate this dependence can lead to invalid point estimates, primarily through distorted estimates of the true standard error. This, in turn, will have adverse consequences for any CIs or hypothesis tests that are based on the invalid point estimates. Taking the dependence between groups into account can actually yield more powerful statistical tests and narrower CIs that are more likely to include the true value of the unknown parameter. In Section 4.4.2.1, we illustrate the close relationship between the paired and "unpaired" t-test and provide an example in which taking the pairing into account actually yields a much lower p-value for the comparison of means. Similarly, in Section 4.9.4.4, we provide an example in which the "matched pair" analysis for the OR yields a lower p-value for the test that the true OR is equal to one. The bottom line is that the analyst should always make full use of all the salient features of the data in hand; failure to do so will result in inefficient analyses that may lead to erroneous conclusions.

4.4.2 Comparing Two Dependent Means

4.4.2.1 Paired t-test In Chapter 3, we considered the study by Faupel-Badger et al. (2006), who examined the research question "Does the breast cancer prevention drug raloxifene affect the serum estradiol levels of premenopausal women at high risk for developing breast cancer?" To address this question, the researchers measured the serum estradiol levels of premenopausal women at baseline upon enrollment into their study, and then again after taking 60 mg raloxifene daily for 12 months. In Section 3.6.2, we used this example to introduce the concepts of hypothesis testing and CI estimation for a single population mean, μ, where $\mu =$ the true mean change in serum estradiol levels for these women after taking raloxifene. We indicated out that the *one-sample t-test* could be used to test the hypotheses

$$H_0 : \mu = 0 \text{ vs. } H_\text{a} : \mu \neq 0;$$

the appropriate test statistic would be

$$t_0 = \frac{\bar{x}}{s/\sqrt{n}}, \tag{4.37}$$

where $\bar{x} =$ the sample mean change in serum estradiol levels, $s =$ the sample standard deviation of the change, and $n =$ the sample size. The absolute value of t_0 would then be evaluated against the Student t-distribution with $(n - 1)$ degrees of freedom in order to calculate a two-tailed p-value.

As we pointed out in Section 3.6.2, performing a one-sample t-test on the mean change (after – before) in serum estradiol levels is equivalent to using the paired t-test to compare the subjects' serum estradiol levels before and after taking raloxifene. This is an example of the comparison of "dependent means," in the sense that we are not comparing the means of two independent groups of subjects, but rather the means of the same group of subjects before and after some treatment has been applied. In that sense, the "before and after" observations on each female patient in Faupel-Badger et al. are "paired" with each other.

In this section, we introduce new notation so that we can more clearly describe the relationship between the paired t-test and the independent samples t-test. Let $\mu_\text{d} =$ the true mean of the paired differences. To determine if there is a significant change in the response variable from "before" to "after," we test the hypotheses

$$H_0 : \mu_\text{d} = 0 \text{ vs. } H_\text{d} : \mu_\text{d} \neq 0. \tag{4.38}$$

(Note that we could test the null hypothesis that the true mean paired difference is equal to some non-zero value μ_{d0}; in this case, (4.38) becomes $H_0 : \mu_d = \mu_{d0}$ vs. $H_a : \mu_d \neq \mu_{d0}$. However, the null value to be tested in the paired t-test is almost always $\mu_{d0} = 0$.)

Let $\{x_1, x_2, \ldots x_n\}$ denote the sample of "before" biomarker values and let $\{y_1, y_2, \ldots y_n\}$ denote the sample of "after" biomarker values and let $\{d_1, d_2, \ldots d_n\}$ denote the sample of paired differences, where $d_i = x_i - y_i,\ i = 1,\ 2,\ \ldots,\ n$. To test (4.38) using the paired t-test, we calculate the following test statistic:

$$t_{p0} = \frac{\bar{d}}{s_d/\sqrt{n}}, \tag{4.39}$$

where $\bar{d}$ = the sample mean of the paired differences, s_d = the sample standard deviation of the paired differences, and n = the number of pairs. The absolute value of t_{p0} would then be evaluated against the Student t-distribution with $(n - 1)$ degrees of freedom in order to calculate a two-tailed p-value.

Another way to think of the paired t-test is as a "dependent" or "correlated" two-sample t-test. This is equivalent to the equal-variance two-sample t-test that we discussed in Section 3.7.1 when there is no pairing or dependence in the data. Recall that the test statistic for comparing the means of two groups using the equal-variance t-test is given by

$$t_0 = \frac{\bar{x}_1 - \bar{x}_2}{s_p\sqrt{\frac{1}{n_1} + \frac{1}{n_2}}}, \tag{4.40}$$

where $\bar{x}_1$ and $\bar{x}_2$ are the sample means in the two groups, n_1 and n_2 are the sample sizes, and s_p is the "pooled" sample standard deviation (see Equation 3.11):

$$s_p = \sqrt{\frac{(n_1 - 1)s_1^2 + (n_2 - 1)s_2^2}{n_1 + n_2 - 2}}.$$

In this formula, s_1^2 and s_2^2 denote the sample variances for groups 1 and 2, respectively. Note that if $n_1 = n_2$, as would be the case in the paired t-test setting, the "pooled" sample standard deviation becomes

$$s_p = \sqrt{\left(s_1^2 + s_2^2\right)/2}. \tag{4.41}$$

If the two groups being compared are not independent (as would be the case with the paired t-test), then the covariance between the "before" value and the "after" value must be incorporated into (4.41). This yields:

$$s_p = \sqrt{\left(s_1^2 + s_2^2 - 2s_{12}\right)/2}, \tag{4.42}$$

where s_{12} denotes the sample covariance between the before and after scores. Using the definition of covariance, s_p given in (4.42) can be rewritten as

$$s_p = \sqrt{\left(s_1^2 + s_2^2 - 2rs_1s_2\right)/2}, \tag{4.43}$$

where r denotes the sample correlation between the "before" and the "after" values. Using a result from statistical theory (Wilcox 1987, p. 114), it can be shown that:

$$s_d = \sqrt{s_1^2 + s_2^2 - 2rs_1s_2}, \tag{4.44}$$

where s_d is the standard deviation of the paired differences, which appears in the formula for the test statistic for the paired t-test in (4.39). Recalling once again that $n_1 = n_2$ in the paired t-test setting and rewriting s_p in (4.43) as $s_p = \sqrt{s_d^2/2} = s_d/\sqrt{2}$, the test statistic for the two-sample equal-variance t-test in (4.40) becomes:

$$t_0 = \frac{\bar{x}_1 - \bar{x}_2}{\left(s_d/\sqrt{2}\right)\left(\sqrt{2/n}\right)} = \frac{\bar{x}_1 - \bar{x}_2}{s_d/\sqrt{n}}, \tag{4.45}$$

which is equivalent to the formula for the paired t-test in (4.39) since $\bar{d} = \bar{x}_1 - \bar{x}_2$; in other words, the mean of the paired differences is equal to the "before mean" minus the "after mean."

Another way to say this is that the paired t-test is a generalized version of the two-sample equal-variance t-test in which the dependence between the "before" and "after" groups being compared is taken into account. If there is no correlation between the before and after biomarker levels (i.e., $r = 0$ in (4.44)), then the paired t-test is identical to the equal-variance t-test when $n_1 = n_2$. Note that if $r > 0$ in (4.44) (as is almost always the case with biomarker data), the estimated standard deviation will be less than what it would be if the dependence between groups were ignored. This means that the standard error, which appears in the denominator of the t-test statistic, will also be smaller, which will result in a larger value of the test statistic. This generally will lead to a smaller p-value; a complicating factor is that $df = n - 1$ for the paired t-test, whereas, $df = 2(n - 1)$ for the corresponding unpaired t-test. (For the same value of the test statistic, smaller degrees of freedom yield larger p-values.) However, provided that r is sufficiently large, the effect of smaller degrees of freedom will be offset by the increase in the value of the test statistic. This phenomenon is illustrated for the data in Table 4.14 following Example 4.16.

Note that the paired t-test is applicable only when the paired differences can be assumed to constitute a sample from a normal distribution. It is *not* necessary for either the "before" biomarker levels or the "after" biomarker levels to also follow a normal distribution. Thus, when verifying the underlying distributional assumption prior to applying the paired t-test, one need only test the sample of paired differences for normality using the methods described in Section 4.2.2. If the assumption of normality appears to be violated for the paired differences, then the distribution-free methods described in Sections 4.4.2.2 and 4.4.2.3 should be considered.

The paired t-test can be performed using the TTEST procedure in SAS. It can also be performed by applying the UNIVARIATE procedure to the paired differences. (As discussed before, the UNIVARIATE procedure can also be used to assess the normality of the paired differences.) SAS code that can be used to apply the paired t-test to the data in Table 4.14 is provided following Example 4.16.

4.4.2.2 Wilcoxon Signed Ranks Test We wish to test the same hypotheses as in the paired t-test (Equation 4.38):

$$H_0 : \mu_{\mathrm{d}} = 0 \text{ vs. } H_{\mathrm{a}} : \mu_{\mathrm{d}} \neq 0,$$

where μ_{d} = population mean difference between X and Y. Like the paired t-test, the application of the Wilcoxon signed ranks (WSR) test focuses on the paired differences of the dependent observations. Let $\{x_1, x_2, \ldots x_n\}$ denote the sample of "before" biomarker levels and let $\{y_1, y_2, \ldots y_n\}$ denote the sample of "after" biomarker levels and let $\{d_1, d_2, \ldots d_n\}$ denote the sample of paired differences, where $d_i = x_i - y_i$, $i = 1, 2, \ldots, n$. The first step in performing the WSR test is to calculate the absolute value of each paired difference: $|d_i| = |x_i - y_i|$, $i = 1, 2, \ldots, n$. Omit from further consideration all pairs with a difference of zero, that is, any pairs for which $d_i = x_i - y_i = 0$. Denote the number of non-zero paired differences by n'. Next, order the n' non-zero differences from smallest to largest, and assign a rank of 1 to the smallest absolute difference and a rank of n' to the largest absolute difference. In the case of tied absolute differences, mid-ranks are assigned to each of the tied differences (see Example 4.6). Now define R_i, the *signed rank*, for each pair as follows:

$$R_i = \left\{ \begin{array}{l} \text{rank assigned to } |d_i| \text{ if } d_i > 0 \\ \text{negative of rank assigned to } |d_i| \text{ if } d_i < 0. \end{array} \right\}$$

The test statistic for the WSR test is given by sum of the positive signed ranks: $T_0^+ = \sum_{\text{all } d_i > 0} R_i$. Exact percentage points for T_0^+ are widely available when there are no ties in the absolute ranks and $n \leq 50$ (e.g., Table A12 in Conover (1999, pp. 545–546)). If ties are present in the absolute ranks and/or $n > 50$, then a normal approximation is available for the signed rank test statistic, but a different test statistic is used:

$$T_0 = \left(\sum_{i=1}^{n} R_i \right) \bigg/ \sqrt{\sum_{i=1}^{n} R_i^2}. \tag{4.46}$$

Note that T_0, unlike T_0^+, makes use of all of the signed ranks, with their + or − signs attached. The value of T_0 in (4.46) is compared against the standard normal distribution to obtain an approximate p-value.

The WSR test can be performed using SAS by applying the UNIVARIATE procedure to the paired differences. The approximate and exact versions of the WSR test are also available in StatXact. SAS code that can be used to apply the WSR test to the data in Table 4.14 is provided following Example 4.16.

Just as the M-W-W test statistic is directly related to the equal-variance two-sample t-test statistic (Section 4.2.3.3), the WSR test statistic can also be shown to be an monotonic function of the paired t-test statistic (Conover and Iman 1981). In fact, the t-test approximation to the distribution of the WSR test statistic is more accurate than the standard normal approximation under most conditions, and the t-approximation is used by SAS when $n > 20$. When $n \leq 20$, SAS uses the exact distribution of T_0^+.

4.4.2.3 Sign Test The WSR test described in the previous section is based on the assumption that the difference $D = X - Y$ has a symmetric distribution in the population (Conover 1999, p. 353). However, for biomarker data, there may very well be situations in which the "before minus after" differences do not appear to be symmetrically distributed. (See Example 4.16.) In this case, it would be useful to have an alternative testing procedure that does not depend on the symmetry assumption. One such alternative is the sign test, which is the oldest of all nonparametric tests, dating to 1710 (Conover 1999, p. 157).

As in our discussion of the WSR test in the previous section, let $\{x_1, x_2, \ldots x_n\}$ denote the sample of "before" biomarker values and let $\{y_1, y_2, \ldots y_n\}$ denote the sample of "after" biomarker values. Within each pair (x_i, y_i), a comparison is made and the pair is classified as "plus" (+) if $x_i < y_i$, "minus" (−) if $x_i > y_i$, and "tie" (0) if $x_i = y_i$. Let P(+) and P(−) denote the probabilities that $X < Y$ and $X > Y$ in the population, respectively. The sign test gives us a way to test the following hypotheses:

$$H_0 : P(+) = P(-) \text{ vs. } H_1 : P(+) \neq P(-). \tag{4.47}$$

The test statistic for the sign test is given by the number of "plus" pairs; that is, T_0 = total number of +s resulting from the within-pair comparison of x_i with y_i. If the null hypothesis H_0 in (4.47) is true, then the null distribution of T is binomial with $p = 1/2$ and n = number of non-tied (x_i, y_i) pairs. Thus, any software package that can calculate binomial probabilities can be used to perform the exact version of the sign test. As with the paired t-test and WSR test, the sign test can be performed by applying the UNIVARIATE procedure in SAS to the paired differences. The exact version is also available in StatXact. SAS code for performing the paired t-test, WSR test, and sign test for the data in Table 4.14 is given following Example 4.16.

Example 4.16 Paired *t*-Test, Wilcoxon Signed Ranks Test, and Sign Test

Consider the data in Table 4.14 taken from Naylor et al. (1976). The authors were interested in the use of ES concentration as a potential biomarker for the response to lithium treatment in patients with bipolar illness. The ES levels were measured in 10 bipolar patients before and after treatment with lithium (mean plasma value

TABLE 4.14 Erythrocyte Sodium Concentrations (mmol/L) in Bipolar Patients

Phase	Erythrocyte Sodium Concentration (mmol/L)
Ill ("before")	5.67, 5.89, 5.46, 7.30, 6.74, 5.80, 8.30, 6.01, 5.37, 5.45
On lithium ("after")	6.02, 5.87, 7.42, 7.50, 6.24, 6.55, 8.65, 6.27, 5.64, 6.38
Difference	0.35, −0.02, 1.96, 0.20, −0.50, 0.75, 0.35, 0.26, 0.27, 0.93

over 1 year = 0.26 mEq/L). The ES levels before and after treatment with lithium, as well as the after − before differences are given in Table 4.14. A box plot suggests that the paired differences are not symmetrically distributed, with an apparent outlier of 1.96 mmol/L (Figure 4.8). The difference between the mean (0.455 mmol/L) and median (0.310 mmol/L) is fairly substantial relative to the magnitude of the paired differences. The apparent departure from symmetry for the paired differences is not so evident from a histogram (Figure 4.9).

To apply the WSR test to the data in Table 4.14, we must first arrange the absolute differences in order from smallest to largest, and then assign "signed" ranks (Table 4.15). The sum of the "positive ranks" (including mid-ranks for the two tied differences at 0.35) is given by $T_0^+ = \sum_{\text{all } d_i > 0} R_i = 2 + 3 + 4 + 5.5 + 5.5 + 8 + 9 + 10 = 47$. The exact p-value, obtained using either SAS or StatXact, is $p = 0.0449$.

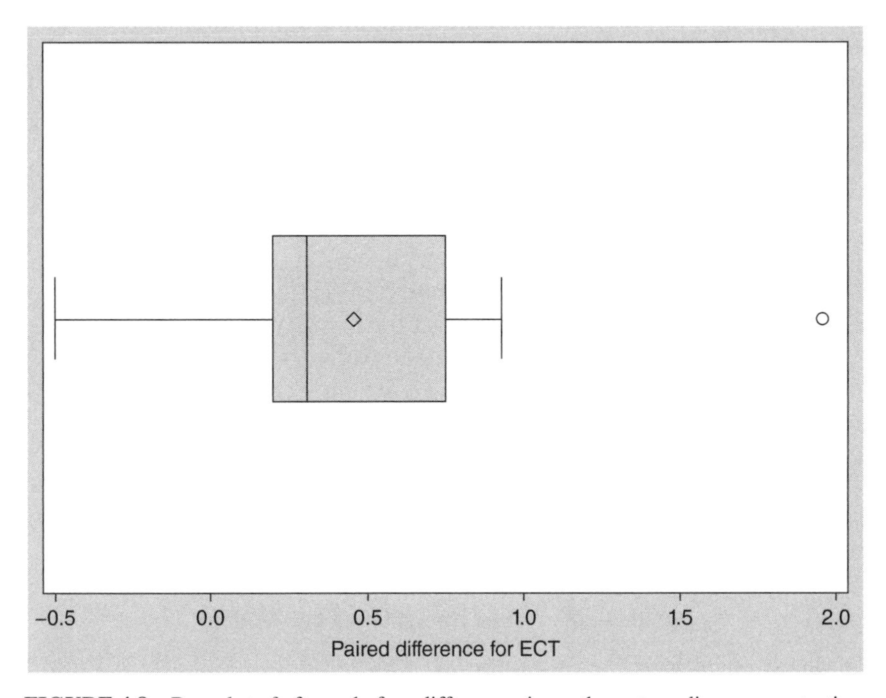

FIGURE 4.8 Box plot of after − before differences in erythrocyte sodium concentration.

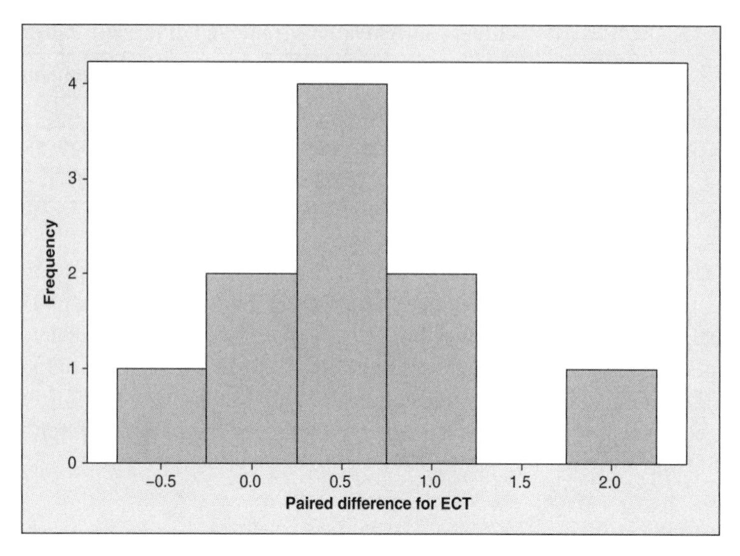

FIGURE 4.9 Histogram of after − before differences in erythrocyte sodium concentration.

The mid-P value, obtained using StatXact, is given by $2[0.02245 - {}^1/_2(0.0029)] = 0.0421$.

To apply the sign test to the data in Table 4.14, one simply counts the number of positive differences, yielding $T_0 = 8$. The exact two-tailed p-value based on the binomial distribution with $n = 10$ and $p = {}^1/_2$ is $2\,\Pr(X \geq 8|n = 10, p = 0.5) = 0.1094$, with a mid-$P$ value of $2[0.0547 - {}^1/_2\ (0.0439)] = 0.0654$. For the paired t-test, the test statistic is given by $t_{p0} = \frac{\bar{d}}{s_d/\sqrt{n}} = \frac{0.455}{0.656/\sqrt{10}} = 2.19$, with $df = 9$ and a two-tailed p-value of 0.0560. Thus, the WSR test yields a significant result, whereas the sign test and paired t-test do not.

After applying the methods described in Section 4.2.2 for assessing the normality of the paired differences in Table 4.14, there is some evidence of a departure from the normality assumption: $\sqrt{b_1} = 1.24$, and $g_2 = 2.82$, indicating positive skewness and much heavier tails than the normal. Furthermore, a probability plot indicates a departure from normality (Figure 4.10), and the CC test for normality is significant at the 0.10 level of significance after using linear interpolation in Table 4.1 ($r_{cc0} = 0.931$, $p = 0.091$). The S-W test is not significant ($W_0 = 0.889$, $p = 0.166$). However, assessing normality in samples as small as $n = 10$ is difficult because of the low power of goodness-of-fit tests (Razali and Wah 2011). Taking all of these results together, we conclude that there is

TABLE 4.15 Signed Ranks of Erythrocyte Sodium Concentrations

Sorted absolute differences	0.02, 0.20, 0.26, 0.27, 0.35, 0.35, 0.50, 0.75, 0.93, 1.96
Signed ranks	−1, 2, 3, 4, 5.5, 5.5, −7, 8, 9, 10

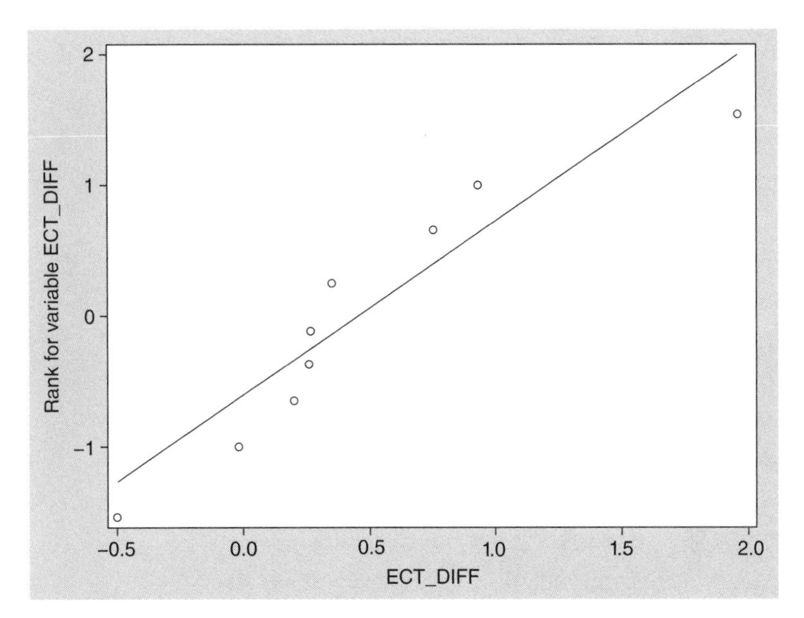

FIGURE 4.10 Normal probability plot of after − before differences in erythrocyte sodium concentration.

some indication of a violation of the normality assumption, as well as a departure from the assumption of symmetry, for the paired differences in Table 4.14, even though the evidence is rather weak. At the risk of being overly cautious, we recommend that the sign test be used to analyze these data. We would therefore conclude that ES concentration does not appear to be significantly elevated in patients with bipolar illness following treatment with lithium (mid-P value = 0.0655).

The following SAS code can be used to perform the paired t-test, WSR test, and sign test for the data in Table 4.14. Note that the measures of skewness and kurtosis are provided as part of the standard output from the UNIVARIATE procedure. Use of the option `"normal"` in the PROC UNIVARIATE statement will produce the results for the S-W test applied to the paired differences.

```
/*
     This code performs the paired t-Test, Wilcoxon signed ranks
     test, and sign test for the paired differences. It also
     tests them for normality.
*/

data ILL;
input ECT_ILL @@;
datalines;
5.67 5.89 5.46 7.30 6.74 5.80 8.30 6.01 5.37 5.45
;
```

```
data TRT;
input ECT_TRT @@;
datalines;
6.02 5.87 7.42 7.50 6.24 6.55 8.65 6.27 5.64 6.38
;

data DIFF;
input ECT_DIFF @@;
datalines;
0.35 -0.02 1.96 0.20 -0.50 0.75 0.35 0.26 0.27 0.93
;

data ATPase;
       merge ILL TRT DIFF;

proc univariate normal data = ATPase;
     var ECT_DIFF;
     title 'Tests of Paired Differences';
     run;
```

The following SAS code can be used to perform the exact version of the sign test and calculate a mid-*P* value (see Section 4.9.4.1):

```
data ATPase;
     SET ATPase;
     if ect_diff > 0 then pos = 1;  else pos = 0;

proc freq data = ATPase;
     output out = sign_test binomial;
     tables pos / binomial (p = .5 level = '1');
     exact binomial / point;
     run;

data sign_test;
     set sign_test;
     p_hat = _BIN_;
     successes = p_hat * N;
     point_prob = pdf('BINOM',successes,.5,N);
     if p_hat < .5 then exact_p_1 = xpl_bin;
     if p_hat > .5 then exact_p_1 = xpr_bin;
     exact_p_2 = xp2_bin;
     mid_p_1 = exact_p_1 - .5 * point_prob;
     mid_p_2 = 2 * mid_p_1;
     if mid_p_2 > 1 then mid_p_2 = 1;
```

```
     keep N successes p_hat exact_p_1 exact_p_2 point_prob
     mid_p_1 mid_p_2;
proc print  data = sign_test;
     var N successes p_hat exact_p_1 exact_p_2 point_prob mid_p_1
     mid_p_2;
     title1 'Exact and mid-P Values for Sign Test';
     run;
```

Example 4.16 provides yet another illustration of a situation in which a nonparametric test yields a significant result but the corresponding normal-theory method does not, contrary to the widely held belief that normal-theory methods are always more powerful. While it is true that the paired t-test is slightly more powerful than the WSR test when the paired difference data do, in fact, come from a normal distribution; this is not necessarily the case if the data are from a non-normal distribution. If the data are normally distributed, the ARE of the WSR relative to the paired t-test is 95.5%; roughly speaking, this means that if $n = 100$ is required to achieve the desired power (usually 80%) for the WSR test, then $n = 96$ would be required for the paired t-test to achieve the same level of power. However, if the data come from a uniform distribution, the ARE of the WSR relative to the paired t-test is 100%; if the data come from a double exponential distribution, this ARE is 150%. Regardless of the true parent population, the ARE of the WSR to the paired t-test is never less than 86.4% (Conover 1999, p. 363). Since the power advantage of the paired t over the WSR is relatively small when the data do arise from a normal distribution, some would argue that one should always use the WSR test for the dependent two-sample problem, especially since there is no infallible method for determining if the paired differences are truly normally distributed.

Complicating the issue even further is the fact that the sign test can, in fact, be more powerful than either the WSR or the paired t-test under certain conditions. For example, if the true distribution of the paired differences is double exponential, the ARE of the sign test relative to the t-test is 200%; relative to the WSR test, the relative efficiency is 133.3%. However, for other distributions, the ARE of the sign test relative to the t-test and the WSR test is quite poor: if the differences are normally distributed, the ARE of the sign test vs. the paired t-test is only 63.7%, and vs. the WSR test it is only 66.7%. If the differences follow a uniform distribution, the ARE of the sign test is only 33.3% vs. both the paired t-test and the WSR test (Conover 1999, p. 364). Since the proper application of the WSR tests depends on the assumption that the paired differences follow a symmetric distribution, some would argue that one should always use the sign test for the dependent two-sample problem. We believe that this is an extreme position because of the obvious inferiority of the sign test under certain distributions; however, as we saw in Example 4.16, it can be very difficult to determine if, in fact, the paired differences are symmetrically distributed.

Note what the effect would be on the analyses of these data in Example 4.16 if the dependence were ignored. For the data in Table 4.14, let Group 1 consist of the patients when they were on lithium, and let Group 2 consist of the patients when they were ill. Then $\bar{x}_1 = 6.654$, $s_1^2 = 0.8596$, $n_1 = 10$; and $\bar{x}_2 = 6.199$, $s_2^2 = 0.9204$, $n_2 = 10$. Using the formula for the test statistic for the equal-variance t-test (Equation 4.40), we have:

$$t_0 = \frac{\bar{x}_1 - \bar{x}_2}{s_p\sqrt{\frac{1}{n_1} + \frac{1}{n_2}}} = \frac{6.654 - 6.199}{(0.9434)\sqrt{\frac{1}{10} + \frac{1}{10}}} = 1.08, \tag{4.48}$$

where s_p is the "pooled" sample standard deviation (Equation 3.11):

$$s_\text{p} = \sqrt{\frac{(n_1 - 1)s_1^2 + (n_2 - 1)s_2^2}{n_1 + n_2 - 2}} = \sqrt{\frac{(10 - 1)(0.8596) + (10 - 1)(0.9204)}{10 + 10 - 2}} = 0.9434.$$

Thus, with $df = 10 + 10 - 2 = 18$, the test statistic in (4.48) yields a two-tailed p-value of 0.2951. The unequal-variance t-test (Section 4.3.2.1) yields almost identical results: $t_{\text{ou}} = 1.08$, $df = 17.98$, two-tailed $p = 0.2951$. Note that the paired t-test results were quite different and almost yielded a statistically significant result at the 0.05 level: $t_{\text{p0}} = 2.19$, $df = 9$, two-tailed p-value $= 0.0560$. This illustrates the importance of taking the correlation between paired observations into account then comparing the group means. The large discrepancy between the "paired" and "unpaired" analyses for this example is not surprising, given that the correlation between the before and after ES concentrations in Table 4.14 was $r = 0.76$. This large value of r resulted in t_{p0} being over twice as large as t_o, which offset the difference in degrees of freedom between the paired ($df = 9$) and unpaired ($df = 18$) t-test and reduced the p-value by a factor of 5.3. (See Section 4.4.2.1.)

4.4.3 Tests of Dependent Proportions

4.4.3.1 McNemar's Test In research studies involving biomarkers, it is often of interest to compare the accuracies of two or more biomarkers or to compare the accuracy of a biomarker with those of other diagnostic tests (Section 5.4.2.1). One may wish to determine which of several newly proposed biomarkers is the most accurate, or to compare one or more newly proposed biomarkers with an existing gold standard test of whatever outcome the biomarker is intended to detect. For example, Qiao et al. (1997) compared the accuracy of a new biomarker they were proposing with that of two "routine clinical detection methods" for lung cancer (sputum cytology and chest x-ray). Since the new biomarker, sputum cytology, and chest x-ray were all applied to the same study subjects in order to assess their respective classification accuracies, a formal statistical comparison of each of the "routine" methods with the new biomarker would require the use of a test for dependent proportions. The preferred method for performing such a comparison is McNemar's test (Agresti 2007, pp. 245–246). Qiao et al. (1997) did not present sufficient data in their article for us to be able to perform McNemar's test. Therefore, to illustrate the method, we constructed a hypothetical 2 × 2 table for the comparison of their new biomarker

TABLE 4.16 Hypothetical 2 × 2 Table for Comparing the Sensitivities of a New Biomarker for Lung Cancer Versus Chest X-Ray

	Chest X-Ray		
Biomarker	Correct	Incorrect	Total
Correct	19	23	42
Incorrect	5	10	15
Total	24	33	57

with chest x-ray in terms of sensitivity (Table 4.16). This table yields approximately the same test statistic for the chi-square approximation to McNemar's test ($\chi^2 = 11.6$) as that presented in their article ($\chi^2 = 12.0$). (Note, however, that Qiao et al. (1997) referred to the statistical method they used as the "paired χ^2 test," so it is unclear if they used McNemar's test.)

It is important to note the special structure of Table 4.16, which is often referred to as the "canonical form" for the comparison of two dependent proportions. The rows and columns are each labeled "correct" and "incorrect." Each cell entry in the 2 × 2 table represents the number of specimens which the newly proposed biomarker *and* the more traditional method of chest x-ray both correctly classified into that category. Out of the 57 confirmed cases of lung cancer in Qiao et al. (1997), 42 were correctly classified by the new biomarker and 24 were correctly classified by chest x-ray. Under our hypothetical scenario, the biomarker and x-ray agreed on a correct diagnosis for only 19 of 57 confirmed cases, and they agreed on an incorrect negative diagnosis for 10 of 57. These "concordant" cases of the disease are irrelevant as far as the statistical analysis is concerned, since the test statistic for McNemar's test is calculated using only the "discordant" cases of lung cancer; that is, those for which the biomarker and chest x-ray disagreed: 23 cases out of the 57 which the biomarker correctly identified as lung cancer, but chest x-ray did not, and the 5 cases out of the 57 which chest x-ray correctly identified as lung cancer, but the biomarker did not.

*Technical Description of McNemar's Test** In Table 4.16, for $i, j = 1, 2$, let n_{ij} = number of subjects in cell (i, j), and let π_{ij} = true probability that a subject falls into cell (i, j). The true probabilities of accurate lung cancer diagnoses by the two methods are then given by π_{1+} and π_{+1}, respectively, where a "+" sign indicates summation over that subscript. So, for example, π_{1+} indicates the true probability that a subject falls into row 1 of the 2 × 2 table. If $\pi_{1+} = \pi_{+1}$, we say that *marginal homogeneity* is present. Since $\pi_{1+} - \pi_{+1} = \pi_{12} - \pi_{21}$, marginal homogeneity in a 2 × 2 table like the one in Table 4.16 is equivalent to equality of the "off-diagonal" probabilities, that is, $\pi_{12} = \pi_{21}$. Let $n^* = n_{12} + n_{21}$ denote the sum of the counts in the two off-diagonal cells. Conditional on the value of n^*, the allocation of the n^* observations to one of the two off-diagonal cells can be modeled using a binomial random variable (RV) with n^* trials and probability of "success" equal to π. Under the null hypothesis H_0: $\pi_{12} = \pi_{21}$, each of the n^* observations has probability $1/2$ of being in cell (1, 2) and probability $1/2$ of being in cell (2, 1). So, n_{12} and n_{21} are the number of "successes" and "failures" for a binomial RV based on n^* trials and probability of success $\frac{1}{2}$ Thus, an exact conditional test of H_0: $\pi_{12} = \pi_{21}$ can be performed by calculating the exact p-value using the binomial distribution.

SAS and StatXact are both capable of performing the approximate and exact versions of McNemar's test. SAS code that can be used to analyze the data in Table 4.16 is provided following Example 4.17.

Example 4.17 McNemar's Test

In Table 4.16, $n_{12} = 23$, $n_{21} = 5$, and $n^* = 28$. The reference distribution (conditional on the value of n^*) is a binomial with $n^* = 28$ and $\pi = 0.5$. First, consider testing H_0: $\pi_{12} = \pi_{21}$ vs. the one-sided alternative hypothesis H_a: $\pi_{12} > \pi_{21}$ (or, equivalently, H_0: $\pi_{1+} = \pi_{+1}$ vs. H_a: $\pi_{1+} > \pi_{+1}$). For the data in Table 4.16, the exact p-value for this one-sided alternative is Pr $(n_{12} \geq 23 \mid n^* = 28, \pi = 0.5) = 0.000456$. For the two-sided alternative H_a: $\pi_{12} \neq \pi_{21}$ (or, equivalently, H_a: $\pi_{1+} \neq \pi_{+1}$), the two-tailed p-value would be twice the upper-tailed p-value, or 0.000912. The one-tailed mid-P value is Pr $(n_{12} \geq 23 \mid n^* = 28, \pi = 0.5) - \frac{1}{2}$Pr $(n_{12} = 23 \mid n^* = 28, \pi = 0.5) = 0.000456 - \frac{1}{2}(0.000366) = 0.000273$, yielding a two-tailed mid-P value of $2(0.00273) = 0.000546$. Thus, there is very strong evidence of a difference in diagnostic accuracy between the new biomarker and chest x-ray. (For a general discussion of mid-P values, see Section 4.9.4.1.)

McNemar's test, as originally formulated, was based on the normal approximation to the binomial. For the exact version of the test, as described above, the reference distribution is a binomial with parameters n^* and $\pi = 0.5$. Thus, the normal approximation to this binomial would have a mean of $n^*\pi = n^*/2$, and variance $n^*\pi(1-\pi) = n^*\left(\frac{1}{2}\right)\left(\frac{1}{2}\right) = n^*/4$, and the approximate test statistic for testing H_0: $\pi_{1+} = \pi_{+1}$ vs. H_a: $\pi_{1+} > \pi_{+1}$ would be given by

$$z_0 = \frac{n_{12} - (n^*/2)}{\sqrt{n^*/4}} = \frac{n_{12} - n_{21}}{\sqrt{n_{12} + n_{21}}}, \tag{4.49}$$

after some algebra. The square of the test statistic in (4.49) has a chi-squared distribution with one degree of freedom, so the test statistic for McNemar's test as originally proposed is given by

$$\chi_0^2 = \frac{(n_{12} - n_{21})^2}{n_{12} + n_{21}}. \tag{4.50}$$

The test statistic in (4.50) is evaluated against a chi-squared distribution with one *df* to obtain an approximate p-value. For the data in Table 4.16, the test statistic in (4.50) is equal to $\chi_0^2 = \frac{(n_{12} - n_{21})^2}{n_{12} + n_{21}} = \frac{(23-5)^2}{23+5} = 11.57$. Based on a chi-square with one *df*, the p-value is 0.000670, an almost identical result to the mid-P value for the exact test (0.000546).

The following SAS code can be used to perform the approximate and exact versions of McNemar's test for the data in Table 4.16, as well as calculate the two-tailed mid P-value.

```
data lung_CA;
input biomarker x_ray count @@;
cards;
1 1 19   1 0 23
0 1 5    0 0 10
;

proc format;
value casefmt
     1='correct'
     0='incorrect';

proc format;
value cntlfmt
      1='correct'
      0='incorrect';

proc freq data = lung_CA order = data; weight count;
     format x_ray casefmt.;
     format biomarker cntlfmt.;
     tables biomarker * x_ray / nocol norow;
     exact  mcnem / point;
     output out = mcnemar mcnem;
     title1 'McNemar''s Test';
     run;

data mcnemar;
     set mcnemar;
     exact_p_2 = xp_mcnem;
     pprob = xpt_mcnem;
     mid_p_2 = exact_p_2 - .5 * pprob;
     keep exact_p_2 pprob mid_p_2;

proc print data = mcnemar;
     title2 'Exact and mid-P Results';
     run;
```

If one ignores the dependence between the proportions in Example 4.17, then one obtains the 2×2 table in Table 4.17.

Applying Fisher's exact test to the data in Table 4.17, we obtain an upper-tailed mid-P value of $0.0006 - {}^1/_2(0.0004) = 0.0004$ and a two-tailed mid-P value of $2(0.0004) = 0.0008$. Recall that the two-tailed mid-P value for the exact test was

TABLE 4.17 Hypothetical 2 × 2 Table for Comparing the Sensitivities of a New Biomarker for Lung Cancer Versus Chest X-Ray, Ignoring Dependence

Diagnostic Test	Correct	Incorrect	Total
Biomarker	42	15	57
Chest X-Ray	24	33	57
Total	66	48	114

0.0005, a stronger result. Although there is no difference in the conclusion if one ignores the dependence between the proportions in this example, one can see that failure to account for this dependence could easily yield a different conclusion.

4.4.3.2 Cochran's Q test Sometimes, we wish to compare more than two dependent proportions. For example, in the study described in Brown (1980), the investigators evaluated a biomarker (serum acid phosphatase, SAP) and four other preoperative variables in terms of their usefulness in determining whether prostate cancer had spread to the neighboring lymph nodes. A total of 53 prostate cancer patients participated in the study; 20 had nodal involvement and 33 did not. The investigators wished to compare the five preoperative variables in terms of their true probabilities of correctly classifying a prostate cancer patient as having nodal involvement. When comparing $k > 2$ dependent proportions, as in this study, Cochran's Q test (Cochran 1950), which is an extension of McNemar's test, can be used.

Let π_i = true probability that Classifier i correctly identifies a subject as a "success," $i = 1, 2, \ldots, k$. Note that each classifier is applied to each subject in the study. The hypotheses we wish to test are

$$H_0 : \pi_1 = \pi_2 = \cdots = \pi_k \text{ vs. } H_\text{a}\text{: at least two of the } \pi_i\text{s are different.} \quad (4.51)$$

To perform Cochran's Q test, let n denote the number of biological specimens under study, and let k denote the number of biomarkers being compared. Let y_{ij} denote the determination (usually "positive" or "negative") based on the jth biomarker for the ith specimen, where $y_{ij} = 1$ for "positive" and $y_{ij} = 0$ for "negative," and let

$$y_{i.} = \sum_{j=1}^{k} y_{ij}$$

denote the total number of positive findings for the ith specimen. Similarly, let

$$y_{.j} = \sum_{i=1}^{n} y_{ij}$$

denote the total number of specimens that are classified as positive by the jth biomarker.

TABLE 4.18 Accuracy Results for Five Diagnostic Tests for Nodal Involvement in Prostate CA

Accuracy Pattern[a]	Frequency
1 1 1 1 1	25
1 0 1 1 1	8
0 1 1 1 1	2
1 1 1 0 1	1
0 1 0 1 1	3
1 0 1 1 0	3
1 0 0 1 1	2
0 1 0 0 1	3
1 0 1 0 0	1
0 0 0 1 0	1
0 1 0 0 0	1
0 0 0 0 0	3

[a]The first value in each pattern indicates the accuracy result for x-ray alone, the second value indicates the result for the biomarker (serum acid phosphatase) alone, the third value indicates the result for x-ray plus the biomarker, the fourth value indicates the result for the "majority rule" based on the five predictors, and the fifth value indicates the result of a multiple logistic regression model based on all five predictors. (See text for more details.) The pattern 1 0 1 1 1, for example, indicates that the biomarker classified the specimen incorrectly, whereas the other four classifiers were all correct.

The test statistic for Cochran's Q test is given by

$$Q_0 = \frac{k(k-1)\sum_{j=1}^{k}\left(y_{.j} - \frac{y_{..}}{k}\right)^2}{ky_{..} - \sum_{i=1}^{n} y_{i.}^2}, \tag{4.52}$$

where $y_{..}$ denotes the total number of specimens that are classified as positive by any of the k biomarkers being compared. The test statistic Q_0 is asymptotically distributed as χ^2_{k-1}, so an approximate p-value is given by $p = \Pr(\chi^2_{k-1} \geq Q_0)$, where Q_0 is the value of the test statistic in (4.52) calculated from the data. The exact p-value for Cochran's Q test can be obtained using the permutation approach, as described by Mehta and Patel (2010, p. 253). Both StatXact and SAS can perform the approximate version of Cochran's Q test and StatXact can perform the exact version (with mid-P correction). SAS code that can be used to perform Cochran's Q test for the data in Table 4.18 is provided following Example 4.18.

Example 4.18 Cochran's Q Test

As stated previously, of the 53 prostate cancer patients in the study described in Brown (1980), 20 had nodal involvement and 33 did not. This determination was based on the gold standard of laparotomy, that is, surgery to examine the lymph nodes and remove tissue samples to examine microscopically for evidence that the cancer had spread. The five dichotomous preoperative variables, all of which were scored as either positive or negative, were: (1) x-ray reading; (2) pathology reading (grade) of a tumor biopsy obtained before surgery; (3) a rough measure of the size and location of the tumor (stage) obtained by palpation with the fingers via the rectum; (4) age <60; and (5) the result for the biomarker (SAP) with SAP $\geq$ 60 indicating nodal involvement. Five classifiers based on these preoperative variables were compared in terms of their consistency, that is, their agreement with the lymph node biopsy gold standard: (C1) x-ray alone; (C2) SAP alone; (C3) x-ray plus SAP (both had to be positive); (C4) "majority rule" (the patient was classified as "positive" for nodal involvement if three or more of the five predictors were positive and "negative" if three or more of the predictors were negative); and (C5) a multiple logistic regression (MLR) model based on all the five predictors.

Table 4.18 gives the overall accuracy results for each of the five classifiers. A "1" indicates that the classifier correctly classified that patient as either having nodal involvement or not, whereas a "0" indicates that the classifier incorrectly classified the patient. Note that for 25 of the 53 patients, all 5 classifiers were correct; for 3 of the patients, all 5 classifiers were incorrect. Based on the results in Table 4.18, we see that the overall accuracy of the five classifiers was as follows: C1 (40/53, 75%), C2 (35/53, 66%), C3 (40/53, 75%), C4 (44/53, 83%), C5 (44/53, 83%).

We can apply Cochran's Q test to test the null hypothesis in (4.51) that all the five classifiers have the same degree of overall accuracy. Using Equation (4.52), the value of Cochran's Q for these data is $Q_0 = 8.90$ and, with $df = 4$, the approximate chi-squared p-value is 0.0636. The exact p-value is 0.0634 with point probability 0.0035 and mid-P value of $0.0634 - 0.0035 = 0.0599$. Even though these results do not reach our usual criterion of 0.05 for statistical significance, they are suggestive of possible differences among the five classifiers in terms of overall accuracy. In fact, if one performs all 10 possible pairwise comparisons among the 5 classifiers using McNemar's test, one finds that there are two differences that are significant at the usual 0.05 level of significance: Classifier 2 vs. Classifier 4 ($\chi_0^2 = 4.26$, $df =$ 1, approximate p-value = 0.0389, mid-P = 0.0414) and Classifier 2 vs. Classifier 5 ($\chi_0^2 = 7.36$, $df = 1$, approximate p-value = 0.0067, mid-P = 0.0064). (Note, however, that neither of these would be significant after applying the Bonferroni adjustment for all 10 pairwise comparisons since the Bonferroni-adjusted significance level for each comparison would be $\alpha' = 0.05/10 = 0.005$.) Thus, there is some evidence that use of acid phosphatase alone does not perform as well as the "majority rule" or the MLR model in terms of overall accuracy. Perhaps a larger study with more prostate cancer patients is needed to fully evaluate the usefulness of SAP as a biomarker for nodal involvement in prostate cancer.

The following SAS code can be used to perform the approximate version of Cochran's Q test for the data in Table 4.18. The code for performing the exact and approximate versions of McNemar's for the comparison of Classifier 2 vs. Classifiers 4 and 5 is also provided. Note that the SAS code provided following Example 4.17 could be applied to calculate the mid-P value for these comparisons as well.

```
data prostate;
input classifier1-classifier5 count;
cards;
1 1 1 1 1 25
0 1 1 1 1 2
1 0 1 1 1 8
1 1 1 0 1 1
0 1 0 1 1 3
1 0 0 1 1 2
1 0 1 1 0 3
1 0 1 0 0 1
0 1 0 0 1 3
0 0 0 1 0 1
0 1 0 0 0 1
0 0 0 0 0 3
;

data classifiers;
     set prostate;
     keep patient classifier correct;
     retain patient 0;
     do i = 1 to count;
     patient = patient + 1;
     classifier = 1; correct = classifier1; output;
     classifier = 2; correct = classifier2; output;
     classifier = 3; correct = classifier3; output;
     classifier = 4; correct = classifier4; output;
     classifier = 5; correct = classifier5; output;
     end;

proc freq data = prostate;
     tables
classifier1*classifier2*classifier3*classifier4*classifier5 /
     agree noprint;
     weight count;
     title1 'Cochran''s Q';
     run;

proc freq data = prostate;
     tables classifier2*classifier4 / agree noprint;
     weight Count;
     exact mcnem;
     title 'McNemar''s Test';
     run;
```

TABLE 4.19 2 × 2 Table for Comparing Classifier 2 with Classifier 4

	Classifier 4		
Classifier 2	Incorrect	Correct	Total
Incorrect	4	14	18
Correct	5	30	35
Total	9	44	53

```
proc freq data = prostate;
    tables classifier2*classifier5 / agree noprint;
    weight Count;
    exact mcnem;
    title 'McNemar''s Test';
    run;
```

It is important to note that Example 4.18 illustrates an aspect of Cochran's Q test (and other tests of dependent proportions) that may be confusing to some data analysts. Note that Classifiers 4 and 5 both have the same degree of classification accuracy (44/53, 83%). However, when compared with Classifier 2 (35/53, 66% accuracy), the p-values for McNemar's test are quite different ($p = 0.0389$ vs. Classifier 4 and $p = 0.0067$ vs. Classifier 5). This can be explained by the fact that McNemar's test is based only on the discordant cases in the data. Table 4.19 contains the "canonical form" for the 2 × 2 table comparing Classifier 2 with Classifier 4, and Table 4.20 contains the corresponding table for comparing Classifier 2 with Classifier 5. Note that the ratio of discordant cases in Table 4.19 is 14/5 = 2.8, whereas the corresponding ratio in Table 4.20 is 10/1 = 10.0. The discrepancy in these ratios accounts for the lower p-value when comparing Classifiers 2 and 5 vs. the comparison of Classifiers 2 and 4. These ratios of discordant cases are also related to estimating the OR in the presence of paired data (see Section 4.9.4.4).

4.4.3.3 Sample Size and Power Considerations As discussed in Section 4.4.3.1, McNemar's test is used to test for marginal homogeneity with paired dichotomous outcomes. Numerous methods have been developed to estimate sample size requirements for McNemar's test. Lachin (1992) compared four of these methods and found that the method due to Connor (1987) provides accurate and "slightly conservative" sample size estimates. The formula for Connor's sample size calculation is

TABLE 4.20 2 × 2 Table for Comparing Classifier 2 with Classifier 5

	Classifier 5		
Classifier 2	Incorrect	Correct	Total
Incorrect	8	10	18
Correct	1	34	35
Total	9	44	53

given by

$$n = \frac{\left\{ z_\alpha \sqrt{\pi_{12} + \pi_{21}} + z_\beta \sqrt{(\pi_{12} + \pi_{21}) - (\pi_{12} - \pi_{21})^2} \right\}^2}{(\pi_{12} - \pi_{21})^2}, \qquad (4.53)$$

where z_α and z_β represent the upper α-and β-percentage points, respectively, from the standard normal distribution, and n denotes the number of paired observations needed to achieve $100(1-\ \beta)\%$ power to reject H_0: $\pi_{12} = \pi_{21}$ vs. H_a: $\pi_{12} > \pi_{21}$ at significance level α. For a two-tailed test, one simply replaces z_α by $z_{\alpha/2}$.

Example 4.19 Sample Size for Dependent Proportions

Suppose that the investigators in the study described in Example 4.18 wish to plan a larger study in which the SAP biomarker will again be compared with the "majority rule" and the MLR model in terms of overall accuracy. Once the new study has been completed, McNemar's test will be used to compare SAP (Classifier 2) vs. majority rule (Classifier 4) and SAP vs. MLR (Classifier 5) in an effort to confirm the findings in the small study of 53 patients in Example 4.18. A Bonferroni adjustment will be used to control the overall family-wise error rate at 0.05; thus, each application of McNemar's test will be performed at a two-sided significance level of 0.05/2 = 0.025. To determine the appropriate sample size for this new study, we use the formula in Equation (4.53) to determine the sample size required to achieve 80% power to detect a difference between SAP (Classifier 2) and majority rule (Classifier 4) at least as large as that observed in the study described in Example 4.18 using a two-tailed McNemar's test with a significance level of 0.025. Note that this sample size will also yield at least 80% power for the comparison of Classifier 2 vs. Classifier 5 since the observed difference for this comparison was greater than that for Classifier 2 vs. Classifier 4. From the results in Table 4.19, we obtain the planning values $\pi_{12} = 14/53 = 0.26415$ and $\pi_{21} = 5/53 = 0.09434$. We have $z_{0.0125} = 2.24$, $z_{0.20} = 0.84$. Substituting these values into (4.53), we obtain $n = 116$.

The following SAS code can be used to calculate the required sample size for McNemar's test in Example 4.19:

```
%let pi_12 = .26415;
%let pi_21 = .09434;
%let alpha = .025;
%let power = .80;

proc  power;
      pairedfreq dist = normal method = connor
      discproportions = &pi_12 | &pi_21
      npairs = .
      power = &power;
      sides = 2
      alpha = &alpha
      run;
```

4.5 CORRELATED OUTCOMES

When analyzing data from research studies involving biomarkers, we are often interested in examining the association between two continuous or ordinal variables, at least one of which is the numerical value of a particular biomarker. For example, Salmi et al. (2002) correlated observed levels of sVAP-1 with risk factors for coronary heart disease (CHD), measures of liver dysfunction, diabetic parameter levels, etc. If both variables involved in the association are normally distributed, then the appropriate measure of association is the PCC, denoted by r (Section 3.8). However, if the data for either variable are non-normally distributed, then a distribution-free measure of association such as Spearman's r_S should be used instead (Siegel and Castellan, 1988, pp. 224–225). For example, in the study by Buss et al. (2003), the authors correctly used Spearman correlation in their evaluation of 3-chlorotyrosine in tracheal aspirates from preterm infants as a biomarker for protein damage by myeloperoxidase; they stated that they used Spearman's r_S "because the data were not normally distributed" (p. 5). (Note, however that the authors provided no justification for how they determined that their data violated the normality assumption.)

In the following sections, we consider five challenges frequently encountered when one uses CCs in the analysis of biomarker data: (1) choice of the appropriate measure of association, (2) recommended methods of statistical analysis, (2) recommended methods for interpreting the statistical results, (4) sample size determination, and (5) comparison of CCs.

4.5.1 Choosing the Appropriate Measure of Association

In Section 2.3.1, we discussed the importance of selecting the appropriate measure of association during the design stage of a study. Table 2.1 can be helpful in determining the appropriate technique to use, depending on the characteristics of the variables whose association is of interest (both variables are ordinal, one variable is ordinal and one is dichotomous, etc.). As stated previously, if both variables appear to be normally distributed (after applying the methods discussed in Section 4.2.2), the PCC is the appropriate measure to use (see Section 3.8). If the data for either variable appear to be non-normally distributed, then a distribution-free method for measuring association should be considered. In the following sections, we describe the two most commonly used distribution-free measures of association: Spearman's rho and Kendall's tau-b.

4.5.1.1 Spearman's rho *Spearman's rank correlation coefficient* (SCC), denoted by ρ_S in the population and by r_S in the sample, measures the "agreement in rankings" between two sets of data values (one labeled "X" and the other labeled "Y"), after the measurements have been ordered ("ranked") from smallest to largest. Like other CCs, the SCC ranges between 1 (perfect agreement in rankings) and -1 (perfect disagreement in rankings). This method is particularly useful, and to be preferred over Pearson's correlation, when examining the agreement between two continuous variables that do not follow a bivariate normal distribution (i.e., either X or Y or both

TABLE 4.21 Hypothetical Rankings of the Levels of Four Biomarkers for Nine Specimens

Specimen Number	1 2 3 4 5 6 7 8 9
Rank by Biomarker A	1 2 3 4 5 6 7 8 9
Rank by Biomarker B	1 2 3 4 5 6 7 8 9
Rank by Biomarker C	9 8 7 6 5 4 3 2 1
Rank by Biomarker D	2 4 6 8 1 3 5 7 9

are non-normally distributed). It is also appropriate when either X or Y or both are measured on an ordinal scale.

To illustrate the concepts underlying the SCC, suppose $n = 9$ and that the levels of Biomarker A for the nine specimens have been arranged in order from smallest to largest, with the smallest receiving rank 1 and the largest receiving rank 9. The same ordering is repeated for the nine specimens for the levels of Biomarkers B and C. The specimens are first arranged in order of their rankings according to Biomarker A, and then the respective ranks for the specimens using the levels of Biomarkers B and C are also noted, as in Table 4.21.

Biomarkers A and B have perfect agreement in rankings ($r_s = 1$), whereas Biomarkers A and C have perfect disagreement in rankings ($r_s = -1$). (Note that strong disagreement in rankings between Biomarkers A and C does not necessarily indicate lack of agreement; it could be that the specimens were inadvertently scored in the wrong direction for Biomarker C. If the biomarker readings for Biomarker C were "reversed scored" in some way, there would be perfect agreement in rankings between Biomarker A and the "new" version of Biomarker C.) Biomarkers A and D have an intermediate degree of agreement in rankings, yielding a value of $r_s = 0.5$.

The sample value of the SCC for Biomarkers A and D, for example, would be calculated as follows:

$$r_s = 1 - \frac{6 \sum_{i=1}^{n} (u_i - v_i)^2}{n(n^2 - 1)}, \tag{4.54}$$

where u_i = the rank of specimen i according to Biomarker A, v_i = the rank of specimen i according to Biomarker D, and n = the number of specimens. Note that this formula should be used to calculate the SCC only if there are no ties in the data values for either Biomarker A or Biomarker D. Using the ranks for Biomarkers A and D in Table 4.21,

$$\sum_{i=1}^{9} (u_i - v_i)^2 = (1-2)^2 + (2-4)^2 + (3-6)^2 + (4-8)^2 + (5-1)^2$$
$$+ (6-3)^2 + (7-5)^2 + (8-7)^2 + (9-9)^2 = 60.$$

Thus,

$$r_s = 1 - \frac{6 \sum_{i=1}^{9} (u_i - v_i)^2}{9(9^2 - 1)} = 1 - \frac{6(60)}{9(80)} = 0.5.$$

If there had been any ties in the values for either Biomarker A or Biomarker D, the value of the SCC would be obtained by calculating the Pearson correlation between the ranks of the values for Biomarkers A and D. The *mid-rank* (i.e., the average of all the ranks for the tied values) would be used for the ranks of any tied values (see Example 4.6). Using the same notation as above, let $\{u_1, u_2, \ldots, u_n\}$ denote the ranks of the n observed levels of Biomarker A, and let $\{v_1, v_2, \ldots, v_n\}$ denote the ranks of the n observed values of Biomarker D, including any mid-ranks. Then the sample value of the SCC is calculated using Equation (3.17), which yields:

$$r_s = \frac{\sum_{i=1}^{n} (u_i - \overline{u})(v_i - \overline{v})}{\sum_{i=1}^{n} (u_i - \overline{u})^2 \sum_{i=1}^{n} (v_i - \overline{v})^2}, \tag{4.55}$$

where $\overline{u}$ and $\overline{v}$ denote the mean ranks of the levels of Biomarkers A and D, respectively. If there are no ties in the biomarker levels for either Biomarker A or D, then Equations (4.54) and (4.55) will yield identical values for the SCC. The calculation of the SCC is illustrated in Example 4.20.

As previously mentioned, the SCC should be used instead of the PCC when at least one of the variables is not normally distributed. In practice, the SCC is often used when one or both variables are ordinal. Hwang et al. (2009) used the SCC to examine "the correlation between the serum levels of (five) biomarkers and ovarian cancer stage" and found that "only the mean serum CA-125 level showed a significant positive correlation with cancer stage" ($r_s = 0.242$, $p = 0.002$). The use of the SCC was appropriate for these data since cancer stage (I, II, IIIA, IIIB, IV, etc.) is an ordinal variable.

4.5.1.2 Kendall's tau-b Kendall's coefficient of concordance (KCC), denoted by τ_b in the population and by t_b in the sample, is not as commonly used as the SCC, but has been applied in many research studies involving biomarkers, especially in the analysis of environmental data (Helsel 2012). For example, Helsel (2012, pp. 227-228) used Kendall's tau to determine if the concentrations of dissolved iron (DI) collected from the Brazos River, Texas, during summers from 1977–1985 followed a trend. Out of a sample of $n = 9$ summers, there were 3 summers that had complete DI data, 4 for which the DI data were right censored at 10 (i.e., the measuring equipment could not register any concentrations of DI greater than 10), and 2 summers for which the DI data were left censored at 3 (i.e., the measuring equipment could not register any concentrations of DI less than 3). This is an example of correlating variables that are subject to a limit of detection (LOD); this topic covered more fully in Section 4.8.

The KCC is computed for a bivariate sample of data by first arranging the (x, y) data pairs in ascending order of x. Then, one counts the number of "concordant" and "discordant" pairs. The pairs (x_i, y_i) and (x_j, y_j) are concordant if $y_i < y_j$ and discordant if $y_i > y_j$ (assuming, of course, that $x_i < x_j$). The pair is neither concordant or discordant if $x_i = x_j$ or $y_i = y_j$. Pairs that are neither concordant nor discordant do not contribute to the calculation of the KCC. The value of τ_{b} is the difference in the number of concordant and discordant pairs divided by their sum:

$$t_{\text{b}} = \frac{n_{\text{c}} - n_{\text{d}}}{n_{\text{c}} + n_{\text{d}}}, \tag{4.56}$$

where n_{c} denotes the number of concordant pairs and n_{d} denotes the number of discordant pairs. Thus, if all pairs are concordant (discordant) t_{b} will be 1 (-1), and if the numbers of concordant and discordant pairs are the same, τ_{b} will be 0. A quick calculation will verify that $t_{\text{b}} = 1$ using the ranks for Biomarkers A and B in Table 4.21 (since all of the pairs are concordant), and $t_{\text{b}} = -1$ using the ranks for Biomarkers A and C (since all of the pairs are discordant). It is important to note that the original biomarker levels are not required for calculation of either the KCC or the SCC; only their relative rankings are needed.

Consider once again the ranks obtained according to the levels of Biomarkers A and D for the nine specimens given in Table 4.21:

Specimen Number	1 2 3 4 5 6 7 8 9
Rank by Biomarker A	1 2 3 4 5 6 7 8 9
Rank by Biomarker D	2 4 6 8 1 3 5 7 9

For Specimen 1 (i.e., the specimen with the smallest value (Rank 1) according to Biomarker A and the specimen with the second smallest value (Rank 2) according to Biomarker D), there are a total of eight pairs (i.e., Specimen 1 is paired with each of Specimens 2–9). Of these eight pairs, seven are concordant; the only discordant pair is (2, 1). Proceeding to Specimen 2 (Rank 2 according to Biomarker A and Rank 4 according to Biomarker D), there are seven unique pairs not previously considered; five are concordant and two are discordant ((4,1) and (4,3)). For Specimen 3, there are six pairs not previously considered; three are concordant and three are discordant. For Specimen 4, there are five new pairs; only one is concordant and four are discordant. For Specimens 5, 6, 7, and 8 there are four, three, two, and one new pairs, respectively, and all are concordant. Thus, $n_{\text{c}} = 7 + 5 + 3 + 1 + 4 + 3 + 2 + 1 = 26$, $n_{\text{d}} = 1 + 2 + 3 + 4 = 10$, and applying the formula for Kendall's coefficient given in (4.56), $t_b = \frac{n_{\text{c}} - n_{\text{d}}}{n_{\text{c}} + n_{\text{d}}} = \frac{26-10}{36} = 0.44$.

As an example of the use of the KCC with biomarker data, consider the study by Heist et al. (2010), who investigated the use of bevacizumab as a chemotherapeutic agent for the treatment of advanced non-small-cell lung cancer. They found that, after a single induction dose of bevacizumab, the patients' mean tumor blood flow decreased and there was a significant association between blood flow and the Response Evaluation Criteria in Solid Tumor (RECIST) results for the tumors ($t_b = 0.58$, $n = 12$, $p < 0.01$). The use of the KCC with these data was appropriate since one of the variables was ordinal; namely, the RECIST result, which indicated whether the patient's cancer improved, stayed the same, or worsened.

The CORR procedure in SAS can be used to compute any of the three sample CCs discussed in this section, with the PCC being the default coefficient, while the SPEARMAN and KENDALL options can be used to obtain the SCC and the KCC, respectively. The CORR procedure produces the sample estimate of the requested CC and a p-value corresponding to the null hypothesis that the population correlation is equal to 0. It is also possible to obtain CIs for the PCC and the SCC (but not the KCC), and to test hypothesized values other than 0 using the CORR procedure. However, the CORR procedure does not incorporate recent advances in statistical inference for the SCC (Bonett and Wright 2000). SAS code that can be used to perform these improved analyses for the SCC, as well as for the PCC and KCC, is provided following Example 4.20.

As noted above, either the SCC or the KCC should be used when one or both of the variables are not normally distributed. When computed on the same data, $|r|$ is generally larger than $|r_s|$, which is generally larger than $|t_b|$; however, the significance tests usually yield very similar results (Conover, 1999). Since the width of a CI for any CC depends on both the magnitude of the sample correlation and the sample size, CIs based on the same set of data will generally be narrowest for the PCC, followed by those for the SCC and the KCC, especially for smaller values of n. However, there are exceptions, as seen in Example 4.20.

4.5.2 Recommended Methods of Statistical Analysis for Correlation Coefficients

An example of the use of Pearson correlation in the analysis of biomarker data can be found in Hwang et al. (2009). The authors claimed to find a significant negative correlation between serum prolactin and leptin levels ($r = -0.182$), and a significant positive correlation between serum prolactin and osteopontin levels ($r = 0.195$) in their study of 56 newly diagnosed epithelial ovarian cancer patients. However, the p-values for the tests that their correlations are significantly different from zero do not achieve statistical significance: $p = 0.1794$ for the PCC between serum prolactin and leptin levels, and $p = 0.1498$ for the PCC between serum prolactin and osteopontin. Furthermore, the correlation matrix presented in their article (Table 3, p. 172) is not symmetric (Table 4.22). For any two variables X and Y, it must always be the case that $\text{Corr}(X, Y) = \text{Corr}(Y, X)$, where "Corr" denotes correlation. Note also that the p-values for the correlations with leptin do not appear in the correct columns in their correlation matrix (Table 4.22).

In terms of hypothesis testing for the PCC, there is an exact test of $H_0 : \rho = 0$ based on the t-distribution. The test statistic is given by

$$t_0 = \frac{r\sqrt{n-2}}{\sqrt{1-r^2}}, \tag{4.57}$$

TABLE 4.22 Correlation Matrix for Epithelial Ovarian Cancer Patients

	Leptin	Prolactin	OPN	IGF-II	CA-125
Leptin					
CC	1	−0.182*	−0.022	0.102	−0.125
Significance	0.021	0.779	0.197	0.116	
Prolactin					
CC	−0.182*	1	0.195*	0.061	0.133
Significance	0.021		0.014	0.442	0.093
OPN					
CC	−0.022	0.195*	1	−0.020	0.072
Significance	0.779	0.014		0.798	0.363
IGF-II					
CC	0.102	0.061	−0.020	1	0.109
Significance	0.197	0.442	0.798		0.217
CA-125					
CC	−0.125	0.133	0.072	0.028	1
Significance	0.116	0.093	0.363	0.722	

OPN: osteopontin, IGF-II insulin-like growth factor-II, CC correlation coefficient.
*Correlation is significant at the 0.05 level (2-tailed).
Source: Reprinted from Table 3 of Hwang et al. (2009, p. 172) with permission from the Korean Society of Gynecologic Oncology.

which is compared with the Student's t-distribution with $n - 2$ degrees of freedom to obtain the exact p-value. The problem with using this approach to obtain the exact p-value for the PCC is that the test statistic in (4.57) can be used to test only the null value $\rho_0 = 0$. This means that there is no corresponding CI procedure that will yield a conclusion identical to that obtained when (4.57) is used as the test statistic. Instead, the *Fisher z-transformation* can be used to transform the sample correlation r to a new random variable that is approximately normally distributed. This transformed random variable can then be used to derive a test statistic for testing $H_0 : \rho = \rho_0$, where ρ_0 is any hypothesized value of the PCC (zero, negative, positive). This transformed random variable can also be used to derive an approximate CI for the true value of the PCC.

The Fisher's z-transformed PCC is given by

$$z(r) = \frac{1}{2} \log \frac{1+r}{1-r}, \tag{4.58}$$

where r is the sample value of the PCC. This new random variable has an approximate normal distribution with mean 0 and variance $1/(n - 3)$. This result can be used to derive a test statistic for testing $H_0 : \rho = \rho_0$:

$$z_0 = \frac{z(r) - z(\rho_0)}{1/\sqrt{n-3}}, \tag{4.59}$$

where n is the sample size, $z(r)$ is the Fisher z-transformation applied to the sample value of the PCC, and $z\left(\rho_0\right)$ is the Fisher z-transformation applied to the hypothesized value (usually 0, in which case $z\left(\rho_0\right) = z(0) = 0$). The value of z_0 in (4.59) is then compared with the standard normal distribution to obtain an approximate p-value. Unless n is very small, there will be very little difference in the p-values obtained when using the test statistics in (4.57) and (4.59).

The Fisher z-transformation can also be used to derive an approximate $100(1 - \alpha)\%$ CI for ρ that will always yield conclusions consistent with those obtained using the hypothesis test based on (4.59). To derive the formula for the CI for ρ, one must first derive a Wald-type approximate CI for the Fisher z-transformed value of the population correlation $z(\rho) = \frac{1}{2}\log\frac{1+\rho}{1-\rho}$. This CI is given by

$$z(r) \pm z_{\alpha/2}\sqrt{1/(n-3)}, \tag{4.60}$$

where $z_{\alpha/2}$ is the upper $\alpha/2$-percentage point of the standard normal.

Next, the endpoints of the CI in (4.60) are "back-transformed" using the inverse of the Fisher z-transformation. (In other words, Equation (4.58) is solved for r in terms of z.) This yields the following approximate $100(1 - \alpha)\%$ for ρ:

$$\left(\frac{\exp[2(\mathrm{LCL}) - 1]}{\exp[2(\mathrm{LCL}) + 1]}, \frac{\exp[2(\mathrm{UCL}) - 1]}{\exp[2(\mathrm{UCL}) + 1]}\right), \tag{4.61}$$

where

$$\mathrm{LCL} = z(r) - z_{\alpha/2}\sqrt{1/(n-3)} \tag{4.62}$$

and

$$\mathrm{UCL} = z(r) + z_{\alpha/2}\sqrt{1/(n-3)}.$$

Fisher's z-transformation can also be applied to Spearman's and Kendall's coefficients. The test statistic for testing $H_0 : \rho_s = \rho_{s0}$ is given by

$$z_{s0} = \frac{z(r_s) - z(\rho_{s0})}{\sqrt{(1 + \rho_{s0}^2/2)/(n-3)}}, \tag{4.63}$$

and the test statistic for testing $H_0 : \tau_b = \tau_{b0}$ is given by

$$z_{t0} = \frac{z(t_b) - z(\tau_{b0})}{\sqrt{0.437/(n-4)}}. \tag{4.64}$$

Approximate confidence limits for the true values of ρ_s and τ_b can be derived using the same approach used in deriving the confidence limits in (4.61) for the PCC. Thus, an approximate $100(1-\alpha)\%$ CI for $z(\rho_s)$ is given by

$$z(r_s) \pm z_{\alpha/2}\sqrt{(1 + r_s^2/2)/(n - 3)} \quad (4.65)$$

and an approximate $100(1-\alpha)\%$ CI for $z(\tau_b)$ is given by

$$z(t_b) \pm z_{\alpha/2}\sqrt{0.437/(n - 4)}. \quad (4.66)$$

Approximate confidence limits for ρ_s and τ_b are obtained by applying the "back-transform" in (4.61) to the limits obtained in (4.65) and (4.66). For additional details in these approaches, see Bonett and Wright (2000). All of these methods are illustrated in Example 4.20.

Example 4.20 Pearson, Spearman, and Kendall's Coefficients

In an unpublished Masters thesis, Stuart (2013) evaluated several potential biomarkers for severity of symptoms of dry mouth (xerostomia). As part of her assessment of criterion validity (Section 5.4.4), she examined the associations of one of the potential biomarkers, p21, with measures of quality of life and severity of symptoms for patients with xerostomia. Severity of symptoms was measured using five items measured on a visual analog scale (VAS). A sample item is Question 5 (Q5): "How difficult is it for you to speak without drinking liquids"; the possible response ranged from 1 (Very difficult) to 100 (Not difficult), depending on where the respondent placed a mark on a 100 mm line. The scores of the 5 items on the VAS were totaled to yield an overall score, which ranged from 5 to 500. Table 4.23 contains the values for item Q5 on the VAS, the total VAS score, and the p21 levels for 20 patients currently suffering from xerostomia. Scatterplots of p21 vs. Q5 and VAS are given in Figures 4.11 and 4.12, respectively. Table 4.24 contains a summary of the analyses described above for the Pearson, Spearman, and Kendall coefficients, considered as measures of the association of p21 with each of Q5 and VAS. SAS code for performing these analyses is provided below. As stated previously, the results for the Fisher z-transformed Spearman's coefficient produced by the CORR procedure in SAS do not incorporate the improved Fisher z-transformation proposed by Bonett and Wright (2000). Furthermore, CIs for Kendall's coefficient are not available from the CORR procedure. Thus, we have written our own SAS code to perform these analyses.

```
data Table4_23;
input Patient  Q5  VAS p21;
datalines;
```

```
1       4       47      0.4831
2       24      59      0.6234
3       6       24      0.5885
4       24      83      0.5886
5       46      315     0.5193
6       11      85      0.7022
7       15      93      0.5665
8       0       9       0.3120
9       20      211     0.6340
10      11      81      0.5609
11      42      226     0.7317
12      23      91      0.5763
13      36      126     0.5134
14      12      31      0.4056
15      2       17      0.3472
16      0       0       0.4860
17      23      113     0.5226
18      21      257     0.5051
19      6       69      0.3523
20      7       68      0.5140
;
run;

proc corr data = Table4_23 pearson spearman kendall
fisher(biasadj=no);
  var Q5 VAS;
  with p21 ;
  title 'Results for Spearman Using This Fisher z Not Recommended';
/*   This code requires that values of Spearman (rs) and Kendall
     (rk) coefficients (calculated using PROC CORR) and sample
     size be input using the %let macro statement
*/

%let rs = .56949;
*%let rs = .47669;
%let n = 20;

data fisher_rs;

rs_fisher=0.5*(log((1+&rs)/(1-&rs)));
low_rsz=rs_fisher-1.96*sqrt(1+(&rs**2)/2)/(sqrt(&n-3));
up_rsz=rs_fisher+1.96*sqrt(1+(&rs**2)/2)/(sqrt(&n-3));
low_rs=(exp(2*low_rsz)-1)/(exp(2*low_rsz)+1);
up_rs=(exp(2*up_rsz)-1)/(exp(2*up_rsz)+1);
se_rs = sqrt((1+(&rs**2)/2)/(&n-3));
```

```
z_rs = rs_fisher/se_rs;
p_val_rs = 2*(1-probnorm(abs(z_rs)));
run;

proc print data=fisher_rs;
title 'Spearman Coefficient Using Bonett and Wright Transforma-
tion';
run;

%let rk = .42137;
*%let rk = .31579;
%let n = 20;

data fisher_rk;
rk_fisher=0.5*(log((1+&rk)/(1-&rk)));
low_rkz=rk_fisher-1.96*sqrt(0.437)/(sqrt(&n-4));
up_rkz=rk_fisher+1.96*sqrt(0.437)/(sqrt(&n-4));
low_rk=(exp(2*low_rkz)-1)/(exp(2*low_rkz)+1);
up_rk=(exp(2*up_rkz)-1)/(exp(2*up_rkz)+1);
se_rk = sqrt((0.437)/(&n-4));
z_rk = rk_fisher/se_rk;
p_val_rk = 2*(1-probnorm(abs(z_rk)));
run;

proc print data=fisher_rk;
title 'Kendall Coefficient Using Fieller et al. (1957) Transfor-
mation';
run;
```

Contrary to popular belief, the sample value of Spearman's rho for the correlation of p21 with VAS in Table 4.24 is actually larger than the sample value of Pearson's coefficient ($r_s = 0.477$ vs. $r = 0.402$). (The most likely explanation for this is that the true relationship between p21 and VAS is nonlinear rather than linear.) Furthermore, Spearman's coefficient is significantly different from zero (p = 0.043), whereas Pearson's is not (p = 0.079). Even though Kendall's coefficient is smaller than Pearson's ($t_b = 0.316$ vs. $r = 0.402$), it does achieve statistical significance at the 0.05 level (p = 0.048), unlike the Pearson coefficient. As far as determining the correct measure of association to use for these data, given that there is strong evidence of a violation of normality for the VAS data (Table 4.25), either the SCC or the KCC would be preferable to the PCC for measuring the association between p21 and VAS.

Note that the results for the SCC are also stronger than those for the PCC for the correlation between p21 and Q5 (Table 4.24). Even though the data for both p21 and Q5 appear to be normally distributed (Table 4.25), the SCC and the KCC

TABLE 4.23 Unpublished Data on Biomarkers and Quality of Life for Xerostomia Patients

Patient	Q5	VAS	p21
1	4	47	0.4831
2	24	59	0.6234
3	6	24	0.5885
4	24	83	0.5886
5	46	315	0.5193
6	11	85	0.7022
7	15	93	0.5665
8	0	9	0.3120
9	20	211	0.6340
10	11	81	0.5609
11	42	226	0.7317
12	23	91	0.5763
13	36	126	0.5134
14	12	31	0.4056
15	2	17	0.3472
16	0	0	0.4860
17	23	113	0.5226
18	21	257	0.5051
19	6	69	0.3523
20	7	68	0.5140

Source: Data courtesy of Dr. Mary Stuart.

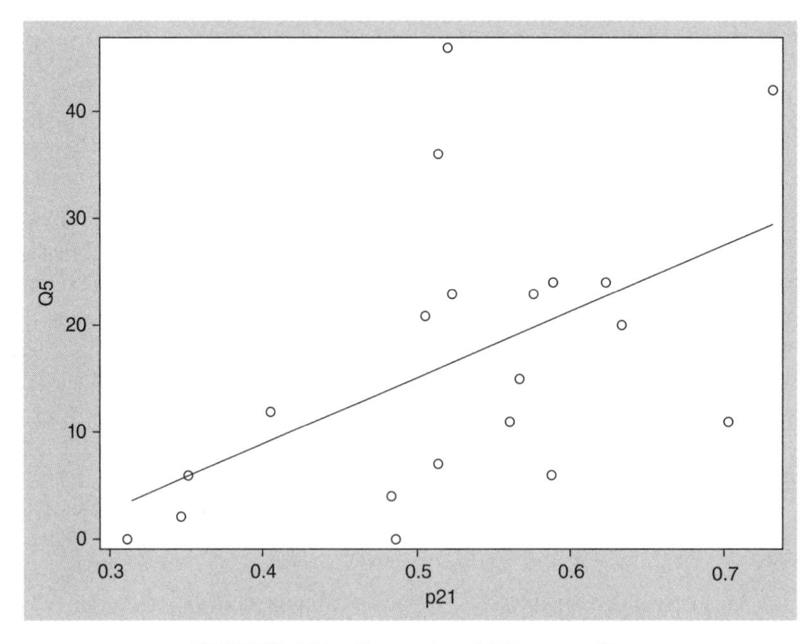

FIGURE 4.11 Scatterplot of Q5 versus p21.

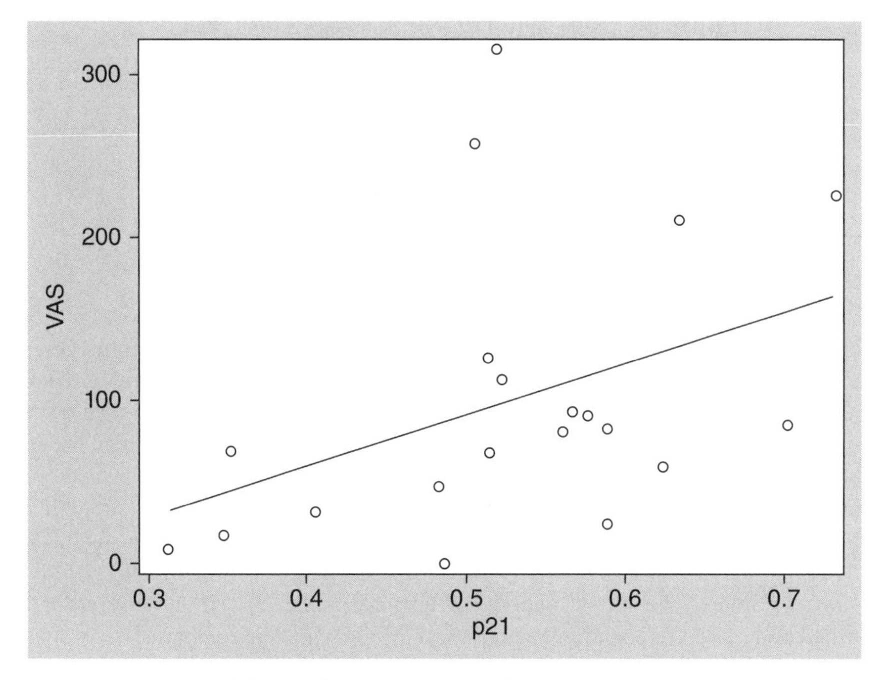

FIGURE 4.12 Scatterplot of VAS versus p21.

both produce lower p-values than the PCC (Table 4.24). In general, we recommend that Spearman's coefficient (and, under certain conditions, Kendall's coefficient) be considered as viable alternatives to Pearson's correlation, especially when one is interested primarily in measuring the strength of association between two variables, not just the strength of the linear relationship between them. If one is only interested in a linear relationship between two variables (as in linear regression), then Pearson's coefficient is preferred, but only if X and Y are both normally distributed.

TABLE 4.24 Results for Fisher z-Transformed Correlations of p21 Level with Two Measures of Quality of Life in Dental Patients with Xerostomia

Correlate	Measure of Association	Estimated Coefficient	95% CI for ξ	p-value for Test of H_0: $\xi = 0$
Q5	Pearson	0.511	(0.089, 0.778)	0.020[a]
	Spearman	0.569	(0.134, 0.821)	0.013
	Kendall	0.421	(0.125, 0.649)	0.007
VAS	Pearson	0.402	(-0.049, 0.717)	0.079[a]
	Spearman	0.477	(0.017, 0.770)	0.043
	Kendall	0.316	(0.003, 0.572)	0.048

ξ, Population value of measure of association ($\xi = \rho$ for Pearson's, $\xi = \rho_s$ for Spearman's, and $\xi = \tau_b$ for Kendall's).

[a]Exact p-values obtained from SAS: 0.021 (p21 vs. Q5); 0.079 (p21 vs. VAS).

TABLE 4.25 Normality Test Results for Xerostomia Data

Variable	Skewness	Kurtosis-3	Shapiro–Wilk p-value
p21	−0.26	−0.08	0.581
Q5	0.77	−0.07	0.099
VAS	1.23	0.82	0.010

4.5.3 Recommended Methods for Interpreting Correlation Coefficient Results

Generally speaking, in any statistical inference setting, it is preferable to present both the p-value for the appropriate hypothesis test *and* the corresponding CI. This is especially true when performing inference for a CC; without the CI, the reader has no direct way to ascertain the precision of the sample result, or to get an idea of what reasonable upper and lower bounds might be for the true value of the unknown parameter. Without the p-value, the reader is unable to ascertain the strength of evidence against the null hypothesis. Of course, CIs are always appropriate, regardless of whether it is of interest to test any particular hypothesized value or not.

An example of the use of hypothesis testing for the PCC in a study utilizing biomarker data can be found in Murphy et al. (2004). In their comparison of urinary biomarkers for tobacco and carcinogen exposure in smokers, the authors found a significant positive correlation between percentage NNAL glucuronidation and percentage cotinine glucuronidation in their sample of $n = 47$ smokers ($r = 0.310$, $z(r) = 0.321$, $z_0 = 2.13$, $p = 0.0335$). (Note that the exact test results are almost identical: $t_0 = 2.19$, $df = 45$, $p = 0.0340$.)

Although not presented in Murphy et al., an approximate 95% CI for the true correlation between percentage NNAL glucuronidation and percentage cotinine glucuronidation based on the Fisher z-transformation is given by (0.025, 0.548). Note that this CI is so wide that it provides very little useful information about the true magnitude of the PCC; essentially, it says that the true correlation could be any value between 0 and 0.55. Some methods for dealing with this problem are described in Section 4.5.4.

In another example of the use of the PCC with biomarker data, Salmi et al. (2002) assessed the "significance" of the PCCs for the sVAP-1 biomarker in their study by testing the null hypothesis $H_0 : \rho = 0$. However, there are several problems with this approach, the main one being that correlations of no practical significance may be declared to be "significant" simply because the p-value is less than 0.05 (Looney, 1996). For example, in their sample of 411 Finnish men, Salmi et al. (2002) found a "significant" correlation of 0.108 between sVAP-1 and carbohydrate-deficient transferrin, a measure of liver dysfunction. While this correlation is statistically significant ($p = 0.029$), it has questionable practical significance, especially when one considers that the proportion of variability in transferrin that is explained by the variability in sVAP-1 is only $(0.108)^2 = 0.012$ (i.e., 1.2%).

We feel that published guidelines can be extremely useful when interpreting the practical significance of CCs. In particular, we have found the classification scheme presented by Morton et al. (1996, p. 92) to be helpful in interpreting the magnitude of CCs. They classify correlations between 0.0 and 0.2 in absolute value as "negligible," between 0.2 and 0.5 as "weak," between 0.5 and 0.8 as "moderate," and between 0.8 and 1.0 as "strong." Thus, while the correlation of 0.108 that Salmi et al. (2002) found between sVAP-1 and carbohydrate-deficient transferrin may be statistically significant, it still would be considered "negligible" according to the Morton et al. criteria, thereby raising doubt about the practical significance of the result. Of course, there is nothing sacred about the Morton et al. criteria, and other criteria specific to the field of application may be more appropriate. For example, Cohen (1988, p. 79–80) provided guidelines for interpreting the magnitude of the correlation between two variables in terms of effect size, with a PCC of 0.1 indicating a "small" effect size, 0.3 a "medium" effect size, and 0.5 a "large" effect size. Using these criteria, the "significant" correlation of 0.108 between sVAP-1 and carbohydrate-deficient transferrin that Salmi et al. found in their study would be considered to be "small." The cutoffs proposed by Cohen were used by Ansari et al. (2013) to interpret the magnitude of the PCCs in their study.

As is the case with most statistical analyses (see Section 2.4), one should always provide the appropriate CI in addition to the p-value for the hypothesis test of interest whenever analyzing CCs. In the example taken from Salmi et al. (2002) mentioned above, the 95% CI for ρ is $(0.011 - 0.203)$. Thus, the entire CI essentially falls within the "negligible" range according to the Morton et al. criteria; we feel this provides even more convincing evidence of the lack of practical significance of the observed correlation.

Another problem that arises when one declares a correlation to be "significant" simply because $p < 0.05$ is that smaller correlations can be declared to be significant even when n is fairly small. Basing a CI on such a small sample often results in CIs that are too wide to be of any practical use (Looney 1996). In the study by Salmi et al. (2002), the Pearson correlation between sVAP-1 and ketone bodies in a sample of 38 diabetic children and adolescents was $r = 0.34$ ($p = 0.037$), a statistically significant result. However, the 95% CI for ρ based on this sample of $n = 38$ is $(0.02 - 0.60)$, which indicates that the population correlation ρ could be anywhere between "negligible" and "moderate," according to the Morton et al. criteria (or a small, medium, or large effect size according to the Cohen criteria). We contend that a CI this wide provides very little useful information about the magnitude of the population correlation, especially when one thinks in terms of practical significance.

4.5.4 Sample Size Issues in Correlation Analysis

One way to avoid the difficulties described in the previous section is to perform a sample size calculation prior to beginning the study, which should be done as a matter of routine practice in biomarker research studies. (See Section 2.3.3.) Salmi et al. (2002) provided no justification for the sample sizes used in their study, so one must assume that no power analysis or sample size calculation was performed. For a study in which the primary statistical analysis will be based on CCs, the standard approach is to determine the sample size required for the study so that adequate power is achieved for testing $H_0 : \rho = 0$; in other words, the null hypothesis that the population correlation is zero. However, as pointed out by Looney (1996), this approach is flawed for several reasons. One is that it is usually of no interest to test $H_0 : \rho = 0$, especially in the context of a method comparison study involving biomarkers (see Section 5.4.3). In fact, Strike (1996, p. 170) goes so far as to say that the test of $\rho = 0$ is "utterly redundant" in that context. Similarly, Shoukri (2011, p. 92) says that a test of $H_0 : \rho = 0$ is "meaningless." Another problem with basing the sample size calculation for a correlation study on the test of $H_0 : \rho = 0$ is that it can lead to small sample sizes that yield CIs that are too wide to be of any practical use once the study data have been collected. Looney describes several alternative approaches for determining the required n; typically, these approaches yield sample sizes that provide more useful information about the true value of the population correlation and the practical significance of the sample correlation. These approaches include basing the sample size calculation on (1) achieving a specified width of the CI for the population correlation, and/or (2) tests of null hypotheses that incorporate null values other than zero for the population correlation. For example, one might test $H_0 : \rho \leq .2$; rejecting this null hypothesis would indicate that the population correlation is "non-negligible" according to the Morton et al. criteria.

If one wishes to base a sample size calculation for the PCC on the test of some hypothesized value for the true correlation (i.e., $H_0 : \rho = \rho_0$, where ρ_0 could be zero), we recommend that one use the procedure in which the Fisher z-transformed value of r is used as the test statistic (Equation 4.59):

$$z_0 = \frac{z(r) - z(\rho_0)}{1/\sqrt{n-3}},$$

(One could base the sample size calculation on the exact test statistic given in (4.57), but then the only null value that could be tested is $\rho_0 = 0$.) For limitations of this approach, see Ogus et al. (2007).

If one plans to use the Fisher z-based testing procedure, then the following formula can be used to determine the minimum sample size n required for achieving power of $100(1 - \beta)\%$ (usually, at least 80%) for detecting an alternative value ρ_1 of the true correlation ($\rho_1 > \rho_0$) in the upper-tailed test of $H_0 : \rho \leq \rho_0$ vs. $H_1 : \rho > \rho_0$, where $\rho_0 \neq 0$:

$$n = 3 + \left[\frac{(z_\alpha + z_\beta)}{z(\rho_1) - z(\rho_0)}\right]^2. \tag{4.67}$$

In this formula, α denotes the desired significance level (usually 0.05), z_γ denotes the upper γ-percentage point of the standard normal and $z(\rho)$ denotes the Fisher z-transformed value of ρ. The corresponding formula for the SCC is as follows:

$$n = 3 + \left(1 + \frac{\rho_{s1}^2}{2}\right)\left[\frac{(z_\alpha + z_\beta)}{z(\rho_{s1}) - z(\rho_{s0})}\right]^2, \tag{4.68}$$

where ρ_{s0} and ρ_{s1} are the null and alternative hypothesized values of the Spearman correlation ($\rho_{s1} > \rho_{s0}$). Similarly, for the KCC,

$$n = 4 + 0.437 \left[\frac{(z_\alpha + z_\beta)}{z(\tau_{b1}) - z(\tau_{b0})} \right]^2, \tag{4.69}$$

where τ_{b0} and τ_{b1} are the null and alternative values of Kendall's coefficient ($\tau_{b1} > \tau_{b0}$).

Note that in the sample size formula for the SCC in Equation (4.68), the more accurate approximation to the distribution of $z(r_s)$ proposed by Bonett and Wright (2000) has been incorporated into the sample size formula. In the more traditional approach, $1 + \frac{\rho_{s1}^2}{2}$ in Equation (4.68) would be replaced by 1.06 (Fieller et al. 1957). For a two-tailed test (e.g., $H_0 : \rho = \rho_0$ vs. $H_1 : \rho \neq \rho_0$, the formulas in (4.67), (4.68), and (4.69) would be modified by replacing z_α by $z_{\alpha/2}$.

If one wished to base the sample size calculation on achieving a specified width of the CI for ρ (or ρ_s or τ_b) rather than on achieving a pre-specified level of power against some alternative hypothesis, one could use Table 2 in Looney (1996), or the more general method proposed by Bonett and Wright (2000). Table 4.26, adapted from Table 2 in Looney (1996), can be used to obtain the appropriate sample size under a variety of conditions.

The Bonett and Wright (2000) approach for determining the appropriate sample size for a future study in which CI estimation of a CC is to be the primary statistical analysis is based on a two-stage approach. It can be used to determine the appropriate n to use for CI estimation of Pearson's, Spearman's, or Kendall's coefficients. Adapting their method to any of the three coefficients requires that one specify the appropriate values of two quantities, which they denote by b and c^2. Table 4.27 provides these values for each of the three coefficients.

TABLE 4.26 Minimum Sample Size Required to Yield a 95% CI(ρ) of Specified Width

r ↓ Width of 95% CI(ρ) →	0.10	0.20	0.30	0.40
0.1	1507	378[a]	168[a]	95[a]
0.2	1418	355	159	90[a]
0.3	1275	320	143	81
0.4	1087	273	123	70
0.5	868	219	99	57
0.6	634	161	74	43
0.7	404	105	49	30
0.8	205	56	28	19
0.9	63	20	14	10

[a]Confidence intervals based on these values of n and r will contain $\rho = 0$, resulting in a failure to reject $H_0 : \rho = 0$.

TABLE 4.27 Constants Required for Fisher *z*-Transformation of Measures of Association

Measure of Association	b	c^2	Source
Pearson	3	1	Fieller et al. (1957)
Spearman	3	$1 + \frac{r_s^2}{2}$	Bonett and Wright (2000)
Spearman	3	1.06	Fieller et al. (1957)
Kendall	4	0.437	Fieller et al. (1957)

The value r_s is a planning estimate for the Spearman coefficient ρ_s that could be based on expert opinion or obtained from previous research.

Let ξ denote the true value of the measure of association to be used (either the PCC, SCC, or KCC). The first step in the process proposed by Bonett and Wright is to calculate the "first stage" sample size approximation:

$$n_0 = 4c^2\left(1 - \widehat{\xi^2}\right)\left(\frac{z_{\alpha/2}}{w}\right)^2 + b, \tag{4.70}$$

where w is the desired width of the Fisher z-based CI for ξ with limits given in Equation (4.61), $\hat{\xi}$ is a planning estimate of ξ, and b and c are obtained from Table 4.27. Round the value of n_0 in (4.70) up to the nearest integer and set $n_0 = 10$ if Equation (4.70) produces a value less than 10.

The next step in the Bonett and Wright approach is to calculate w_0, the width of the Fisher z CI for ξ based on the value of n_0 obtained from Equation (4.70). This is done by applying the "back-transform" in (4.61) to the limits for the PCC, SCC, and KCC given in (4.60), (4.65), and (4.66), respectively. It is important to compare the value of w_0 with the desired width of the CI; if $w_0 \leq w$, then the desired CI width can be achieved using n_0 as the sample size and it is not necessary to apply the second stage of the Bonett–Wright approach. However, a smaller value of n can be obtained by applying the second stage.

If $w_0 > w$, the desired CI width cannot be achieved using n_0 as the sample size, so the second stage is required. The required sample size n for the desired CI estimation of ξ is then given by

$$n = (n_0 - b)\left(\frac{w_0}{w}\right)^2 + b, \tag{4.71}$$

where the appropriate value of b is obtained from Table 4.27.

Example 4.21 Sample Size Determination for Pearson, Spearman, and Kendall's Coefficients Based on Confidence Interval Estimation

In this example, we assume that CI estimation of a CC will be the primary statistical analysis to be performed in a study that is being planned. We illustrate the application of Equations (4.70) and (4.71) in finding the required sample size for studies in which the PCC, SCC, or KCC will be used as the measure of association.

Pearson Correlation Coefficient Suppose that one wishes to plan a study to examine the association of the sVAP-1 biomarker described by Salmi et al. (2002) with the level of ketone bodies in diabetic adults. (Note that Salmi et al. examined this association in diabetic children and adolescents only.) In their 2002 study, Salmi et al. found a Pearson correlation of $r = 0.34$ in their sample of $n = 38$ children and adolescents. Even though this correlation was statistically significant ($p = 0.037$), the 95% CI for ρ was too wide to be of any practical use (0.02–0.60). Thus, in the future study of adults that is being planned, the investigators want to use a sample size that is large enough to yield a meaningful CI once the study data are collected and analyzed. Suppose that it is determined that a 95% CI will be appropriate for the proposed study, and that the Fisher z-based interval for ρ is to be no wider than $w = 0.2$. (Roughly speaking, this means that the sample estimate r will differ from the true value ρ by no more than 0.1). The value of the sample PCC obtained by Salmi et al. (2002) ($r = 0.34$) is to be used as the "planning estimate." Applying (4.70) with $c^2 = 1$, $\hat{\xi} = 0.34$, $z_{\alpha/2} = 1.96$, $w = 0.2$, and $b = 3$, the "first stage" sample size approximation is $n_0 = 304$ (after rounding up). The width of the CI for ρ based on Fisher z using on $\hat{\xi} = 0.34$ and $n_0 = 304$ is $w_0 = 0.19927$, which is slightly less than the desired width of 0.200 for the planned study. Applying (4.71) with $n_0 = 304$, $b = 3$, $w_0 = 0.19927$, and $w = 0.2$ yields the desired sample size for the planned study of $n = 302$. (Note that one could use the "first stage" sample size estimate of $n_0 = 304$ without any harm.)

Spearman Correlation Coefficient Next, consider the study of $n = 20$ patients with xerostomia by Stuart (2013), who found p21 to be a promising biomarker for severity of symptoms of xerostomia due to its statistically significant correlations with item Q5 and the overall score on the VAS for severity of symptoms (see Table 4.24). The investigators now wish to design a much larger multi-center study of patients with xerostomia in order to confirm these encouraging findings. Even though the correlation of Q5 with p21 was statistically significant ($r_s = 0.569$, $p = 0.037$), the 95% CI for ρ_s was too wide to be of any practical use (0.134, 0.821). Thus, in the future study that is being planned, the investigators want to use a sample size that will be large enough to yield a meaningful CI for the SCC once the study data have been collected and analyzed. Suppose that it is determined that a 95% CI will be appropriate for the proposed study, and that the Fisher z CI for ρ_s is to be no wider than $w = 0.2$. The value of the sample SCC obtained by Stuart ($r = 0.57$) is to be used as the "planning value." Note that, according to Table 4.27, $b = 3$ and $c^2 = 1 + \frac{r_s^2}{2} = 1 + \frac{(0.57)^2}{2} = 1.1625$. Applying (4.70) with $c^2 = 1.1625$, $\hat{\xi} = 0.57$, $z_{\alpha/2} = 1.96$, $w = 0.2$, and $b = 3$, the "first stage" sample size approximation is $n_0 = 207$ (after rounding up). The width of the CI for τ_b based on Fisher z using $\hat{\xi} = 0.57$ and $n_0 = 207$ is $w_0 = 0.19972$, the desired width (after rounding) of the CI to be obtained from the study that is being planned. Therefore, there is no need to apply (4.71) and the required sample size for the future study is $n = 207$. If the Fieller value of c^2 (= 1.06) were used instead of the Bonett and Wright value ($c^2 = 1.1625$), the required sample size would be quite a bit lower: $n = 189$ instead of $n = 207$.

Kendall Concordance Coefficient Consider now the promising study ($n = 12$) on the use of bevacizumab as a chemotherapeutic agent for the treatment of advanced non-small-cell lung cancer (Heist et al. 2010) considered in Section 4.5.1.2. Another team of investigators wishes to plan a multi-center study to further examine the effectiveness of this agent. Despite the statistically significant results for the KCC in the Heist et al. study ($t_b = 0.58, p = 0.005$), the 95% CI (0.20, 0.81) is very wide and of no practical use. (This is not surprising given that the sample size in Heist et al. was only $n = 12$.) Thus, in the study being planned, the investigators wish to select a sample size that will be large enough to yield a meaningful CI for τ_b. Suppose that it is determined that a 95% CI will be appropriate for the proposed study, and that the Fisher z-interval for τ_b is to be no wider than $w = 0.2$. The value of t_b obtained in the study by Heist et al. (0.58) is to be used as the "planning value." Applying (4.70) with $c^2 = 0.437$, $\hat{\xi} = 0.58$, $z_{\alpha/2} = 1.96$, $w = 0.2$, and $b = 4$, the "first stage" sample size approximation is $n_0 = 78$ (after rounding up). The width of the Fisher z CI for τ_b based on $n_0 = 78$ is $w_0 = 0.19991$, the desired width (after rounding) of the CI to be obtained from the future study. Therefore, there is no need to apply (4.71) and the desired sample size for the future study is $n = 78$.

The following SAS code can be used to carry out the Bonett and Wright approach to sample size calculation for the PCC, SCC, and KCC for Example 4.21.

```
/*
    This code requires that the following input be supplied using
    %let macro statements:
    (a) planning values of Pearson (rp), Spearman (rs)and Kendall
        (rk)coefficients,
    (b) desired width of 95% confidence interval (w),
    (c) values of constants for Pearson (b=3, c^2=1),
        Spearman (b=3) and Kendall (b=4, c^2=.437),
*/

/*   Pearson     */

%let rp = .34;
%let w = .2;
%let b = 3;
%let c_sq = 1;

data fisher_rp_sample;
n_0_1 = 4*(&c_sq)*((1-&rp**2)**2)*((1.96/&w)**2)+&b;
if n_0_1 < 10 then n_0 = 10;
if int(n_0_1) < n_0_1 then n_0 = int(n_0_1)+1; else n_0 = n_0_1;
rp_fisher=0.5*(log((1+&rp)/(1-&rp)));
low_rpz=rp_fisher-1.96*sqrt(&c_sq)/(sqrt(n_0-&b));
up_rpz=rp_fisher+1.96*sqrt(&c_sq)/(sqrt(n_0-&b));
```

```
low_rp=(exp(2*low_rpz)-1)/(exp(2*low_rpz)+1);
up_rp=(exp(2*up_rpz)-1)/(exp(2*up_rpz)+1);
w_0 = up_rp -low_rp;
n_1 = (n_0 - &b)*(w_0/&w)**2+&b;
if int(n_1) < n_1 then n = int(n_1)+1; else n = n_1;
run;

proc print data=fisher_rp_sample;
title 'Sample Size Calculation';
title2 'Pearson';
run;

/*    Spearman using the Bonett-Wright value of c2 calculated from
      the planning value of r_s      */

%let rs = .57;
%let w = .2;
%let b = 3;

data fisher_rs_sample;
c_sq = 1+(&rs**2)/2;
n_0_1 = 4*(c_sq)*((1-&rs**2)**2)*((1.96/&w)**2)+&b;
if n_0_1 < 10 then n_0 = 10;
if int(n_0_1) < n_0_1 then n_0 = int(n_0_1)+1; else n_0 = n_0_1;
rs_fisher=0.5*(log((1+&rs)/(1-&rs)));
low_rsz=rs_fisher-1.96*sqrt(c_sq)/(sqrt(n_0-&b));
up_rsz=rs_fisher+1.96*sqrt(c_sq)/(sqrt(n_0-&b));
low_rs=(exp(2*low_rsz)-1)/(exp(2*low_rsz)+1);
up_rs=(exp(2*up_rsz)-1)/(exp(2*up_rsz)+1);
w_0 = up_rs -low_rs;
n_1 = (n_0 - &b)*(w_0/&w)**2+&b;
if int(n_1) < n_1 then n = int(n_1)+1; else n = n_1;
run;

proc print data=fisher_rs_sample;
title 'Sample Size Calculation';
title2 'Spearman Using Bonett-Wright Value of c^2';
run;

/*    Spearman using the Fieller et al. value of c^2 = 1.06    */

%let c_sq = 1.06;
%let rs = .57;
%let w = .2;
%let b = 3;
```

```
data fisher_rs_sample;
n_0_1 = 4*(&c_sq)*((1-&rs**2)**2)*((1.96/&w)**2)+&b;
if n_0_1 < 10 then n_0 = 10;
if int(n_0_1) < n_0_1 then n_0 = int(n_0_1)+1; else n_0 = n_0_1;
rs_fisher=0.5*(log((1+&rs)/(1-&rs)));
low_rsz=rs_fisher-1.96*sqrt(&c_sq)/(sqrt(n_0-&b));
up_rsz=rs_fisher+1.96*sqrt(&c_sq)/(sqrt(n_0-&b));
low_rs=(exp(2*low_rsz)-1)/(exp(2*low_rsz)+1);
up_rs=(exp(2*up_rsz)-1)/(exp(2*up_rsz)+1);
w_0 = up_rs -low_rs;
n_1 = (n_0 - &b)*(w_0/&w)**2+&b;
if int(n_1) < n_1 then n = int(n_1)+1; else n = n_1;
run;

proc print data=fisher_rs_sample;
title 'Sample Size Calculation';
title2 'Spearman Based on Fieller et al. Value of c^2 = 1.06';
run;

/*    Kendall     */

%let rk = .58;
%let w = .2;
%let b = 4;
%let c_sq = .437;

data fisher_rk_sample;
n_0_1 = 4*(&c_sq)*((1-&rk**2)**2)*((1.96/&w)**2)+&b;
if n_0_1 < 10 then n_0 = 10;
if int(n_0_1) < n_0_1 then n_0 = int(n_0_1)+1; else n_0 = n_0_1;
rk_fisher=0.5*(log((1+&rk)/(1-&rk)));
low_rkz=rk_fisher-1.96*sqrt(&c_sq)/(sqrt(n_0-&b));
up_rkz=rk_fisher+1.96*sqrt(&c_sq)/(sqrt(n_0-&b));
low_rk=(exp(2*low_rkz)-1)/(exp(2*low_rkz)+1);
up_rk=(exp(2*up_rkz)-1)/(exp(2*up_rkz)+1);
w_0 = up_rk -low_rk;
n_1 = (n_0 - &b)*(w_0/&w)**2+&b;
if int(n_1) < n_1 then n = int(n_1)+1; else n = n_1;
run;

proc print data=fisher_rk_sample;
title 'Sample Size Calculation';
title2 'Kendall';
run;
```

Example 4.22 Sample Size Determination for Pearson, Spearman, and Kendall's Coefficients Based on Hypothesis Testing

It could very well be that the sample sizes obtained in Example 4.21 for the PCC ($n = 302$), SCC ($n = 240$), and KCC ($n = 78$) are too large; in other words, the available resources are not sufficient to carry out studies of this magnitude. In that case, an alternative approach that generally yields much smaller sample sizes could be to determine the minimum sample size n required to achieve power of $100(1 - \beta)\%$ for detecting an alternative value ρ_1 of the true correlation. The most economical way to do this is to state the hypotheses to be tested as one sided (e.g., either $H_0 : \rho \leq \rho_0$ vs. $H_1 : \rho > \rho_0$ or $H_0 : \rho \geq \rho_0$ vs. $H_1 : \rho < \rho_0$, where $\rho_0 \neq 0$ is the desired null value). However, one-sided hypotheses are controversial (Freedman 2008; Lombardi and Hurlbert 2009) and may not always be appropriate. Furthermore, in order to obtain a conclusion from the CI that is consistent with the results of a one-sided test, one must use a one-sided CI. However, these are not widely used in practice. For purposes of illustration, we will present both one-sided and two-sided CIs in this section.

In the standard approach to determining the appropriate sample size for a study in which correlation will be the primary statistical analysis, the value of n is based on achieving the desired level of power (typically 80%) to detect some alternative value $\rho_1 > 0$ in the test of $H_0 : \rho = 0$ vs. $H_1 : \rho \neq 0$. However, as pointed out by Looney (1996) and discussed elsewhere in this section, the sample size obtained using this approach may be too small to provide a meaningful CI.

In this example, we assume that an hypothesis test of a CC will be the primary statistical analysis to be performed in a study that is being planned and illustrate the application of Equations (4.67), (4.68), and (4.69) in finding the required sample size for studies in which the PCC, SCC, or KCC will be used as the measure of association.

Pearson Correlation Coefficient Suppose again that it is desired to plan a study to examine the association of the sVAP-1 biomarker described by Salmi et al. (2002) with the level of ketone bodies in diabetic adults. The investigative team determined that the sample size of $n = 302$ obtained using the CI approach in Example 4.21 would require more than the available resources for the study. A decision was made to base the sample size calculation on an appropriate hypothesis test involving the true correlation ρ between the sVAP-1 biomarker and the level of ketone bodies in adult diabetics. The traditional approach would be to base the determination of n on the test of $H_0 : \rho = 0$ vs. $H_1 : \rho \neq 0$. For planning purposes, assume that the true correlation ρ_1 is equal to 0.38, the value obtained in the Salmi et al. study of 38 children. We apply Equation (4.67) with $z_{\alpha/2} = z_{0.025} = 1.96$ (since we will perform a two-tailed test), $z_\beta = z_{0.2} = 0.84$, $z(\rho_1) = z(0.34) = 0.354$, and $z(\rho_0) = z(0) = 0$, and obtain $n = 66$. For the sake of argument, suppose that the study is done with $n = 66$ adults and that the sample value of the PCC is exactly equal to 0.34, the alternative value ρ_1 that we wished to detect. This yields a statistically significant result ($p = 0.005$), but the 95% CI is (0.11, 0.54). This interval is too wide to draw any meaningful conclusions about the true magnitude of ρ. Based on this interval, the true correlation could be small (0.1), medium (0.3), or large (0.5), according to Cohen's criteria. Using the Morton et al. criteria, the true correlation could be anywhere between "negligible" and "moderate" (see Section 4.5.3).

Suppose instead that we base the sample size calculation for the new study on achieving adequate power for a test of $H_0 : \rho \leq 0.2$ vs. $H_1 : \rho > 0.2$. Rejecting H_0 would at least tell the investigators that the true correlation is not "negligible" ($0 \leq \rho \leq 0.2$) according to the Morton et al. criteria. Applying Equation (4.67) with $z_\alpha = z_{0.05} = 1.645$ (since we will perform an upper-tailed test), $z_\beta = z_{0.2} = 0.84$, $z(\rho_1) = z(0.34) = 0.354$, and $z(\rho_0) = z(0.2) = 0.203$, we obtain $n = 273$, which is somewhat smaller than the value obtained using the CI approach ($n = 302$). Again, for the sake of argument, suppose that the study is done with $n = 273$ adults and that the sample value of the PCC is exactly equal to the alternative value ρ_1 that we wished to detect (0.340). This yields a statistically significant result (upper-tailed $p = 0.006$), with a 95% two-sided CI of (0.23, 0.44) and a one-sided CI of (0.25, 1.00). Note that we can conclude that the true correlation between sVAP-1 and ketone bodies in diabetic adults is not negligible. Furthermore, based on the two-sided CI, the true correlation cannot be considered moderate or strong. Morton et al. would classify it as "weak" since it is likely to fall between 0.2 and 0.5, based on the 95% CI.

Spearman Correlation Coefficient Now, let us again consider planning a multi-center study of patients with xerostomia in order to confirm the encouraging findings in the study of $n = 20$ patients by Stuart (2013), who found p21 to be a promising biomarker for severity of symptoms of xerostomia. Suppose that the sample size of $n = 207$ obtained using the CI approach (Example 4.21) would require more resources than are available for the new study. As in the newly proposed study of diabetic adults described above, the decision is made to base the sample size calculation on achieving adequate power for an appropriate hypothesis test involving the true Spearman correlation ρ_s between the level of the p21 biomarker and the response to Q5 on the VAS. The traditional approach would be to base the determination of n on the test of $H_0 : \rho_s = 0$ vs. $H_1 : \rho_s \neq 0$. For planning purposes, assume that the true correlation ρ_{s1} is equal to 0.57, the value obtained by Stuart in her study of $n = 20$ xerostomic patients. We apply Equation (4.68) with $z_{\alpha/2} = z_{.025} = 1.96$ (since we will perform a two-tailed test), $z_\beta = z_{0.2} = 0.84$, $z(\rho_{s1}) = z(0.57) = 0.648$, and $z(\rho_{s0}) = z(0) = 0$, obtaining $n = 25$. (If we use the Fieller et al. value of $c^2 = 1.06$ in Equation (4.68), we obtain $n = 23$.) For the sake of argument, suppose that the new multi-center study is done with $n = 25$ adults and that the sample value of the SCC is exactly equal to 0.57, the alternative value ρ_1 that we wished to detect. This yields a statistically significant result ($p = 0.005$), but the 95% CI is (0.19, 0.80). This interval is too wide to draw any meaningful conclusions about the true magnitude of ρ_s. Using the Morton et al. (1996) criteria, based on this interval, the true Spearman correlation could be anything from "negligible" to "strong."

Suppose instead that we base the sample size calculation for the new study on achieving adequate power for a test of $H_0 : \rho_s \geq 0.8$ vs. $H_1 : \rho_s < 0.8$. Rejecting H_0 would at least tell the investigators that the true correlation cannot be considered to be "strong" ($0.8 \leq |\rho| \leq 1.0$) according to the Morton et al. (1996) criteria. Applying Equation (4.68) with $z_\alpha = z_{.05} = 1.645$ (since we will perform an upper-tailed test), $z_\beta = z_{0.2} = 0.84$, $z(\rho_{s1}) = z(0.57) = 0.648$, and $z(\rho_{s0}) = z(0.8) = 1.099$, we obtain $n = 39$, which is substantially smaller than the value obtained using the CI approach ($n = 207$). (If we use the Fieller et al. value of $c^2 = 1.06$ in Equation (4.68), we obtain $n = 36$.) Again, for the sake of argument, suppose that the study is done with $n = 39$ adults and that the sample value of the SCC is exactly equal to the alternative value ρ_{s1} that we wish to detect (0.57). This yields a statistically significant result (lower-tailed $p = 0.006$), with a two-sided 95% CI of (0.29, 0.76) and a one-sided 95% CI of (−1.00, 0.74). Although this CI is still rather wide, we can safely conclude that the true correlation between p21 and Q5 is not large enough to be classified as "strong." The best we can say is that it is between "weak" and "moderate" according to the Morton et al. criteria.

Kendall Concordance Coefficient Finally, consider once again the design of a larger study to examine further the encouraging results on the use of bevacizumab as a chemotherapeutic agent for the treatment of advanced non-small-cell lung cancer (Heist et al. 2010) considered in Section 4.5.1.2. Suppose that the sample size of $n = 78$ obtained using the CI approach (Example 4.21) was felt to be manageable given the available resources, but the study team decided to also consider the hypothesis testing approach in determining the sample size for the new study. The decision was made to base the sample size calculation on achieving adequate power for an appropriate hypothesis test involving the true value of τ_b between tumor blood flow (the biomarker) and score on the RECIST scale. The traditional approach would be to base the determination of n on the test of $H_0 : \tau_b = 0$ vs. $H_1 : \tau_b \neq 0$. It was decided that the alternative value to be detected with the new study would be $\tau_{b1} = 0.58$, the value obtained by Heist et al. in their study of $n = 12$ lung cancer patients. We apply Equation (4.69) with $z_{\alpha/2} = z_{.025} = 1.96$ (since we will perform a two-tailed test), $z_\beta = z_{0.2} = 0.84$, $z(\tau_{b1}) = z(0.58) = 0.662$, and $z(\tau_{b0}) = z(0) = 0$, obtaining $n = 12$. Note that this is the same sample size as that used in the pilot study by Heist et al. Assuming that the value of t_b obtained in the new study is not that much different from 0.58, we know that the CI will be too wide to be of any use (0.20, 0.81).

Suppose instead that the investigators decide to base the sample size calculation for the new study on achieving adequate power for a test of $H_0 : \tau_b \leq \tau_{b0}$ vs. $H_1 : \tau_b > \tau_{b0}$ for some appropriately chosen null value τ_{b0}. After careful consideration, the decision was made to choose $\tau_{b0} = 0.30$ since this corresponds to a medium effect size based on Cohen's criteria for the PCC. Applying Equation (4.69) with $z_\alpha = z_{.05} = 1.645$ (since we will perform an upper-tailed test), $z_\beta = z_{0.2} = 0.84$, $z(\rho_1) = z(0.58) = 0.662$, and $z(\rho_0) = z(0.30) = 0.310$, we obtain $n = 26$. Again, for the sake of argument, suppose that the new study is done with $n = 26$ and that the sample value of the KCC is exactly equal to the alternative value we wish to detect ($\tau_{b1} = 0.58$). This yields a statistically significant result (upper-tailed $p = 0.006$), with a two-sided 95% CI of (0.37, 0.73) and a one-sided 95% CI of (0.41, 1.00). Thus, we can safely conclude that the true KCC between tumor blood flow and RECIST score is significantly larger than 0.30 and would be classified as a "large" effect size according to the Cohen criteria.

The following SAS code can be used to carry out the sample size calculations for the PCC, SCC, and KCC for Example 4.22.

```
/*
     This code requires that the following input be supplied using
     %let macro statements:
     (a) alternative hypothesized values of Pearson (rho_1),
         Spearman (rho_s_1) and Kendall (tau_1) coefficients,
     (b) null hypothesized values of Pearson (rho_0), Spearman
         (rho_s_0) and Kendall (tau_0) coefficients,
     (c) desired significance level (alpha),
     (d) desired probability of Type II error or 1-power (beta),
     (e) values of constants for Pearson (b=3, c^2 =1),
         Spearman (b=3) and Kendall (b=4, c^2=.437).
*/

/*    Pearson      */

%let rho_1=.34;
%let rho_0=0;
*%let rho_0=.2;
%LET alpha=.025;
*%LET alpha=.05;
%LET beta=.20;
%let b=3;
%let c_sq=1;

data fisher_rho_sample;
z_alpha=probit(1 - &alpha);
z_beta=probit(1 - &beta);
rho_1_z=0.5*(log((1+&rho_1)/(1-&rho_1)));
rho_0_z=0.5*(log((1+&rho_0)/(1-&rho_0)));
n=& b + sqrt(&c_sq)*((z_alpha + z_beta) / (rho_1_z -
rho_0_z))**2;
if int(n) > n then n=int(n)+1;
run;

proc print data=fisher_rho_sample;
title 'Sample Size Calculation';
title2 'Pearson';
title3 'Based on Hypothesis Test';
run;
```

```
/*    Spearman using the Bonett-Wright value of c^2 calculated
      from the planning value of r_s_1     */

%let rho_s_1=.57;
*%let rho_s_0=.8;
%let rho_s_0=0;
%LET alpha=.025;
*%LET alpha=.05;
%LET beta=.20;
%let b=3;

data fisher_Spearman_sample;
c_sq=1 + (&rho_s_1**2)/2;
*c_sq=1.06;
z_alpha=probit(1 - &alpha);
z_beta=probit(1 - &beta);
rho_s_1_z=0.5*(log((1+&rho_s_1)/(1-&rho_s_1)));
rho_s_0_z=0.5*(log((1+&rho_s_0)/(1-&rho_s_0)));
n=& b + c_sq*((z_alpha + z_beta) / (rho_s_1_z - rho_s_0_z))**2;
if int(n) > n then n=int(n)+1;
run;

proc print data=fisher_Spearman_sample;
title 'Sample Size Calculation';
title2 'Spearman Using Bonett-Wright Value of c^2';
title3 'Based on Hypothesis Test';
run;

/*    Spearman using the Fieller et al. value of c^2=1.06    */

%let rho_s_1=.57;
*%let rho_s_0=.8;
%let rho_s_0=0;
%LET alpha=.025;
*%LET alpha=.05;
%LET beta=.20;
%let b=3;
%let c_sq=1.06;

data fisher_Spearman_sample;
z_alpha=probit(1 - &alpha);
z_beta=probit(1 - &beta);
rho_s_1_z=0.5*(log((1+&rho_s_1)/(1-&rho_s_1)));
rho_s_0_z=0.5*(log((1+&rho_s_0)/(1-&rho_s_0)));
```

```
n=& b + &c_sq*((z_alpha + z_beta) / (rho_s_1_z - rho_s_0_z))**2;
if int(n) > n then n=int(n)+1;
run;

proc print data=fisher_Spearman_sample;
title 'Sample Size Calculation';
title2 'Spearman Using Fieller et al. Value of c^2=1.06';
title3 'Based on Hypothesis Test';
run;

/*    Kendall     */

%let tau_1=.58;
*%let tau_0=.30;
%let tau_0=0;
%LET alpha=.025;
*%LET alpha=.05;
%LET beta=.20;
%let b=4;
%let c_sq=.437;

data fisher_Kendall_sample;
z_alpha=probit(1 - &alpha);
z_beta=probit(1 - &beta);
tau_1_z=0.5*(log((1+&tau_1)/(1-&tau_1)));
tau_0_z=0.5*(log((1+&tau_0)/(1-&tau_0)));
n=& b + &c_sq*((z_alpha + z_beta) / (tau_1_z - tau_0_z))**2;
if int(n) > n then n=int(n)+1;
run;

proc print data=fisher_Kendall_sample;
title 'Sample Size Calculation';
title2 'Kendall';
title3 'Based on Hypothesis Test';
run;
```

The sample size results for all the three coefficients using the CI and hypothesis testing approaches are summarized in Table 4.28. A comparison of the sample size results for the SCC and KCC in this table illustrates the phenomenon described by Helsel (2012, p. 224) that, all other things (including sample size) being equal, smaller values of t_b relative to r and r_s are required to yield a given degree of statistical significance. Put another way, the same value of the KCC as for the PCC and SCC in a sample of size n will yield stronger results. For example, when $n=50$ and $r=0.4$, the p-value for the two-tailed test of $H_0: \rho = 0$ based on the Fisher z-transformed

TABLE 4.28 Sample Size Results Using Various Methods

Measure of Association	Study	Primary Analysis	Design Parameters	Sample Size
Pearson	Salmi et al. (2002)	CI	$w = 0.20$	302
			$\hat{\rho} = 0.34$	
		Test H_0: $\rho = 0$	$\rho_1 = 0.34$	66
		Test H_0: $\rho \leq 0.2$	$\rho_1 = 0.34$	273
Spearman	Stuart (2013)	CI	$w = 0.20$	207
			$\hat{\rho}_s = 0.57$	
		Test H_0: $\rho_s = 0$	$\rho_{s1} = 0.57$	25
		Test $H_0 : \rho_s \geq 0.8$	$\rho_{s1} = 0.57$	39
Kendall	Heist et al. (2010)	CI	$w = 0.20$	78
			$\hat{\tau}_b = 0.58$	
		Test $H_0 : \tau_b = 0$	$\tau_{b1} = 0.58$	12
		Test $H_0 : \tau_b \geq 0.3$	$\tau_{b1} = 0.58$	26

value of r is 0.0037, with a 95% CI (ρ) of (0.14, 0.61). When $n = 50$ and $r_s = 0.40$, the results for the two-tailed test of $H_0 : \rho_s = 0$ using the Fisher z-transformed version of r_s ($c^2 = 1.06$) are not quite as strong but are almost identical to those for the PCC: $p = 0.0048$, 95% CI (0.13, 0.62). However, when $n = 50$ and $t_b = 0.40$, for the two-tailed test of $H_0 : \tau_b = 0$ using the Fisher z-transformed version of t_b, the results are much stronger: $p = 0.00001$, 95% CI (0.23, 0.55).

4.5.5 Comparison of Correlation Coefficients

In this section, we describe general approaches that can be used to compare two population CCs. These comparisons can generally be classified as either (1) comparison of "independent" CCs, or (2) comparison of "dependent" correlations. By "independent" correlations, we mean two sample CCs between the same variables X and Y that are calculated from independent samples of data. For example, we may wish to determine if the true correlation between urinary cotinine (X) and environmental cigarette smoke exposure (Y) is the same for male workers in the service industry as it is for female workers in the service industry. Let $\rho_{xy}^{(m)}$ denote the true correlation between X and Y for males and let $\rho_{xy}^{(f)}$ denote the true correlation between X and Y for females. We wish to test:

$$H_0 : \rho_{xy}^{(m)} = \rho_{xy}^{(f)} \text{ vs. } H_0 : \rho_{xy}^{(m)} \neq \rho_{xy}^{(f)}. \tag{4.72}$$

To test these hypotheses, we would obtain a sample of male service workers and an independent sample of female service workers, measure urinary cotinine and environmental cigarette smoke exposure in both samples, calculate the sample Pearson coefficients $r_{xy}^{(m)}$ and $r_{xy}^{(f)}$, and then calculate an appropriate test statistic based on $r_{xy}^{(m)}$ and $r_{xy}^{(f)}$.

Alternatively, the correlations we wish to compare may be "dependent," in the sense that both of them are based on the same sample of data. Correlations such as these can best be thought of as elements of a correlation matrix, and Steiger (1980) proposed several efficient statistical test procedures for comparing elements of such a matrix. We describe these procedures in Section 4.5.5.2.

4.5.5.1 Comparison of Independent Correlation Coefficients It may be of interest to compare the correlation of X with Y between two independent groups. For example, in the unpublished Masters thesis by Stuart (2013), another biomarker that was evaluated in addition to p21 was PCNA. As part of her assessment of criterion validity (Section 5.4.4), Stuart examined the association between p21 and PCNA in two independent samples: (1) a sample of $n_{\mathrm{h}} = 19$ healthy subjects and (2) a sample of $n_{\mathrm{x}} = 20$ patients with xerostomia (see Example 4.20). In the healthy subjects, she obtained a Spearman's correlation of $r_{\mathrm{sh}} = 0.049$, and in the xerostomic patients, she obtained a Spearman's correlation of $r_{\mathrm{sx}} = 0.357$. One might naturally ask: "Does the correlation of p21 with PCNA differ significantly between healthy and xerostomic patients?" The hypotheses to be tested are

$$H_0 : \rho_{\mathrm{sh}} = \rho_{\mathrm{sx}} \text{ vs. } H_{\mathrm{a}} : \rho_{\mathrm{sh}} \neq \rho_{\mathrm{sx}} \tag{4.73}$$

where ρ_{sh} denotes the true Spearman correlation between p21 and PCNA among healthy individuals and ρ_{sx} denotes the true Spearman correlation between p21 and PCNA among those with xerostomia. Denote by $z(r_{\mathrm{sh}})$ and $z(r_{\mathrm{sx}})$ the Fisher z-transformed values of the sample Spearman's coefficients r_{sh} and r_{sx}, respectively. Based on the results presented in Section 4.5.2, it can be shown that, under the null hypothesis H_0 in (4.73), the random variable $z(r_{\mathrm{sh}}) - z(r_{\mathrm{sx}})$ has a normal distribution with mean 0 and variance $1.06\left(\frac{1}{n_{\mathrm{h}}-3} + \frac{1}{n_{\mathrm{x}}-3}\right)$. (Note that, for purposes of comparing Spearman correlations, we recommend using the Fisher z-transformation of r_{s} proposed by Fieller et al. (1957).) Therefore, a Wald-type test statistic (Equation 3.9) for testing the null hypothesis in (4.73) is given by

$$z_0 = \frac{\left[z(r_{\mathrm{sh}}) - z(r_{\mathrm{sx}})\right]}{\sqrt{1.06\left(\frac{1}{n_{\mathrm{h}}-3} + \frac{1}{n_{\mathrm{x}}-3}\right)}}. \tag{4.74}$$

The resulting value of z_0 is then compared with the standard normal to obtain an approximate p-value. For comparing independent Pearson and Kendall coefficients, a similar approach is used. The general version of the test statistic that can be used with any one of the three coefficients is given by

$$z_0 = \frac{\left[z(\hat{\xi}_{\mathrm{sh}}) - z(\hat{\xi}_{\mathrm{sx}})\right]}{\sqrt{c^2\left(\frac{1}{n_{\mathrm{h}}-b} + \frac{1}{n_{\mathrm{x}}-b}\right)}}, \tag{4.75}$$

where $\hat{\xi}$ denotes the estimated coefficient (either Pearson's, Spearman's, or Kendall's) and the appropriate values of b and c^2 are obtained from Table 4.27.

Example 4.23 Test of Independent Correlation Coefficients

Using the results obtained by Stuart (2013), $r_{\mathrm{sh}}=0.049$, $r_{\mathrm{sx}}=0.357$, $n_{\mathrm{h}}=19$, and $n_{\mathrm{x}}=20$. The formula in (4.74) yields $z_0=0.91$ and $p=0.365$, indicating that the Spearman correlation of p21 with PCNA does not differ significantly between healthy subjects and xerostomic patients.

The following SAS code can be used to perform the Wald test for the data in Example 4.23.

```
/*
    This code requires that values of Spearman's coefficient
    (rs) and sample sizes (n) from two independent samples be
    input using %let macro statements. The constants b
    and c^2 from Table 4.27 must also be input.
*/

%let rs_h=.04912;
%let n_h=19;

%let rs_x=.35728;
%let n_x=20;

%let c_sq=1.06;
%let b=3;

data fisher_rs_ind;
rsh_fisher=0.5*(log((1+&rs_h)/(1-&rs_h)));
se_rs_h=sqrt((&c_sq)/(&n_h-&b));
rsx_fisher=0.5*(log((1+&rs_x)/(1-&rs_x)));
se_rs_x=sqrt((&c_sq)/(&n_x-&b));
se_rs_ind=sqrt(((se_rs_h)**2) + ((se_rs_x)**2));
z_rs_ind=(rsh_fisher - rsx_fisher)/se_rs_ind;
p_val_rs_ind=2*(1-probnorm(abs((z_rs_ind))));
run;

proc print data=fisher_rs_ind;
title1 'Comparison of Independent Spearman Correlations';
title2 'Using Fieller et al. (1957) Transformation';
run;
```

Note that the SAS code given above can be easily modified to perform the test comparing two independent Pearson correlations or two independent Kendall coefficients. All that is required is to input the appropriate values of b and c^2 taken from Table 4.27 using the %let statements.

TABLE 4.29 Correlation Matrix for Systolic and Diastolic Blood Pressure in Diabetics Before (BL) and After (F/U) 6 Months of Treatment with an Anti-Hypertensive Drug

Variable	$X1$	$Y1$	$Z1$	$X2$	$Y2$	$Z2$
$X1$	—					
$Y1$	ρ_{12}	—				
$Z1$	ρ_{13}	ρ_{23}	—			
$X2$	ρ_{14}	ρ_{24}	ρ_{34}	—		
$Y2$	ρ_{15}	ρ_{25}	ρ_{35}	ρ_{45}	—	
$Z2$	ρ_{16}	ρ_{26}	ρ_{36}	ρ_{46}	ρ_{56}	—

$X1$, sVAP-1 at BL; $X2$, sVAP-1 at F/U; $Y1$, systolic BP at BL; $Y2$, systolic BP at F/U; $Z1$, diastolic BP at BL; $Z2$, diastolic BP at F/U.

4.5.5.2 Comparison of Dependent Correlation Coefficients Suppose that, in a longitudinal study, we wish to examine the correlations of the sVAP-1 biomarker described in Salmi et al. (2002) with systolic and diastolic blood pressure in diabetics before (baseline, BL) and after (follow-up, F/U) 6 months of treatment with an anti-hypertensive drug. Let $X1$ and $X2$ denote the levels of sVAP-1 at BL and F/U, respectively. Similarly, let $Y1$ and $Y2$ will denote systolic blood pressure at BL and F/U, and $Z1$ and $Z2$ will denote the two diastolic blood pressure readings. Then we can represent all of the pairwise correlations among these variables in the correlation matrix given in Table 4.29.

Thus, if we wished to determine if the correlation between sVAP-1 and systolic blood pressure at BL was the same as the correlation between sVAP-1 and diastolic blood pressure at BL, we would test

$$H_0 : \rho_{12} = \rho_{13} \text{ vs. } H_a : \rho_{12} \neq \rho_{13}. \tag{4.76}$$

Since the two population correlations have a subscript in common (namely, "1"), we would refer to this as a comparison of "related dependent correlations" or "dependent correlations with a variable in common." On the other hand, if we wished to determine if the correlation between sVAP-1 and systolic blood pressure was the same at F/U as at BL, we would test

$$H_0 : \rho_{12} = \rho_{45} \text{ vs. } H_a : \rho_{12} \neq \rho_{45}. \tag{4.77}$$

This is still a comparison of "dependent" correlations since the estimates of ρ_{12} and ρ_{45} would be obtained from the same sample of longitudinal data, but we would call them "unrelated" since they do not share a subscript in common. (We might also refer to them as "dependent correlations with no variables in common.") In the next two sections, we describe methods for comparing "related dependent," and "unrelated dependent" correlations.

Comparison of Related Dependent Correlation Coefficients In some research studies in which biomarkers are used, it is of interest to compare "related" CCs; that is, the correlation of X with Y vs. the correlation of X with Z. For example, Salmi et al. (2002) found statistically significant correlations of sVAP-1 with both glucose ($r=0.57$, $p < 0.001$) and ketone bodies ($r=0.34$, $p=0.037$) using their sample of $n=38$ diabetic children and adolescents. They concluded that there was a "less marked" correlation of sVAP-1 with ketone bodies than with glucose. However, they gave no indication that a formal statistical test had been performed to determine if, in fact, the corresponding population CCs were different from each other. Had they performed such a test, as described in Steiger (1980), they would have found no significant difference between the two correlations ($p=0.093$). The method we recommend for performing this test is described below.

The hypotheses to be tested when comparing related dependent correlations can be stated as:

$$H_0 : \rho_{uv} = \rho_{uw} \text{ vs. } H_a : \rho_{uv} \neq \rho_{uw}, \tag{4.78}$$

where ρ_{uv} denotes the population correlation between the random variables U and V and ρ_{uw} denotes the population correlation between the random variables U and W. In the example taken from Salmi et al. described above, $U=$ sVAP-1, $V=$ glucose, and $W=$ ketone bodies. Let r_{uv} and r_{uw} denote the sample correlations between U and V and between U and W, respectively, and let $\bar{r}_{uv,uw}$ denote the mean of r_{uv} and r_{uw}. Denote by z_{uv} and z_{uw} the Fisher's z-transformed values of r_{uv} and r_{uw}, respectively. Then the test statistic recommended by Steiger (1980) for testing the hypotheses in (4.78) is given by

$$z_0 = \frac{(z_{uv} - z_{uw})\sqrt{n-3}}{\sqrt{2(1 - \bar{s}_{uv,uw})}}, \tag{4.79}$$

where $\bar{s}_{uv,uw}$ is an estimate of the covariance between z_{uv} and z_{uw} given by

$$\bar{s}_{uv,uw} = \frac{\hat{\Psi}_{uv,uw}}{(1 - \bar{r}^2_{uv,uw})^2},$$

where

$$\hat{\Psi}_{uv,uw} = r_{vw}\left(1 - 2\bar{r}^2_{uv,uw}\right) - \left(\bar{r}^2_{uv,uw}\right)\left(1 - 2\bar{r}^2_{uv,uw} - r^2_{vw}\right)/2.$$

The test of the null hypothesis in (4.78) is performed by comparing the sample value of z_0 in (4.79) with the standard normal distribution in order to calculate an approximate p-value. The general version of the test statistic in (4.79) that can be used with any one of the three coefficients is given by

$$z_0 = \frac{(z_{uv} - z_{uw})\sqrt{n-b}}{\sqrt{2c^2(1 - \bar{s}_{uv,uw})}} \tag{4.80}$$

where the appropriate values of b and c^2 are obtained from Table 4.27. (Note that the value of c^2 from Fieller et al. (1957) should be used for Spearman's coefficient.)

Example 4.24 Test of Related Dependent Correlation Coefficients

Using the results given in Salmi et al. (2002), $r_{uv} = 0.57$, $r_{uw} = 0.34$, $r_{vw} = 0.55$, $n = 38$, and $\bar{s}_{jk,jh} = 0.4659$, yielding $z_0 = 1.68$ and $p = 0.093$, as given previously.

The following SAS code can be used to perform Steiger's test for the data in Example 4.24.

```
/*
THIS PROGRAM COMPARES TWO DEPENDENT CORRELATIONS USING THE
METHODS DESCRIBED IN STEIGER JH. TESTS FOR COMPARING ELEMENTS
OF A CORRELATION MATRIX. PSYCHOLOGICAL BULLETIN (1980),
VOL. 87: 245-261.

R1 AND R2 ARE THE DEPENDENT CORRELATIONS TO BE COMPARED.
R12 IS THE CORRELATION BETWEEN THE VARIABLES THAT R1 & R2 DO NOT
HAVE IN COMMON.

FOR EXAMPLE, IF R1 IS THE CORRELATION BETWEEN X1 & X2 AND R2 IS
THE CORRELATION BETWEEN X1 & X3 THEN R12 IS THE CORRELATION
BETWEEN X2 & X3.
*/

%let r1 = 0.57;
%let r2 = 0.34;
%let r12 = 0.55;
%let n = 38;

%let b = 3;
%let c_sq = 1.00;

data dep_related;
z1 = log ((1 + &r1) / (1 - &r1)) / 2;
z2 = log ((1 + &r2) / (1 - &r2)) / 2;
rbar = (&r1 + &r2 ) / 2;
rbart = 1 - 2 * rbar * rbar;
rbart2 = 1 - rbar * rbar;
psi = &r12 * rbart - (rbart - &r12 * &r12) * rbar * rbar / 2;
sbar = psi / (rbart2 * rbart2);

zcal = (z1 - z2) / (sqrt(2) * sqrt (1-sbar)) /
(sqrt (&c_sq / (&n - &b))) ;
pval = 2 * (1 - probnorm(abs(zcal)));
```

```
proc print data=dep_related;
    title 'Dependent Correlations with a Variable in Common';
    run;
```

Note that the SAS code given above can be easily modified to perform the test comparing two dependent Spearman correlations or two dependent Kendall coefficients that share a variable in common. All that is required is to input the appropriate values of b and c^2 from Table 4.27 using the %let statements.

Comparison of Unrelated Dependent Correlation Coefficients Demattos et al. (2002) evaluated biomarkers indicative of brain amyloid burden (a surrogate marker for Alzheimer's disease) by correlating plasma deposition of amyloid-β (Aβ) peptides into amyloid plaques with amyloid burden in the hippocampus and cortex of mice that had been administered a monoclonal antibody to Aβ (m266). They correlated Aβ load and amyloid load with plasma $A\beta_{40}$, $A\beta_{42}$, and $A\beta_{40/42}$ ratio at baseline ("Pre-bleed"), and at 5 minutes, 1 hour, 3 hours, 6 hours, and 24 hours following administration of the monoclonal antibody ("Follow-up," F/U). In their sample of $n=49$ mice, they found a non-significant Pearson correlation between amyloid load and $A\beta_{40/42}$ ratio at baseline ($r=0.129$, $p=0.4393$), and a significant correlation between these same two variables at 5 minutes following administration of the monoclonal antibody ($r=0.483$, $p=0.0004$). Even though the correlations at "pre-bleed" and F/U appear to be quite different, the question naturally arises as to whether the two are *significantly* different in the statistical sense.

The null hypotheses to be tested when comparing unrelated dependent correlations can be stated as

$$H_0 : \rho_{xy} = \rho_{uv} \text{ vs. } H_{\text{a}} : \rho_{xy} \neq \rho_{uv}, \tag{4.81}$$

where ρ_{xy} denotes the population correlation between the random variables X and Y and ρ_{uv} denotes the population correlation between the random variables U and V. In the example taken from Demattos et al. (2002) described above, $X=$ amyloid load and $Y=A\beta_{40/42}$ ratio, both measured at "Pre-bleed," and $U=$ amyloid load and $T=A\beta_{40/42}$ ratio, both measured at 5 minutes F/U. Let r_{xy} and r_{uv} denote the sample correlations between X and Y and between U and V, respectively, and let $\bar{r}_{xy,uv}$ denote the mean of r_{xy} and r_{uv}. Denote by z_{xy} and z_{uv} Fisher's z-transformed values of r_{xy} and r_{uv}, respectively. Then the test statistic recommended by Steiger (1980) for testing the hypotheses in (4.81) is given by

$$z_0 = \frac{(z_{xy} - z_{uv})\sqrt{n-3}}{\sqrt{2(1 - \bar{s}_{xy,uv})}}, \tag{4.82}$$

where $\bar{s}_{xy,uv}$ is an estimate of the covariance between z_{xy} and z_{uv} given by

$$\bar{s}_{xy,uv} = \frac{\hat{\psi}_{xy,uv}}{(1 - \bar{r}^2_{xy,uv})^2},$$

where

$$\hat{\psi}_{xy,uv} = [(r_{xu} - r_{yu}\bar{r}_{xy,uv})(r_{yv} - r_{yu}\bar{r}_{xy,uv}) + (r_{xv} - r_{xu}\bar{r}_{xy,uv})(r_{yu} - r_{xu}\bar{r}_{xy,uv})$$
$$+ (r_{xu} - r_{xv}\bar{r}_{xy,uv})(r_{yv} - r_{xv}\bar{r}_{xy,uv}) + (r_{xv} - r_{yv}\bar{r}_{xy,uv})(r_{yu} - r_{yv}\bar{r}_{xy,uv})]/2.$$

The test of the hypotheses in (4.81) is performed by comparing the value of z_0 in (4.82) calculated from the sample with the standard normal distribution in order to calculate an approximate p-value.

The general version of the test statistic in (4.82) that can be used with any one of the three CCs is given by

$$z_0 = \frac{(z_{xy} - z_{uv})\sqrt{n - b}}{\sqrt{2c^2(1 - \bar{s}_{xy,uv})}}, \tag{4.83}$$

where the appropriate values of b and c^2 are obtained from Table 4.27. (Note that the value of c^2 from Fieller et al. (1957) should be used for Spearman's coefficient.)

Example 4.25 Test of Unrelated Dependent Correlation Coefficients

Using the results given in Demattos et al. (2002), $r_{xy} = 0.1293$, $r_{uv} = 0.4825$, and $\bar{r}_{xy,uv} = 0.3059$. However, the authors did not provide any of the other correlations needed to perform the test of the hypotheses in (4.81) ; namely, r_{xu}, r_{xv}, r_{yu}, and r_{yv}. In the context of this example, these correlations have the following interpretation: r_{xu} = correlation between amyloid load at "Pre-bleed" and at 5 minutes; r_{xv} = correlation between amyloid load at "Pre-bleed" and $A\beta_{40/42}$ ratio at 5 minutes; r_{yu} = correlation between amyloid load at 5 minutes and $A\beta_{40/42}$ ratio at "Pre-bleed"; and r_{yv} = correlation between $A\beta_{40/42}$ ratio at "Pre-bleed" and at 5 minutes. In Table 4.30, we provide the hypothesis testing results under three hypothetical scenarios in order to illustrate the effect that these correlations have on the test of the hypotheses in (4.81). In each scenario, we assume that the correlation between amyloid load and $A\beta_{40/42}$ ratio when each is measured at a different time point is only half of what it is when both are measured at the same time point. When amyloid load and $A\beta_{40/42}$ ratio were both measured at Pre-bleed, the correlation was $r_{xy} = 0.1293$. Therefore, for the correlation between amyloid load measured at Pre-bleed and $A\beta_{40/42}$ ratio measured at 5 minutes, we assume that $r_{xv} = 0.1293/2 = 0.0647$. When amyloid load and $A\beta_{40/42}$ ratio were both measured at 5 minutes, the correlation was $r_{uv} = 0.4825$. For the correlation between amyloid load measured at 5 minutes and $A\beta_{40/42}$ ratio measured at Pre-bleed,

TABLE 4.30 Results of Comparisons of Two Dependent Unrelated Pearson Correlations under Various Inter-Correlation Scenarios

Scenario	Hypothetical Correlations	z_0	p-value
1	$r_{xy}=0.1293$ $r_{uv}=0.4825$ $r_{xu}=0.5000$ $r_{xv}=0.0647$ $r_{yu}=0.2413$ $r_{yv}=0.5000$	−2.18	0.029
2	$r_{xy}=0.1293$ $r_{uv}=0.4825$ $r_{xu}=0.7500$ $r_{xv}=0.0647$ $r_{yu}=0.2413$ $r_{yv}=0.7500$	−3.01	0.003
3	$r_{xy}=0.1293$ $r_{uv}=0.4825$ $r_{xu}=0.2500$ $r_{xv}=0.0647$ $r_{yu}=0.2413$ $r_{yv}=0.2500$	−1.95	0.051

we assume that $r_{yu}=0.4825/2=0.2413$. Next, we examined the effects of the degree of correlation between amyloid load measured at "Pre-bleed" and at 5 minutes, and the correlation between $A\beta_{40/42}$ ratio measured at "Pre-bleed" and at 5 minutes. For purposes of this example only, we assume that these correlations are equal. In the first scenario in Table 4.30, we assume that $r_{xu}=r_{yv}=0.5$, a moderate degree of correlation. In the second scenario, we assume a stronger degree of correlation, $r_{xu}=r_{yv}=0.75$, and, for the third scenario, we assume a weaker degree of correlation, $r_{xu}=r_{yv}=0.25$. As indicated in Table 4.30, changing the degree of correlation in this manner yields quite different p-values. In fact, when a weaker degree of correlation is assumed between the measurements for amyloid load taken at pre-bleed and at 5 minutes, and between the measurements for $A\beta_{40/42}$ ratio taken at the different time points, the null hypothesis H_0 in (4.81) cannot be rejected at the 0.05 level of significance ($z_0=-1.95, p=0.051$). Thus, even though there appeared to be a meaningful difference in the correlations between amyloid load and $A\beta_{40/42}$ ratio at pre-bleed and at 5 minutes (0.129 vs. 0.483), it could have been the case that this difference was not statistically significant. That is why we feel that it is important, whenever possible, to provide the results of a formal statistical test to support any claim that is made with regard to correlations (or any statistical parameters) being different from each other.

The SAS code that was used to perform Steiger's test for these data under the "weaker correlation" Scenario 3 in Table 4.30 is given below. Note that the same code could be used to analyze the data for the "stronger" and "moderate" correlation scenarios simply by changing the values of the macro variables `r_xu` and `r_yv` in the appropriate `%let` statements.

```
/*
THIS PROGRAM COMPARES TWO DEPENDENT CORRELATIONS USING THE
METHODS DESCRIBED IN:
STEIGER JH. TESTS FOR COMPARING ELEMENTS OF A CORRELATION
MATRIX. PSYCHOLOGICAL BULLETIN (1980), VOL. 87: 245-261.

R_XY AND R_UV ARE THE CORRELATIONS TO BE COMPARED.
ALL POSSIBLE INTER-CORRELATIONS AMONG THE VARIABLES MAKING UP
THESE CORRELATIONS MUST ALSO BE SPECIFIED.
*/

%let r_xy=0.1293;
%let r_uv=0.4825;
%let r_xu=0.2500;
%let r_xv=0.0647;
%let r_yu=0.2413;
%let r_yv=0.2500;

%let n=49;

%let b=3;
%let c_sq=1.00;

data dep_unrelated;
z1=log ((1 + &r_xy) / (1 - &r_xy)) / 2;
z2=log ((1 + &r_uv) / (1 - &r_uv)) / 2;
rbar=(&r_xy + &r_uv ) / 2;
rbar_yu=rbar*&r_yu;
rbar_xu=rbar*&r_xu;
rbar_xv=rbar*&r_xv;
rbar_yv=rbar*&r_yv;
psi=(1/2)*((&r_xu-rbar_yu)*(&r_yv-rbar_yu)+
           (&r_xv-rbar_xu)*(&r_yu-rbar_xu)+
           (&r_xu-rbar_xv)*(&r_yv-rbar_xv)+
           (&r_xv-rbar_yv)*(&r_yu-rbar_yv));
rbart2=1 - rbar * rbar;
sbar=psi / (rbart2 * rbart2);
```

```
z2cal = (z1 - z2) / (sqrt(2) * sqrt (1-sbar)) /
      (sqrt (&c_sq / (&n - &b)));
pval2 = 2 * (1 - probnorm(abs(z2cal)));

proc print data = dep_unrelated;
     title 'Dependent Correlations with No Variable in Common';
     run;
```

Note that the SAS code given above can be easily modified to perform the test comparing two dependent Spearman correlations or two dependent Kendall coefficients that do not share a common variable. All that is required is to input the appropriate values of b and c^2 taken from Table 4.27 using the `%let` statements.

4.5.6 Sample Size Issues When Comparing Two Correlation Coefficients

Just as in statistical inference for a single CC (Section 4.5.2), it is important to design a study in which two CCs are to be compared so that the study will have a large enough sample size to yield meaningful statistical results. However, determining the appropriate sample size for the comparison of two CCs is quite a bit more complicated than for a single correlation. We present a method that can be used to determine the sample size needed to compare two independent Spearman coefficients; that is, to test the null hypothesis H_0 in (4.73). Using the appropriate choice of constants from Table 4.27, the method can be easily adapted to determine the sample size required for comparing two independent Pearson or Kendall coefficients.

4.5.6.1 Sample Size Issues When Comparing Independent Correlation Coefficients In order to maximize the power of any statistical test designed to compare two population parameters, the study should be designed such that the samples from each population are equal in size. Let n denote the common sample size from the two populations. Based on the results presented in Section 4.5.2, it can be shown that the random variable $z(r_{s1}) - z(r_{s2})$ has an approximate normal distribution with mean $z(\rho_{s1}) - z(\rho_{s2})$ and variance $\frac{2(1.06)}{n-3}$. (Note that we are once again using the Fisher z-transformation of r_s recommended by Fieller et al. (1957).) Therefore, a Wald-type test statistic for testing the null hypothesis in (4.73) is given by

$$z_0 = \frac{\left[z(r_{s1}) - z(r_{s2})\right]}{\sqrt{\frac{2(1.06)}{n-3}}}, \tag{4.84}$$

which is approximately distributed as standard normal. Using this result, it can be shown that the sample size required to detect a true difference in Fisher z-transformed

Spearman coefficients of $z(\rho_{s1}) - z(\rho_{s2})$ with power $1 - \beta$ using a two-tailed test with significance level α is given by

$$n = 3 + \frac{2(1.06)(z_{\alpha/2} + z_\beta)^2}{\left[z(\rho_{s1}) - z(\rho_{s2})\right]^2}. \tag{4.85}$$

The general formula that can be used with any one of the three coefficients (PCC, SCC, or KCC) is given by

$$n = b + \frac{2c^2(z_{\alpha/2} + z_\beta)^2}{\left[z(\xi_1) - z(\xi_2)\right]^2}, \tag{4.86}$$

where b and c^2 can be found in Table 4.27 and $z(\xi)$ denotes the Fisher z-transformed value of the population parameter ($z(\rho)$ for Pearson's, $z(\rho_s)$ for Spearman's, and $z(\tau_b)$ for Kendall's).

Example 4.26 Sample Size Determination for Comparing Two Independent Spearman Coefficients

In Example 4.23, we presented the results obtained by Stuart (2013) when comparing the Spearman correlation between the biomarkers p21 and PCNA in a sample of 19 healthy subjects ($r_{sh} = 0.049$) with that in a sample of 21 xerostomic patients ($r_{sx} = 0.357$). The difference in the true Spearman coefficients between the two populations was not statistically significant ($p = 0.365$). Suppose that, in a larger study being planned, it will be desired to make the same comparison between healthy and xerostomic patients. The investigators wish to determine the minimum required sample size for this new study. Assuming that the true Spearman correlations are comparable to those found in the small pilot study, we apply (4.85) with $z_{\alpha/2} = z_{.025} = 1.96$, $z_\beta = z_{0.2} = 0.84$, $z(\rho_{sh}) = z(0.049) = 0.049$, and $z(\rho_{sx}) = z(0.357) = 0.373$, obtaining

$$n = 3 + \frac{2(1.06)(1.96 + 0.84)^2}{[z(0.049) - z(0.357)]^2} = 3 + \frac{2(1.06)(z_{\alpha/2} + z_\beta)^2}{[0.049 - 0.373]^2} = 162.$$

Thus, the new study will require 162 healthy subjects and 162 xerostomic patients.

The following SAS code can be used to carry out the sample size calculation in Example 4.26:

```
%let rho_s_1 = 0.049;
%let rho_s_2 = 0.357;

%LET alpha = .025;
%LET beta = .20;
```

```
%let b=3;
%let c_sq=1.06;

data fisher_spearman_two_sample;
z_alpha=probit(1 - &alpha);
z_beta=probit(1 - &beta);
rho_s_1_z=0.5*(log((1+&rho_s_1)/(1-&rho_s_1)));
rho_s_2_z=0.5*(log((1+&rho_s_2)/(1-&rho_s_2)));
n=&b + 2*&c_sq*((z_alpha + z_beta)/(rho_s_1_z - rho_s_2_z))**2;
if int(n) < n then n=int(n)+1;
run;

proc print data=fisher_spearman_two_sample;
title 'Sample Size Calculation';
title2 'Comparison of Two Independent Spearman Coefficients';
run;
```

Note that this SAS code can easily be adapted to situations in which it is desired to compare two independent Pearson coefficients or two independent Kendall coefficients simply by specifying the appropriate values of b and c^2 obtained from Table 4.27.

4.5.6.2 Sample Size Issues When Comparing Dependent Correlation Coefficients

If a study is being planned in which the comparison of dependent CCs is to be the primary analysis, determination of the appropriate sample size is quite a bit more complicated. In fact, we are not aware of any closed-form sample size formulas similar to that for comparisons of independent coefficients (Equation 4.86). However, Aberson (2010) has provided SPSS syntax that can be used to generate power curves for the tests comparing dependent correlations (either related or unrelated) described in Section 4.5.5.2. In order to use this syntax, the analyst much supply "planning values" for each of the correlations that are to be compared in the primary hypothesis tests for the proposed study. For example, consider the comparison of related dependent PCCs in Example 4.24. Salmi et al. (2002) found statistically significant correlations of their biomarker sVAP-1 with both glucose ($r=0.57$, $p < 0.001$) and ketone bodies ($r=0.34$, $p=0.037$) based on their sample of $n=38$ diabetic children and adolescents. In Example 4.24, we compared these two correlations using Steiger's method (Section 4.5.5.2) and obtained $r_{uv}=0.57$, $r_{uw}=0.34$, $r_{vw}=0.55$, $n=38$, and $\bar{s}_{jk,jh} = 0.4659$, yielding $z_0=1.68$, $p=0.093$. Now, we wish to plan a larger study of diabetic adults, and to choose n appropriately large so that we would have a better chance of detecting a significant difference between these two Pearson correlations. Assuming that the sample correlations are reasonable "planning values" for the true correlations in the study to be planned, we used them as input into Aberson's SPSS program, and varied n (the number of diabetic adults) from 40 to 150 in increments

TABLE 4.31 Sample Size and Power Results for Comparing Two Related Dependent Correlations

n	Power
40	0.41
50	0.50
60	0.58
70	0.66
80	0.72
90	0.77
100	0.81
110	0.85
120	0.88
130	0.91
140	0.92

of 10. We specified a two-tailed test with significance level = 0.05. With these input parameters, Aberson's program yielded the results given in Table 4.31.

Thus, a sample size of $n = 100$ diabetic adults would be required to achieve 80% power for detecting a difference similar to that found in the original Salmi et al. study of diabetic children. A sample of $n = 130$ would be required to achieve 90% power.

4.6 CLUSTERED DATA

The term "clustered" or "clustering" has many different meanings in statistics, including cluster analysis, cluster sampling, and cluster randomization. Cluster analysis has to do with identifying group structure among a set of apparently unrelated objects. For example, Iyer et al. (1999) used hierarchical cluster analysis to identify 10 patterns of gene expression in a subset of 517 genes, as part of their time–course experiment on fibroblasts to investigate growth-related changes in RNA products over time. Cluster analysis, as the term is typically used by statisticians, usually has nothing to do with the analysis of clustered data, so we do not consider it further in this textbook.

Cluster sampling refers to sample surveys in which clusters of potential respondents are sampled rather than individual respondents. For example, the National Health and Nutrition Examination Survey (NHANES) is a program of studies conducted by the National Center for Health Statistics that is designed to assess the health and nutritional status of adults and children in the United States. It combines interviews and physical examinations, and data on several biomarkers are collected as part of the survey. One example is blood lead; it has been shown that high levels of lead exposure during pregnancy are associated with adverse birth outcomes and with lower cognitive function test scores in childhood (Jones et al. 2010). NHANES uses cluster sampling as part of the selection process for determining which residents of the United States will be invited to participate. NHANES is based on a multi-stage cluster sampling scheme, in which the primary sampling units (PSUs) are counties or small groups of contiguous counties. Within PSUs, segments are selected; these consist of city blocks or groups of blocks containing a cluster of households. Specific households are selected from within each segment, and study participants are selected from individual households. Thus, there are three levels of clustering—study participants are nested within households, which are nested within blocks, which are nested within counties.

Cluster randomization is used in cluster randomized trials (Section 2.2.7), which are research studies in which clusters of study subjects are randomly assigned to each treatment group, instead of randomly assigning individual subjects to treatments. The process used to assign clusters of study subjects to treatment groups is called "cluster randomization." For example, Grosskurth et al. (1995) performed a randomized trial to evaluate the impact of a sexually transmitted disease (STD) intervention program on the incidence of HIV infection in Tanzania. Six communities (clusters) were randomly assigned to receive the community-based intervention, with six comparison communities serving as the control group. These control communities received the intervention 2 years later. Several biomarkers were used in the study, including an ELISA test for HIV antibodies to ascertain the presence of HIV infection in the community residents who participated in the study.

Data may also be clustered naturally, without any formal structure or intervention imposed by the investigators. For an example of "naturally clustered" biomarker data, consider the study by Chiaradia et al. (1997), who evaluated the impact of occupational exposure to leaded dust from a lead–zinc–copper mine on blood lead concentrations in families of employees of the mine. Eight children of six employees of the mine were studied. Two of the six employees each had two of the children in the study; the remaining four employees had only one child who was included in the study. The data for the children who were siblings should have been treated as nested (or clustered) within their family. The most commonly used terminology for this type of structure would be that the Level 1 data (from the children who were siblings) were nested within the Level 2 data (from their respective families).

In another example of a study that considered naturally clustered biomarker data, Strickland and Kang (1999) considered biomarkers of internal dose to assess recent exposure to polycyclic aromatic hydrocarbons (PAHs). One such biomarker they considered is urinary 1-hydroxypyrene-O-glucuronide (1-OHP-gluc). Strickland and Kang found a significant association between urinary 1-OHP-gluc levels and air particulate measures in six regions in South Korea. Urinary 1-OHP-gluc was assayed in 150 junior high school children (and their mothers, $n = 150$) from 6 schools located in different geographical regions. They found significant differences in urinary 1-OHP-gluc among the six regions studied, with the highest levels occurring in a large urban environment. However, they failed to take into account the fact that each mother–child dyad should be treated as a cluster, despite acknowledging that there was a significant association in 1-OHP-gluc levels between children and their mothers (p. 196).

Any hierarchical or nested structure that is present in the study data should always be taken into account during the statistical analysis; failure to do so can have many adverse consequences, primarily because of the resulting distortions in the standard errors (SEs) of estimates of parameters such as means, proportions, CCs, etc. (Hauck et al. 1991). These inaccurate estimates of the SEs lead to CIs and hypothesis tests that have suboptimal properties. For example, the true coverage probability (CP) of a 95% CI may be much less than 95%, or the true probability of Type I error for an hypothesis test performed at the 0.05 level of significance may be much greater than 0.05. These problems may be avoided by using proper methods of data analysis.

Data that are "naturally nested" are the most common type of clustered data encountered in biomarker studies. However, cluster randomized studies are being used more and more frequently in studies utilizing biomarkers, just as they are becoming more and more popular in clinical and behavioral research. For example, in a study examining the effectiveness of antimicrobial mouthrinses in reducing microbial growth on photostimulable Phosphor (PSP) plates used in making dental x-rays (Hunter et al. 2014), patients were randomly assigned to rinse with one of three test rinses (Listerine®, Decapinol®, or Chlorhexidine oral rinse 0.12%) or to refrain from rinsing prior to receiving a full mouth radiographic survey (FMX). Four PSP plates were sampled from each FMX (i.e., for each patient), the blood agar plates were incubated at 37°C for up to 72 hours, and the number of bacterial colonies per plate were determined following incubation. Thus, the experimental units (PSP plates) from which the colony data were obtained were nested within patients. Thirty subjects were randomly assigned to each of the three rinses, and 40 subjects were randomly assigned to the "no rinse" control group. Thus, there were a total of $n = 120$ data values (4 plates × 30 subjects) in each of the dental rinse groups, and $n = 160$ data values (4 plates × 40 subjects) in the no rinse group. However, these are not the sample sizes to be used in a proper analysis of these data. Rather, the "effective sample size" in each group is the number of clusters (i.e., the number of patients), *not* the number of PSP plates. Failure to properly account for the fact that PSP plates taken from the FMX for a given patient are more likely to be similar than PSP plates taken from the FMXs for different patients leads to improper statistical analysis and incorrect conclusions. Examples 4.27 and 4.28 summarize the results of the analyses of these data.

An in-depth discussion of the analysis of clustered data is beyond the scope of this text. A good non-technical introduction, intended for clinical researchers, can be found in Hauck et al. (1991). The book by Donner and Klar (2010), with the accompanying ACluster software, is an excellent resource for the analysis of data from cluster randomized studies and we highly recommend it. Another very useful resource is Shoukri and Chaudhary (2007), which provides SAS and R code for analyzing clustered data, both naturally occurring and that obtained from cluster randomized trials. Generally speaking, the MIXED procedure in SAS is capable of providing the proper statistical analysis of clustered (or nested) data, but extreme care must be taken to properly specify the appropriate features of the mixed-effects statistical model to be used. We provide SAS code that can be used to analyze the data in Example 4.27, but we encourage those who have little or no experience with fitting mixed-effects models to become familiar with the concepts underlying these models and the appropriate analyses of data that are assumed to follow these models before attempting to use the MIXED procedure. An excellent reference written at a relatively low theoretical level is Singer (1995), who provides technical details as well as SAS code for analyzing data that follow several different types of nested and clustered structures. A comprehensive guide to the use of SAS in analyzing data that have an hierarchical structure that we highly recommend is Littell et al. (2006). Hedeker and Gibbons (2006) is an extremely useful reference for the application of mixed-effects regression models and the companion website http://tigger.uic.edu/~hedeker/long.html provides many examples of the practical application of mixed models, along with SAS code for carrying out these analyses.

Before describing the traditional approach for analyzing clustered data, we must first establish some terminology. By "unit," we mean the Level I entity from which the sample observations are obtained. In the study by Hunter et al., the unit was the PSP plate. By "cluster," we mean the Level II entity that consists of groups of units. In the Hunter et al. study, the cluster was the dental patient. Note that each cluster in this example consists of four units, and that an individual data item (i.e., bacterial colony count) was collected on each of the four units within each cluster. Note that there can also be additional levels of clustering. In the study by Hunter et al., the Level III entity consisted of the treatment group—either "no rinse" or one of the dental rinses. It is assumed that units within a cluster are correlated with regard to the variable being measured (in the example, the number of colonies of bacteria), but that clusters are independent of each other. In the Hunter et al. study, these are reasonable assumptions—the numbers of colonies of bacteria on PSP plates taken from the FMX of the same patient are likely to be correlated since they come from the same person, whereas there is no reason to believe that the patients were not independent of each other. Note that if some of the patients are twins, or share something else in common that could be related to their oral hygiene, then it is very likely that the assumption of independent clusters would be violated for this study.

The basic idea underlying statistical methods traditionally used to adjust for the effects of clustered data (either naturally occurring or by design) is the *intra-cluster correlation coefficient* (ICC). The population version of this parameter is denoted by ρ_{I} and the sample version by r_{I}. It is defined to be the ratio of the variation between clusters divided by the total variation in the data, which is partitioned into the variation between clusters plus the variation within clusters. If there is no variation between clusters, then ICC = 0 and there is no need to adjust for clustering. In this case, the "effective sample size" in the study is the number of units. On the other hand, if all of the variation in the data can be attributed to the variation between clusters (i.e., there is no variation among units within clusters), then there is essentially only one unit in each cluster, so the effective sample size is the number of clusters. In this case, ICC = 1. One way to think of the ICC is the average correlation between any two units selected at random from within any one of the clusters. If ICC = 0, there is no correlation within clusters; if ICC = 1, there is perfect correlation within clusters. With real data, it can happen that ICC < 0. In a cluster randomized study, this would tell us that there was no need to randomly assign clusters to groups; instead, traditional randomization of units to groups could have been used. In this situation, the sample estimate r_{I} should be set equal to zero and the data analyzed as if there were no clustering. With naturally occurring clustering, it can also happen that $r_{\mathrm{I}} < 0$. In this case, the effective sample size will be larger than the actual sample size n. If this occurs, our recommendation is to take the clustering into account when analyzing the data and use the negative value of r_{I}.

There are many possible comparisons that can be made when clustered data are present. For example, in the Hunter et al. study, the investigators were primarily interested in comparing the mean number of colonies of bacteria among dental rinse groups. The group effect in this case would be treated as a fixed effect; hence, the underlying model to be used for the comparison of the four groups would be referred to as a "mixed-effects" model because there is a random effect (patient) as well as a fixed effect (rinse group). Thus, the fixed effect for group would have to be incorporated into the statistical model, in addition to the random effect for patient. Singer (1995) provides examples, along with SAS code, for how this is done.

In the next section, we provide a technical description of the model that is typically assumed to underlie the Level 1 clustered data as we have described it here. This model is commonly referred to as the *one-way random effects model.*

*Technical Details of the Random Effects Model for Clustered Data** Let k denote the number of clusters, and assume that all of the clusters are of size n. (Thus, the total sample size in the study is given by $N = n \cdot k$.) The one-way random effects model for clustered data is then given by

$$Y_{ij} = \mu + b_i + \varepsilon_{ij}, i = 1, 2, \ldots, k;\ j = 1, 2, \ldots, n, \tag{4.87}$$

where Y_{ij} is the jth observation in the ith cluster,

μ is the grand mean,
b_i is a random cluster effect,
ε_{ij} is the within-cluster deviation from the cluster mean.

Note that b_i represents the unique effect due to being in cluster i.

Under the usual assumptions of the model in (4.87), for all $i = 1, 2, \ldots, k;\ j = 1, 2, \ldots, n, E(b_i) = E(\varepsilon_{ij}) = 0,\ \ V(b_i) = \sigma_b^2,\ \ V(\varepsilon_{ij}) = \sigma_\varepsilon^2$, ε_{ij} are independent, b_i and ε_{ij} are independent of each other. (Note that we are assuming that the cluster effects, b_i, constitute a random sample from a normal population of all possible such effects.) Then it follows that $E(Y_{ij}) = \mu$, $Var(Y_{ij}) = \sigma_y^2 = \sigma_b^2 + \sigma_\varepsilon^2$. Under these assumptions, $Cov(y_{ij}, y_{il}) = \sigma_b^2$ and $\rho_I = Corr(y_{ij}, y_{il}) = \frac{\sigma_b^2}{\sigma_b^2+\sigma_\varepsilon^2} = \frac{\sigma_b^2}{\sigma_y^2}$ for all $i = 1, 2, \ldots, k;\ j = 1, 2, \ldots, n;\ \ l = 1, 2, \ldots, n;\ \ j \neq l$. Thus, it can be seen that the intra-cluster correlation ρ_{I} is equal to the proportion of the total variability in Y that can be attributed to the variability between the clusters.

The sample estimate of the ICC is calculated using the following formula:

$$r_{\mathrm{I}} = \frac{\widehat{\sigma_b^2}}{\widehat{\sigma_b^2} + \widehat{\sigma_\varepsilon^2}}, \tag{4.88}$$

where $\widehat{\sigma_b^2}$ and $\widehat{\sigma_\varepsilon^2}$ are estimated variance components obtained by fitting a one-way random effects ANOVA model to the clustered data. If one or more grouping variables are present, these must also be taken into account when estimating the variance components. This is illustrated in Example 4.27.

Once the sample estimate of the ICC has been calculated using (4.88), the next step in the traditional approach to adjusting for the clustered nature of the data is to calculate the *variance inflation factor* (VIF). This is given by VIF $= [1 + (n-1)\rho_\text{I}]$ in the population and $\widehat{\text{VIF}} = [1 + (n-1)r_\text{I}]$ in the sample. As the name implies, the VIF is used to upwardly adjust (or "inflate") the variance estimate obtained when the clustering is ignored. The VIF can also be used to calculate the "effective sample size" that we referred to earlier: $N_\text{eff} = N/\widehat{\text{VIF}}$, where N is the total sample size in the study. (Note that if $r_\text{I} < 0$, $\widehat{\text{VIF}} < 1$ and $N_\text{eff} > N$.) Sometimes the VIF is referred to as the "Design Effect" (DEFF), and represents the relative efficiency of using a cluster randomized sample rather than a "unit" randomized sample, which is a term sometimes used to describe the usual process of randomly assigning units to treatments.

Because of its relationship to the variance (and hence the relationship of $\sqrt{\widehat{\text{VIF}}}$ to the standard error), the estimated VIF can also be used to adjust the value of the test statistic for certain hypothesis tests based on the clustered data. For example, if one wishes to compare the means of two groups in terms of a continuous outcome that is normally distributed, then the usual test statistic for the equal-variance t-test, ignoring the clustering, would be divided by $\sqrt{\widehat{\text{VIF}}}$. We would then say that the equal-variance t-test statistic has been "adjusted for clustering." For the chi-square test comparing two proportions, the usual χ^2 test statistic based on the data ignoring the clustering would be divided by $\widehat{\text{VIF}}$ in order to obtain the "clustering-adjusted χ^2 test statistic."

For example, consider the test statistic for the equal-variance t-test (Equation 3.11):

$$t_0 = \frac{\bar{x}_1 - \bar{x}_2}{s_\text{p}\sqrt{\frac{1}{N_1} + \frac{1}{N_2}}}, \tag{4.89}$$

where $\bar{x}_1$ and $\bar{x}_2$ are the sample means in the two groups, N_1 and N_2 are the sample sizes, and s_p^2 is the "pooled" sample standard variance:

$$s_\text{p}^2 = \frac{(N_1 - 1)s_1^2 + (N_2 - 1)s_2^2}{N_1 + N_2 - 2}. \tag{4.90}$$

(In this formula, s_1^2 and s_2^2 denote the sample variances for Groups 1 and 2, respectively.) The corresponding formula in the situation where the data from both Groups 1 and 2 are clustered is given by

$$t_{0\text{c}} = \frac{\bar{x}_1 - \bar{x}_2}{s_\text{p}\sqrt{\widehat{\text{VIF}}\left(\frac{1}{N_1} + \frac{1}{N_2}\right)}}. \tag{4.91}$$

Note that $t_{0c} = t_0/\sqrt{\widehat{\text{VIF}}}$. This is equivalent to "inflating" the pooled estimate of the population variance, s_p^2 in (4.90) by $\widehat{\text{VIF}}$:

$$t_{0c} = \frac{\bar{x}_1 - \bar{x}_2}{\sqrt{\left(\widehat{\text{VIF}} \cdot s_p^2\right)\left(\frac{1}{N_1} + \frac{1}{N_2}\right)}}. \tag{4.92}$$

If the sample sizes in the two groups are equal, $N_1 = N_2 = N$, the test statistic in (4.92) can also be obtained from the test statistic in (4.89) by dividing N by $\widehat{\text{VIF}}$:

$$t_{0c} = \frac{\bar{x}_1 - \bar{x}_2}{s_p\sqrt{\frac{2}{N/\widehat{\text{VIF}}}}}. \tag{4.93}$$

(Note also that there is also an "adjustment" to the degrees of freedom for the t-test: the df corresponding to the test statistic in (4.89) is $df_t = N_1 + N_2 - 2$, whereas the df for the test statistic in (4.91) is $df_{tc} = k_1 + k_2 - 2$, where k_1 and k_2 are the number of clusters in Groups 1 and 2, respectively. If the sample sizes in the two groups are equal, $N_1 = N_2 = N$, as in (4.93) and the clusters are all of the same size, n, then $k_1 = k_2 = k$; therefore, the degrees of freedom change from $df_t = N_1 + N_2 - 2 = 2(nk - 1)$ to $df_{tc} = 2(k - 1)$.)

Thus, the sample VIF can be used to "adjust" the usual equal-variance t-test by (1) dividing it into the usual t-test statistic, (2) multiplying it times the pooled estimate of the variance, or (3) in the case of equal sample sizes in the two group, dividing it into the common sample size. If VIF > 1 (which it will be in almost all cases), each of these "adjustments" has the net effect of reducing the magnitude of the t-test statistic which, along with the reduction in degrees of freedom, will increase the p-value, thereby making it less likely to reject the null hypothesis. A similar adjustment would be made if one were comparing $k > 2$ means, as in the ANOVA. In this case, MSE, the estimate of the error variance σ^2 in the ANOVA model (see Section 3.7.2) would be multiplied by VIF. (Note that if $r_I < 0$, then VIF < 1, which can lead to a smaller p-value and greater chance of rejecting H_0. One of us (SWL) has encountered this phenomenon more than once in a real-life data analysis problem.)

Example 4.27 Analysis of Clustered Biomarker Data—Comparison of Two Means

We illustrate the basic concepts of analyzing clustered data using a subset of the data from the study of PSP plates by Hunter et al. (2014) mentioned previously. First, we consider the comparison of the no rinse group with the Chlorhexidine oral rinse (CHX) group. For ease of illustration, we consider only those dental patients (28 in the CHX group and 35 in the no rinse group) who had bacterial colony data for all 4 PSP plates. (In other words, there was an equal cluster size of $n = 4$ with $k_1 = 28$ clusters in the CHX group and $k_2 = 35$ clusters in the no rinse group.) The mean

TABLE 4.32 Mean Number of Bacterial Colonies for Each of the 70 Patients (Based on $n = 4$ PSP Plates Per Patient Unless Otherwise Indicated)

CHX	0.00***,	1.00,	0.50,	10.75,	0.75,	26.75,	2.00,	0.50,	6.25,	0.25
($k_l = 30$)	0.50,	0.25,	0.25,	13.25,	0.50,	1.00,	1.00***,	0.75,	1.00,	1.50
	0.25,	0.75,	0.50,	2.00,	2.75,	1.50,	1.50,	4.50,	0.50,	1.25
No Rinse	2.25,	1.00***,	2.00,	1.25,	0.00,	0.00,	1.50,	0.75,	1.00,	0.00
($k_2 = 40$)	0.00,	2.33***,	0.00,	0.50,	12.75,	1.00,	2.25,	1.75,	4.25,	0.00
	20.50,	3.00,	34.25,	14.00,	1.50**,	6.00*,	5.50,	3.50,	0.75,	0.25
	2.75,	10.25,	27.00,	4.00**,	32.50,	40.50,	5.50,	5.00,	0.00,	6.75

*Only one PSP plate was available for this patient.
**Only two PSP plates were available for this patient.
***Only three PSP plates were available for this patient.
Source: Data courtesy of Dr. Allison Hunter Buchanan.

number of colonies per plate in the CHX group was $\bar{x}_1 = 2.97$ and, in the no rinse group, it was $\bar{x}_2 = 6.95$. (Note that the sample means are unaffected by the presence of clustering as long as the clusters are of equal size; in other words, we obtain the same results if we average the number of colonies for all 112 plates in the CHX group and all 140 plates in the no rinse group, or if we average the mean number of colonies for all 28 patients in the CHX group and for all 35 patients in the no rinse group. It is the standard error of the mean that is affected by the presence of clustering in the data.) Table 4.32 contains the mean number of colonies for each of the 70 patients in these two groups; those who had data for fewer than four PSP plates are marked with asterisks to indicate how many plates they had. The present analysis is based only on those patients in these two groups who had bacterial colony data for all four PSP plates.

If we ignore the fact that clustering was present in the data, we obtain $s_1^2 = 70.1164$ in the CHX group, and $s_2^2 = 282.4076$ in the no rinse group. Thus, the "pooled" sample standard deviation is given by

$$s_p = \sqrt{\frac{(N_1 - 1)s_1^2 + (N_2 - 1)s_2^2}{N_1 + N_2 - 2}}$$

$$= \sqrt{\frac{(112 - 1)(70.1164) + (140 - 1)(282.4076)}{112 + 140 - 2}} = 13.72.$$

This yields an equal-variance t-test statistic of

$$t_0 = \frac{\bar{x}_1 - \bar{x}_2}{s_p\sqrt{\frac{1}{N_1} + \frac{1}{N_2}}} = \frac{2.973 - 6.950}{13.717\sqrt{\frac{1}{112} + \frac{1}{140}}} = -2.286,$$

with $df_t = N_1 + N_2 - 2 = 112 + 140 - 2 = 250$. This yields a two-tailed p-value of 0.023, a significant result.

To account for the clustered nature of the data, we first calculate the sample estimate of the ICC:

$$r_{\mathrm{I}} = \frac{\widehat{\sigma_b^2}}{\widehat{\sigma_b^2} + \widehat{\sigma_\varepsilon^2}} = \frac{42.79915}{42.79915 + 146.3783} = 0.22624.$$

(Note that this indicates a rather high degree of clustering within the colony counts for the PSP plates (Adams et al. (2004).) This yields an estimated VIF of $\widehat{\mathrm{VIF}} = [1 + (n-1)r_I] = [1 + (4-1)(0.22624)] = 1.67872$ and a "cluster-adjusted" t-test statistic of

$$t_{0\mathrm{c}} = -2.286/\sqrt{1.67872} = -1.765, \tag{4.94}$$

with $df_{tc} = k_1 + k_2 - 2 = 28 + 35 - 2 = 61$. This yields a two-tailed p-value of 0.083, a non-significant result. Thus, properly adjusting for the clustered nature of the data changed the conclusion from statistical significance to non-significance.

It is important to note that identical results could be obtained by simply performing the usual equal-variance t-test on the 63 cluster means (i.e., the patient-level data) rather than the 252 values for the individual PSP plates. This is called a "cluster-level" analysis, whereas adjusting the analysis based on the individual PCPs using the VIF is called the "cluster-adjusted individual-level" analysis. If we apply the equal-variance t-test to the 63 cluster means of size 4 given in Table 4.32, we obtain the following "cluster-adjusted" pooled standard deviation:

$$s_{\mathrm{pc}} = \sqrt{\frac{(k_1 - 1)s_{1\mathrm{c}}^2 + (k_2 - 1)s_{2\mathrm{c}}^2}{k_1 + k_2 - 2}}$$
$$= \sqrt{\frac{(28-1)(31.4368) + (35-1)(117.4772)}{28 + 35 - 2}} = 8.91,$$

and the following adjusted t-test statistic:

$$t_{0\mathrm{c}} = \frac{\bar{x}_1 - \bar{x}_2}{s_{\mathrm{pc}}\sqrt{\frac{1}{k_1} + \frac{1}{k_2}}} = \frac{2.973 - 6.950}{8.910\sqrt{\frac{1}{28} + \frac{1}{35}}} = -1.762,$$

which differs from the test statistic of $t_0 = -1.767$ that we obtained in the individual-level analysis (Equation 4.94) only in the third decimal place. This discrepancy is due to round-off error in the intermediate results used in the above calculations.

The SAS code used to perform the adjusted individual-level analysis for Example 4.27 using the MIXED procedure is given below and on the companion website. Note that in the DATA step, the data are structured so that the patient identifier is repeated for each PSP plate. In this way, SAS recognizes that the bacterial colony counts for the PSP plates are nested within patients.

```
/*    Input original data      */

data colonies;
input patient group $ plate colonies;
datalines;
31     no_rinse     1     0
31     no_rinse     2     1
31     no_rinse     3     0
31     no_rinse     4     8
32     no_rinse     1     2
32     no_rinse     2     1
32     no_rinse     3     0
32     no_rinse     4     .
...
;

/*   Perform individual level analysis adjusted for
clustering    */

proc mixed data=colonies method=reml ;
     where group='no_rinse' or group='CHX';
     class patient group;
     model colonies=group / solution DDFM=SATTERTHWAITE ;
     random intercept / subject=patient;
     title1 'Mixed Model Analysis';
     title2 'Patients Treated as Clusters';
     run;
```

The following SAS code can be used to calculate the variance components needed to calculate r_{I}, the estimated intra-cluster correlation. It is important to note that, for this calculation, patients must be treated as a nested factor within group.

```
/*     Calculate variance components needed to
estimate the ICC.   */

proc varcomp method=reml data=colonies;
     class patient group;
     model colonies=patient(group) group;
     title1 'Variance Components Needed to Calculate ICC';
     run;
```

The relevant SAS output is as follows:

```
Variance Component        Estimate
Var(Patient(group))       42.79915
```

```
Var(group)          5.35547
Var(Error)        146.37831
```

Thus, as indicated previously, $r_{\mathrm{I}} = \frac{\widehat{\sigma_b^2}}{\widehat{\sigma_b^2}+\widehat{\sigma_\varepsilon^2}} = \frac{42.79915}{42.79915+146.37831} = 0.22624$, which is then used to calculate $\widehat{\mathrm{VIF}}$, the estimated VIF:

$$\widehat{\mathrm{VIF}} = [1 + (n-1)r_{\mathrm{I}}] = [1 + (4-1)(0.22624)] = 1.67872.$$

While $\widehat{\mathrm{VIF}}$ is not needed to perform the adjusted individual-level analysis (since the adjustment is taken care of by using the MIXED procedure), it is useful to know the extent to which the clustering inflated the usual estimate of the standard error.

The SAS code used to perform the cluster-level analysis for Example 4.27 is given below and on the companion website. Note that a new SAS data set must be created that contains the means for each cluster (patient). These cluster means are then analyzed as if they were the original data. They are given in Tables 4.32 and 4.33.

```
/*   Create SAS data set containing cluster means      */

proc sort data=colonies;
     by group patient;

proc means data=colonies mean ;
     by group patient;
     var colonies;
     output  out=patient_means
             mean=colonies_mean
     run;

/*
     Perform cluster-level analysis.  This analysis is
     exact only if all clusters are of equal size.
*/

proc ttest data=patient_means;
     where group='no_rinse' or group='CHX';
     class group;
     var colonies_mean;
     title1 'Cluster-Level Analysis';
     title2 't-test';
     run;
```

As long as the cluster sizes are all equal, clustering can be accounted for simply by applying the "usual" analysis to the cluster means; that is, by treating them as if they were the sample data. This approach works for any number of groups. Thus, the original goal of the Hunter et al. study, which was to compare the mean number of colonies of bacteria per PSP plate among the patients who rinsed with Listerine®, Decapinol®, or Chlorhexidine with those in the no rinse group, could be carried out by applying a one-way ANOVA to the cluster means for the four groups, as long as every patient has complete data (i.e., bacterial colony counts for all four PSP plates). This is illustrated in Example 4.28.

If the cluster sizes are not all equal (as in the original data for the Hunter et al. study), the cluster-level analysis is only approximate, but will be very similar to the exact adjusted individual-level analysis as long as the cluster sizes are not widely discrepant. In this case, the sample VIF can be approximated by $\widehat{\text{VIF}} = [1 + (\bar{n} - 1)r_I]$, where $\bar{n}$ = average cluster size across all k clusters.

In the Hunter et al. study, 2 of the 30 patients in the CHX group had bacterial colony counts for 3 of the 4 PSP plates, while 2 of the 40 patients in the no rinse group had bacterial colony counts for 3 of the 4 plates, 2 had counts for 2 of the 4 plates, and 1 had counts for only 1 PSP plate. (This accounts for the cluster sample sizes of $k_1 = 28$ in the CHX group and $k_2 = 35$ in the no rinse group when we considered only those clusters of size 4 in Example 4.27.) Averaging the cluster sizes in the two treatment groups yields average cluster sizes of 3.93 in the CHX group and 3.78 in the no rinse group. Thus, one would expect very little discrepancy between the results for the approximate cluster-level analysis (an equal-variance t-test on the cluster means from the 2 groups) vs. the exact individual-level analysis based on using the MIXED procedure in SAS to perform a mixed-effects model analysis to account for the clustering. To illustrate this point, we now consider the entire sample of $k_1 = 30$ patients in the CHX group and $k_2 = 40$ patients in the no rinse group. The sample means and variances in the two groups are $\bar{x}_1 = 2.81$, $\bar{x}_2 = 6.45$ and $s_1^2 = 29.6797$, $s_2^2 = 104.6239$, respectively. If we perform the approximate cluster-level t-test, we obtain $t_{0c} = 1.770$, $df_c = 68$, p-value $= 0.0812$. Using the MIXED procedure in SAS, the exact individual-level analysis, adjusted for clustering, yields $t_{0I} = 1.773$, $df_I = 69.1$, p-value $= 0.0807$. Note that there is very little difference between the two sets of results. This can be attributed to the very slight difference in the average cluster sizes in the two groups: $\bar{n}_1 = 3.93$ in the CHX group vs. $\bar{n}_2 = 3.78$ in the no rinse group. Note that, if clustering is ignored, we have $n_1 = 118$, $n_2 = 151$, $\bar{x}_1 = 2.85$, $\bar{x}_2 = 6.62$ and $s_1^2 = 66.8830$, and $s_2^2 = 263.5557$. If we perform the individual-level t-test without adjusting for clustering, we obtain $t_0 = 2.31$, $df = 267$, p-value $= 0.023$. Note that the "mean of the cluster means" is no longer equal to the sample mean in each group when clustering is ignored: 2.81 vs. 2.85 in the CHX group, and 6.45 vs. 6.62 in the no rinse group.

As experienced SAS users will know, for any analysis in which the MIXED procedure is used, the descriptive statistics that should be reported are the "least squares (LS) means" with accompanying standard errors: $\bar{x}_{1LS} = 2.83$, $\bar{x}_{2LS} = 6.55$ and $SE_{1LS} = 1.58$, $SE_{2LS} = 1.39$. These LS means (and corresponding SEs) take into account the hierarchical nature of the data, as well as the unequal cluster sizes.

The equivalence between the exact adjusted individual-level analysis and the cluster-level analysis when the cluster sizes are all equal does not apply when the outcome variable is dichotomous, as would be the case when comparing proportions between two or more groups. In the Hunter et al. study, the investigators were also interested in comparing the four treatment groups in terms of the proportion of PSP plates with at least one bacterial colony. The GLIMMIX procedure in SAS would be appropriate for performing the exact cluster-adjusted individual-level analysis; the outcome of this analysis would be a "cluster-adjusted" chi-square test, just as the application of the MIXED procedure to clustered normally distributed data yields a "cluster-adjusted" t-test in the case of two groups, or a "cluster-adjusted" one-way ANOVA F-test in the case of more than two groups. The cluster-adjusted F-test is illustrated below.

Example 4.28 Analysis of Clustered Biomarker Data—Comparison of More Than Two Means

Returning to the study of the effectiveness of antimicrobial mouthrinses in reducing microbial growth on PSP plates used in making dental x-rays, we now consider all four treatment groups: those who rinsed with either Listerine®, Decapinol®, or Chlorhexidine, plus those who did not rinse. The bacterial colony data for the Listerine® and Decapinol® groups are given in Table 4.33.

As can be seen from Table 4.33, among the patients who rinsed with Listerine®, 2 of the 30 patients had bacterial colony counts for 3 of the 4 PSP plates, and 1 had counts for only 1 of the 4 PSP plates; among those who rinsed with Decapinol®, 2 of the 30 patients had bacterial colony counts for 3 of the 4 plates, and 1 had counts for 2 of the 4 plates. This yields average cluster sizes of 3.83 in the Listerine® group, 3.87 in the Decapinol® group; the average cluster sizes were 3.93 in the CHX group and 3.78 in the no rinse group, as mentioned previously. Thus, one would expect very little discrepancy in the results for the approximate cluster-level analysis (a one-

TABLE 4.33 Mean Number of Bacterial Colonies for Each of the 60 Patients (Based on $n = 4$ PSP Plates Per Patient Unless Otherwise Indicated)

Listerine®	3.00,	8.00,	1.00,	4.33,	4.00***,	7.75,	2.25,	11.00,	0.50,	12.00
($k_3 = 30$)	4.00***,	1.50,	13.00,	7.75,	6.00,	2.25,	4.25,	8.00*,	0.00,	5.50
	4.00,	28.5,	2.25,	22.25,	2.75,	1.50,	3.25,	1.25,	1.00,	0.75
Decapinol®	11.25,	4.75,	3.00,	4.25,	1.50,	3.50,	2.75,	0.50,	1.00,	0.00
($k_4 = 30$)	7.75,	7 .00,	2.25,	2.00,	0.33***,	2.50,	15.25,	7.00,	1.00,	9.33***
	0.00**,	0.50,	0.25,	1.50,	6.25,	1.50,	6.00,	2.50,	3.25,	2.00

*Only one PSP plate was available for this patient.
**Only two PSP plates were available for this patient.
***Only three PSP plates were available for this patient.
Source: Data courtesy of Dr. Allison Hunter Buchanan.

way ANOVA on the cluster means from the four groups) when compared with the exact cluster-adjusted individual-level analysis based on using the MIXED procedure in SAS.

Using the data in Table 4.33, the sample means and variances in the Listerine® and Decapinol® groups were $\bar{x}_3 = 5.79$, $\bar{x}_4 = 3.69$ and $s_3^2 = 40.9429$, $s_4^2 = 13.3141$, respectively. If we perform the approximate cluster-level ANOVA F-test by treating the cluster means as if they were the original data, we obtain $F_{0c} = 1.898$, $df_{c1} = 3$, $df_{c2} = 126$, p-value $= 0.1334$. Using the MIXED procedure in SAS, the exact individual-level analysis, adjusted for clustering, yields $F_{0I} = 1.868$, $df_{I1} = 3$, $df_{I2} = 128$, p-value $= 0.1382$. (Note the difference in degrees of freedom for the exact analysis.) As can be clearly seen, there is very little difference between the results of the two analyses. This can be attributed to the fact that only 13 of the 130 clusters had cluster sizes different from 4, yielding average cluster sizes in the 4 groups of $\bar{n}_1 = 3.93$, $\bar{n}_2 = 3.78$, $\bar{n}_3 = 3.83$, $\bar{n}_4 = 3.87$. If we ignore clustering, we have $n_1 = 118$, $n_2 = 151$, $n_3 = 115$, $n_4 = 116$; $\bar{x}_1 = 2.85$, $\bar{x}_2 = 6.62$, $\bar{x}_3 = 5.76$, $\bar{x}_4 = 3.73$; $s_1^2 = 66.8830$, $s_2^2 = 263.5557$, and $s_3^2 = 116.4841$, $s_4^2 = 53.2410$. The individual-level F-test (with no adjustment for clustering) yields $F_0 = 2.94$, $df_{c1} = 3$, $df_{c2} = 496$, p-value $= 0.0328$. As we saw when we compared the CHX and no rinse groups in Example 4.27, adjusting for clustering leads to a non-significant result, whereas failure to do so yields a statistically significant, but incorrect, result.

SAS code that can be used to perform the adjusted individual-level analyses and the cluster-level analysis for the data in all the four rinse groups is given below and on the companion website. Note that we have used the T-K method to perform pairwise comparisons among the four groups. The MIXED procedure in SAS adjusts these comparisons for the effects of clustering.

```
/*   Perform individual level analysis adjusted for
clustering    */

proc mixed data = colonies method = reml ;
     class patient group;
     model colonies = group / solution ddfm = satterthwaite ;
     random intercept / subject = patient;
     lsmeans group / pdiff adjust = tukey;
     title1 'Mixed Model Analysis';
     title2 'Patients Treated as Clusters';
     run;

/*
     Perform cluster-level analysis. This analysis is
     exact only if each cluster is of equal size.
*/
```

```
proc GLM data=patient_means;
     class group;
     MODEL colonies_mean=GROUP / SS3;
     lsmeans group / pdiff  adjust=tukey;
     title1 'Cluster-Level Analysis';
     title2 '1-way ANOVA';
     run;
```

An issue that we did not address in Example 4.28 is the underlying assumption of normality. The cluster-adjusted individual-level analysis (carried out using PROC MIXED) is based on the assumption that the bacterial colony counts on each plate are normally distributed. Similarly, the cluster-level analysis based on performing a one-way ANOVA on the cluster means (carried out using PROC GLM) is based on the assumption that the mean number of colonies per plate for each patient are normally distributed. However, there is rather strong evidence that these normality assumptions are not supported by the data. In fact, for the cluster means (i.e., the mean number of colonies per plate for each patient), normality is strongly rejected, with $p < 0.001$ using the S-W test in each treatment group. This raises the question of what is the appropriate analysis to perform? One approach would be to perform an adjusted individual-level analysis using a generalized linear mixed model (GLMM) to account for the non-normality of the data. Since the bacterial colony data are given as counts, a reasonable approach would be to use Poisson regression (adjusted for clustering) using the GLIMMIX procedure in SAS (Myers et al. 2010, pp. 369–384). Such an analysis is beyond the scope of this text and, as we pointed out earlier in this section when discussing the use of mixed-effects models in general, one should not undertake an analysis as complex as this unless one has a thorough understanding of GLMMs and experience working with the GLIMMIX procedure.

Since there was not a high degree of variation in the number of PSP plates per patient (i.e., the cluster sizes), a reasonable approximate cluster-level analysis would be to use the distribution-free K-W test (Section 4.2.3.3) to compare the four treatment groups, treating the cluster means as if they were the original data (Donner and Klar 2010, p. 114). If the null hypothesis of no difference among the four groups is rejected, then the Dunn method (Section 4.2.3.3) could be used to identify any significant pairwise differences among the treatment groups. If we apply the K-W test to the cluster means in Tables 4.32 and 4.33, we obtain $\chi_0^2 = 11.81$, $df = 3$, approximate p-value $= 0.0081$. Using the SAS code for performing Dunn's method that we provided with Example 4.10 to analyze the ranks of the cluster means (obtained using the RANK procedure in SAS), we obtain a significant Bonferroni-adjusted p-value for one of the six pairwise comparisons: Listerine® verus CHX: $z_0 = 3.39$, Bonferroni-adjusted Dunn p-value $= 0.004$. Thus, as we have demonstrated elsewhere, contrary to popular belief, the distribution-free method was able to identify a significant difference among the groups, whereas the normal-theory method was not.

4.7 OUTLIERS

4.7.1 The Effects of Outliers

It is often the case that routine examination of a set of biomarker data leads to the discovery of one or more observations that are somehow "removed" from the remaining observations. Usually, an observation is singled out because it is either much larger or much smaller than the remaining observations. In other words, it is *discordant* relative to the other data values in the sample. In statistics, discordant observations are commonly referred to as *outliers*. The presence of outliers in a set of data can have extremely adverse effects on the analysis of those data, leading to invalid point estimates of unknown parameters, distorted estimates of standard errors, inaccurate confidence limits, and incorrect conclusions based on faulty hypothesis tests. Healy (1968) goes so far as to say that rejection of the assumption of normality for a set of data can almost always be attributed to the presence of outliers. Thus, it is important to correctly identify observations that are truly discordant from the remainder of the sample, and then decide on a proper course of action to take with regard to the offending observation; should it be removed from the sample of data and eliminated from further consideration in the statistical analysis, or accommodated in some way so that it remains in the analytic data set, but its adverse effects on the results of the statistical analysis are minimized.

Generally speaking, it is not appropriate to simply remove one or more observations from the analysis simply because they are extreme in some sense. Nor is it considered proper statistical practice to arbitrarily replace apparently extreme values with more representative ones. An example of a biomarker study in which both courses of action were taken can be found in Delfino et al. (2009). In their examination of the association of traffic-related air pollutants with air-pollutant-related increases in systemic inflammation, the authors removed or replaced several outlying values as part of their statistical analysis without appropriate justification: "Four influential high outliers for IL-6 $>$ 10 pg/mL were reset to 10 pg/mL, and one extreme influential outlier for sP-selectin (221 ng/mL) was removed to obtain more representative estimates of association. Residuals for both CRP and TNF-α exhibited a highly skewed distribution, primarily due to a cluster of subjects in the upper quartile of biomarker concentrations, and 2–3 high outliers >3 SD above the mean. Outliers were reset to the next highest values, and secondary subgroup analyses were conducted among subjects in the upper quartile of mean CRP vs. the lower three quartiles" (p. 1234).

In the remainder of this section, we first describe some generally preferred statistical methods for identifying discordant observations in a set of data, and then briefly discuss some methods that can be used to accommodate such observations in a statistical analysis. An in-depth treatment of outlier analysis is beyond the scope of this text; for a thorough discussion, see Barnett and Lewis (1995).

4.7.2 Detection of Outliers

There is no commonly accepted method for detecting outliers in a set of data. Statistical methods for detecting outliers date back at least as far as Chauvenet (1863), who proposed a very simple method. To apply Chauvenet's criterion, the sample mean and standard deviation are computed for the observed data and then the normal cdf is used to calculate the probability of observing a value at least as far from the sample mean as the data point that is farthest, in absolute value, from the mean. The observation is considered to be an outlier if this probability is less than $1/(2n)$, in which case the analyst is instructed to remove the observation and begin the process again by computing the new sample mean and standard deviation using the sample data with the apparent outlier eliminated. As Chauvenet's method is usually applied, the process continues until all outliers have been removed from the sample and none of the remaining observations meet Chauvenet's outlier criterion. However, we do not advise the data analyst to automatically remove an observation simply because it is deemed to be an outlier. Further scrutiny is needed after identifying an extreme observation. First, the analyst should investigate the possibility of a data entry or measurement error. If such causes are ruled out, further inquiry should be made into possible explanations for the unusual value. An observation should be removed from a data set only for a legitimate scientific reason.

Chauvenet's criterion is interesting from an historical point of view, but we do not recommend it when attempting to identify possible discordant observations (see Barnett and Lewis 1995, pp. 28–29). Nor do we recommend the most commonly used method, which is to convert the offending observation to a "z-score"; in other words, to determine how far away the observation is from the sample mean in terms of the sample standard deviation. The apparently discordant observation is then declared to be an outlier if this z-score is greater than some arbitrary cutoff value of 3 or 4. To be more specific, let x^* denote the potentially discordant observation, and let $\bar{x}$ and s denote the mean and standard deviation, respectively, of the entire sample. Let $z^* = \frac{|x^* - \bar{x}|}{s}$ denote the absolute number of standard deviations that x^* is removed from $\bar{x}$. The way in which this *ad hoc* method is usually applied is to declare the offending observation to be an outlier if $z^* > 3$, although other cutpoints have been used. In their study of the traffic-related air pollutants cited earlier, Delfino et al. (2009) identified "2–3 high outliers >3 SD above the mean," which the authors then "reset to the next highest values." However, since the sample mean and sample standard deviation are both calculated using all of the sample data; the "z-score method" cannot be recommended, given how sensitive both the mean and standard deviation are to extreme observations (Wilcox 2012, p. 96). Furthermore, if we let $x_{(n)}$ denote the sample maximum, it can be shown that, for any sample of size n, $z^* = \frac{|x_{(n)} - \bar{x}|}{s}$ can be no larger than $\frac{n-1}{\sqrt{n}}$ (Shiffler 1988, p. 79). (For example, if $n = 9$, the largest value that z* can have is $8/3 = 2.67$. Thus, if one uses the "3 SD Rule" with a sample of size 9, no observation would ever be declared to be discordant, no matter how large.) For further discussion, see Barnett and Lewis (1995, p. 223).

The method that we recommend for identifying possible discordant observations in a sample of normally distributed data is the more sophisticated method proposed by Grubbs (1950). He developed a technique for testing the null hypothesis that the largest or smallest observation in the sample came from the same normally distributed population as the other observations. Let $x_{(i)}$ denote the ith order statistic; in other words, the sample observations have been reordered so that $x_{(1)} \leq x_{(2)} \leq \ldots \leq x_{(n)}$. For the largest observation in the set of data, the Grubbs test statistic is given by

$$\frac{S_n^2}{S^2} = \frac{\sum_{i=1}^{n-1} \left(x_{(i)} - \bar{x}_{(n)}\right)^2}{\sum_{i=1}^{n} \left(x_{(i)} - \bar{x}\right)^2}, \tag{4.95}$$

where $\bar{x}_{(n)} = \left(\sum_{i=1}^{n-1} x_{(i)}\right)/(n-1)$ is the mean of the $n-1$ smallest observations, and $\bar{x}$ is the sample mean of the entire sample $\{x_1, x_2, \ldots, x_n\}$. A similar test statistic for the smallest observation is given by

$$\frac{S_1^2}{S^2} = \frac{\sum_{i=2}^{n} \left(x_{(i)} - \bar{x}_{(1)}\right)^2}{\sum_{i=1}^{n} \left(x_{(i)} - \bar{x}\right)^2}, \tag{4.96}$$

where $\bar{x}_{(1)} = \left(\sum_{i=2}^{n} x_{(i)}\right)/(n-1)$ is the mean of the $n-1$ largest observations. An equivalent way to test whether the observation in question is discordant is to compute the following test-statistic if the observation is the largest in the sample:

$$T_n = \frac{x_{(n)} - \bar{x}}{s}. \tag{4.97}$$

If the apparently outlying observation is the smallest in the sample the test-statistic is given by

$$T_1 = \frac{\bar{x} - x_{(1)}}{s}. \tag{4.98}$$

Grubbs and Beck (1972, pp. 848–850, Table I) provided a table of percentage points for T_1 or T_n that specifies critical values for samples of size 3–147. An abbreviated version of this table ($n = 3(1)50$) is provided in Table 4.34. SAS code that can be used to apply Grubbs test is provided following Example 4.29. The "grubbs.test" function in the "outliers" library in R Version 3.0.1 can also be used to apply Grubbs' test for outliers to any sample of data, as illustrated below for the data in Example 4.29.

The Grubbs test for outliers is based on the assumption that the sample data came from a normally distributed population. Before applying this test, we advise the analyst to test the assumption of normality, as described in Section 4.2.2. If the data are not normally distributed, it may be possible to find a suitable transformation that renders the transformed data approximately normally distributed (See Section 4.2.3.1). The Grubbs test could then be applied to the transformed data.

Alternatively, the Tukey method for identifying outliers (Tukey 1977), which makes no distributional assumptions, can be used. First, the inter-quartile range (IQR), given by the difference between the 75th and 25th percentile, is calculated.

TABLE 4.34 Critical Values of T_1 or T_n for One-Sided Grubbs Test for Outliers

n	$T_{0.001}$	$T_{0.005}$	$T_{0.01}$	$T_{0.025}$	$T_{0.05}$	$T_{0.100}$
3	1.155	1.155	1.155	1.155	1.153	1.148
4	1.499	1.496	1.492	1.481	1.463	1.425
5	1.780	1.764	1.749	1.715	1.672	1.602
6	2.011	1.973	1.944	1.887	1.822	1.729
7	2.201	2.139	2.097	2.020	1.938	1.828
8	2.358	2.274	2.221	2.126	2.032	1.909
9	2.492	2.387	2.323	2.215	2.110	1.977
10	2.606	2.482	2.410	2.290	2.176	2.036
11	2.705	2.564	2.485	2.355	2.234	2.088
12	2.791	2.636	2.550	2.412	2.285	2.134
13	2.867	2.699	2.607	2.462	2.331	2.175
14	2.935	2.755	2.659	2.507	2.371	2.213
15	2.997	2.806	2.705	2.549	2.409	2.247
16	3.052	2.852	2.747	2.585	2.443	2.279
17	3.103	2.894	2.785	2.620	2.475	2.309
18	3.149	2.932	2.821	2.651	2.504	2.335
19	3.191	2.968	2.854	2.681	2.532	2.361
20	3.230	3.001	2.884	2.709	2.557	2.385
21	3.266	3.031	2.912	2.733	2.580	2.408
22	3.300	3.060	2.939	2.758	2.603	2.429
23	3.332	3.087	2.963	2.781	2.624	2.448
24	3.362	3.112	2.987	2.802	2.644	2.467
25	3.389	3.135	3.009	2.822	2.663	2.486
26	3.415	3.157	3.029	2.841	2.681	2.502
27	3.440	3.178	3.049	2.859	2.698	2.519
28	3.464	3.199	3.068	2.876	2.714	2.534
29	3.486	3.218	3.085	2.893	2.730	2.549
30	3.507	3.236	3.103	2.908	2.745	2.563
31	3.528	3.253	3.119	2.924	2.759	2.577
32	3.546	3.270	3.135	2.938	2.773	2.591
33	3.565	3.286	3.150	2.952	2.786	2.604
34	3.582	3.301	3.164	2.965	2.799	2.616
35	3.599	3.316	3.178	2.979	2.811	2.628
36	3.616	3.330	3.191	2.991	2.823	2.639
37	3.631	3.343	3.204	3.003	2.835	2.650
38	3.646	3.356	3.216	3.014	2.846	2.661
39	3.660	3.369	3.228	3.025	2.857	2.671
40	3.673	3.381	3.240	3.036	2.866	2.682
41	3.687	3.393	3.251	3.046	2.877	2.692
42	3.700	3.404	3.261	3.057	2.887	2.700
43	3.712	3.415	3.271	3.067	2.896	2.710
44	3.724	3.425	3.282	3.075	2.905	2.719
45	3.736	3.435	3.292	3.085	2.914	2.727
46	3.747	3.445	3.302	3.094	2.923	2.736
47	3.757	3.455	3.310	3.103	2.931	2.744
48	3.768	3.464	3.319	3.111	2.940	2.753
49	3.779	3.474	3.329	3.120	2.948	2.760
50	3.789	3.483	3.336	3.128	2.956	2.768

Source: Adapted from Table I of Grubbs and Beck (1972) Reprinted with permission of Taylor & Francis LLC.

TABLE 4.35 sTNF RII Levels (pg/mL) in Peripheral Blood Mononuclear Cells of the Patient's Father and Five Healthy Controls

Subject	sTNF RII
Father	1051
Control No. 1	1244
Control No. 2	1253
Control No. 3	1257
Control No. 4	1186
Control No. 5	1202

Source: Data courtesy of Dr. Luis Espinoza.

Then the "inner fences," given by the 25th percentile minus 1.5 times the IQR and the 75th percentile plus 1.5 times the IQR, are computed. Similarly, the "outer fences," given by the 25th percentile minus 3 times the IQR and the 75th percentile plus 3 times the IQR, are calculated. An observation is considered to be an "outlier" if the value falls between the inner fences and the outer fences. The observation is considered an "extreme outlier" if the value falls beyond the outer fences. The Tukey method is illustrated in Example 4.30. SAS code that can be used to apply this method is provided following the example.

Example 4.29 Grubbs Test for Outliers

Lata et al. (2010b) examined gene expression and serologic regulatory biomarkers of bone turnover in the parents of a patient with idiopathic juvenile osteoporosis. The comparison of soluble tissue necrosis factor type II (sTNF RII) expression in peripheral blood mononuclear cells of the patient's father vs. five healthy controls between 25 and 35 years of age was considered (Table 4.35).

First, the null hypothesis that the sTNF RII levels for the five healthy controls were sampled from a normally distributed population was tested using the S-W test, as described in Section 4.2.2.3. This was accomplished via the "shapiro.test" function available within the "stats" package in R Version 3.0.1, as shown below using the sTNF RII levels for the five controls:

```
shapiro.test(c(1244, 1253, 1257, 1186, 1202))
```

The null hypothesis of normality was not rejected ($W_0 = 0.85$, $p = 0.197$) so the "grubbs.test" function from the "outliers" package in R was used to apply the Grubbs test to determine whether or not the sTNF RII level of the father (1051 pg/mL) came from the same normally distributed population as the controls:

```
grubbs.test(c(1051,1244, 1253, 1257, 1186, 1202))
```

The R output indicates that the smallest value of 1051 (i.e., the father's sTNF RII level) is found to be a low outlier: $T_1 = 1.896$, $p = 0.022$. Thus, there is statistical evidence that the father's sTNF RII level is not from the same population as the controls.

Note that by default, the "grubbs.test" function performs a one-sided test on the observation with the largest absolute difference from the mean, but this function is also capable of performing a one-sided test on the most extreme observation in the opposite direction (by specifying "opposite = TRUE" in the R function) or performing a two-sided test (by specifying "two.sided = TRUE"). The "grubbs.test" function can also test for two outliers, either in the same tail or opposite tails. See R help ("?grubbs.test") for details.

The SAS code given below (and also on the companion website) can be used to perform the Grubbs test for the data in Table 4.35. Note that this SAS code implements the equivalent version of the Grubbs test in which the test statistic is transformed into a t-value. It was adapted from Solak (2009) and is presented here with the author's permission.

```
title 'Grubbs Test for Outliers';

%let num=6;
%let ds=grubbs_critval;

%macro grubbs_crit (alpha=0.05, num=, ds=);
data &ds;
t2=tinv(&alpha/(2*&num), (&num-2));
gcrit=((&num- 1) /sqrt (&num)) * sqrt ((t2 * t2) / (&num - 2 +
(t2*t2)));
run;

%mend grubbs_crit;

%grubbs_crit (num=&num, ds=&ds);

data Lata;
input TNF;
datalines;
1051
1244
1253
1257
1186
1202
;

data Lata;
   set Lata;
   TNF_orig=TNF;

proc standard data=Lata mean=0 std=1 out=z_scores;
   var TNF;
   run;
```

```
data z_scores;
   set z_scores;
   g = abs(TNF);
   TNF = TNF_orig;

proc sort data = z_scores ;
   by descending g;

data grubbs;
     merge z_scores Grubbs_critval;
     retain g_crit;
     if _n_ = 1 then do;
     g_crit = gcrit;
     end;
     drop gcrit t2 TNF_orig;
     if g > g_crit then outlier = '*';
     run;

proc print data = grubbs;
     run;
```

Example 4.30 Tukey's Test for Outliers

Lata et al. (2010a) studied bone turnover in spondyloarthropathies (SpA) patients. The serum level of the inflammatory biomarker leptin in a newly diagnosed and untreated SpA patient was compared with the leptin levels of SpA patients treated with disease modifying anti-rheumatic drugs (DMARD) (Table 4.36). The S-W test indicated a significant departure from normality for leptin levels among the six patients treated with DMARD ($W_0 = 0.77$, $p = 0.033$). Thus, the Grubbs test is not appropriate for determining if the leptin level of the untreated patient is discordant with respect to

TABLE 4.36 Leptin Levels (pg/mL) of Six SpA Patients Treated with DMARD and One SpA Patient Naïve to Treatment

Treatment	Leptin
Naïve	3728
DMARD No. 1	4241
DMARD No. 2	6757
DMARD No. 3	17945
DMARD No. 4	4267
DMARD No. 5	5588
DMARD No. 6	8936

Source: Data courtesy of Dr. Luis Espinoza.

the patients treated with DMARD. We recommend that Tukey's (1977) method be used instead.

The 25th and 75th percentiles for the leptin levels of the six patients treated with DMARD are 4241 and 8936, respectively, with an IQR of 4695. Thus, the boundaries for Tukey's inner fence are given by 4241 − 1.5(4695) = −2801.5 pg/mL and 8936 + 1.5(4695) = 15,978.5 pg/mL. Since the leptin level of the treatment-naïve patient (3728 pg/mL) falls within Tukey's inner fence, the value is not considered an outlier. The value for "DMARD #3," 17,945 pg/mL, was also thought to be a possible outlier among the patients treated with DMARD, so Tukey's test was applied to the five remaining DMARD values. (The inner fences based on these five observations are the same as before.) Since 17,945 pg/mL is outside the inner fence, it would be considered to be a possible outlying observation. (Note that the boundaries for the outer fence are −9844 to 23,021, so 17945 would not be considered to be an "extreme" outlier.) Perhaps the individual labeled "DMARD No. 3" had much greater severity of SpA than the other patients in the study, or was not responding well to treatment with DMARD. The following SAS code (also provided on the companion website) can be used to perform Tukey's test for outliers for the data in Table 4.36 after removing the treatment-naïve patient.

```
title1 'Tukey''s Test for Outliers';

%let dsn = Lata;
%let var = leptin;

data Lata;
input leptin;
datalines;
4241
6757
17945
4267
5588
8936
;

proc univariate data=&dsn noprint;
var &var;
output out=qdata q1=q1 q3=q3 qrange=iqr;
run;

data _null_; set qdata;
call symput("q1",q1); call symput("q3",q3); call symput("iqr",iqr);
run;

* save the outliers;
```

```
data outliers;
set &dsn; length severity $2;
severity=" ";
y=&var;
inner_fence_l=(&q1 - 1.5*&iqr);
inner_fence_r=(&q3 + 1.5*&iqr);
outer_fence_l=(&q1 - 3*&iqr);
outer_fence_r=(&q3 + 3*&iqr);
if (y<= inner_fence_l) or (y>= inner_fence_r) then severity="*";
if (y<= outer_fence_l) or (y>= outer_fence_r) then severity="**";
if severity in ("*", "**") then output outliers;
run;

proc print data=qdata;
var q1 q3 iqr;
title2 '1st and 3rd Quantiles and IQR';
run;

proc print data=outliers;
var inner_fence_l inner_fence_r outer_fence_l outer_fence_r;
title2 'Inner and Outer Fences';
run;

proc print data=outliers;
var &var severity;
title2 'Potential Outliers';
run;
```

4.7.3 Methods for Accommodating Outliers

Generally speaking, it is not appropriate to simply discard an apparent outlying observation, even if a formal test for outliers indicates that it is, in fact, discordant from the remaining observations. Once an outlier has been identified, every possible effort must be made to determine if the apparent "error" in the observed value could possibly be explained by an "assignable cause" such as a faulty or miscalibrated instrument used to obtain the data value, a data recording error when the data were transcribed from one source to another, a data entry error when the data were entered into the computer, etc. If one of these "assignable causes" can be identified, then the errant observation should be corrected and all statistical analyses repeated with the corrected data. "Contamination" can also result in discordant observations. For example, suppose that only female subjects were eligible for inclusion in a clinical study that made use of one or more biomarkers. It may be that, due to human error, a male was erroneously admitted to the study and the biomarker data for this one subject was mistakenly combined with the data for the remaining $n - 1$ female subjects. Obviously, it would be appropriate to remove the male subject from further study, and reanalyze only those data for the female subjects.

In Section 4.7.1, we described the study by Delfino et al. (2009), in which several outlying observations were either removed from further analysis or "reset to the next highest value" as part of their examination of the association of traffic-related air pollutants with air-pollutant-related increases in systemic inflammation. Replacing extreme observations with the next highest values has a long history, dating back to at least the 1950s. The term *Winsorization* is used to refer to the process of replacing the largest observation with the next highest value, and replacing the smallest observation with the next smallest. *Trimming* refers to simply ignoring the highest and lowest observations. Note that both of these operations are performed in a symmetric manner; that is, the largest value *and* the smallest value are dealt with simultaneously. (Note that Delfino et al. did *not* deal with their apparent outliers in a symmetric manner.) If either of these methods is used, adjustments must be made to the standard error of whatever is being estimated (mean, CC, regression coefficient, etc.). Wilcox (2012) provides R programs for performing the necessary calculations for these methods, as well as many other robust methods of estimation and hypothesis testing. The UNIVARIATE procedure in SAS can perform trimming and Winsorization, as well as calculate robust estimates of other population parameters.

There is also an entire field of statistics devoted to accommodating apparent outliers and minimizing the effects of violations of the underlying assumptions when performing regression analysis. Various methods are available including robust regression, nonparametric regression, ridge regression, etc. All of these methods are beyond the scope of this text. Wilcox (2012) describes several of these methods and provides R programs for performing many of the calculations. Other texts that deal with outliers in the context of regression analysis include Carroll and Ruppert (1988), Hettmansperger and McKean (1998), and Staudte and Sheather (1990).

4.8 LIMITS OF DETECTION AND NON-DETECTED OBSERVATIONS

In research studies involving biomarker data, there may be specimens for which the concentration of the biomarker is below the analytic LOD. In other words, the measuring device used to determine the level of the analyte present in the biological specimen is such that any concentration below a certain value (the LOD) cannot be detected. All that is known is that the analyte is present, that is, the concentration is not zero. These observations are commonly referred to as non-detects (NDs). In statistical analyses, data below the LOD are usually treated as being "left censored." In statistics, the term "censored" generally refers to observations that the investigator cannot observe. For example, in survival analysis, the lifetimes of subjects who survive until the end of the study period are said to be *right censored*; this is because the study did not last long enough for the death times of these subjects to be observed. Similarly, study subjects who drop out of the study or are lost to follow-up are also classified as being right censored since their death times cannot be observed due to the fact that they are no longer in the study. Non-detects are considered to be left censored because the exact concentration of the analyte, though known to be non-zero, cannot be observed due to limitations of the measuring equipment. If more advanced equipment were available, the concentration of the non-detect might be observable. Analogously, if the duration of a prospective study is extended long enough, eventually the death times of those still alive at the end of the original study could be observed. Similarly, if better follow-up methods were used, it might be possible to determine the death times of subjects who dropped out or were otherwise lost to follow-up. Under both of these scenarios, the lifetimes of these subjects would no longer be treated as censored.

As an example of a biomarker study in which limits of detection were a primary concern, consider Amorim and Alvarez-Leite (1997). The authors examined the concurrent validity (Section 5.4.5) of urinary *o*-cresol as a biomarker of exposure to toluene by correlating the concentration of *o*-cresol in the urine of workers exposed to toluene with their urinary hippuric acid level, which at the time was the most frequently used biomarker for occupational exposure to toluene. Amorim and Alvarez-Leite calculated the correlation between concentrations of *o*-cresol and hippuric acid in urine samples of individuals exposed to toluene in shoe factories, painting sectors of metal industries, and printing shops. In the 54 samples analyzed in their study, the concentration of *o*-cresol was below its LOD (0.2 μg/mL) in 39 (72%); thus, there were only 15 samples with "complete data" for both biomarkers. Out of the 39 urine samples with ND *o*-cresol, the hippuric acid concentration was below its LOD (0.1 mg/mL) in 4 (10%) samples. As another example of a biomarker study in which NDs were a concern, consider Atawodi et al. (1998), in which the investigators evaluated hemoglobin adducts as biomarkers of exposure to tobacco smoke by comparing the adduct levels of 18 smokers and 52 "never smokers." The hemoglobin adduct levels were below the LOD (9 fmol HPB/g Hb) in 7 of the 52 (13%) samples from the "never smokers."

Unfortunately, the methods that are typically used to deal with NDs in biomarker research studies are flawed (Looney and Hagan 2006a; McCracken 2013). Perhaps the most commonly used method is to remove the specimens with NDs and base the statistical analysis on only those specimens that have complete data. Lagorio et al. (1998) used this approach in their evaluation of *trans, trans* muconic acid (*t,t*-MA) as a biomarker for low-level benzene exposure. They examined the intercorrelations among the urinary concentrations of *t,t*-MA obtained using HPLC after three different preanalytical procedures (filtration, methanol dilution, ether extraction) were applied to urine samples from 10 Estonian shale oil workers. Another approach that is commonly used to deal with NDs is to use simple substitution; in other words, replace the missing biomarker levels with some substitute value and then apply the "usual" statistical analysis to the new sample of data that contains the substituted values in place of the NDs. The most commonly substituted values include the LOD (Amorim and Alvarez-Leite 1997; Atawodi et al. 1998) and LOD/2 (Cook et al. 1993).

Another method that has been proposed for dealing with NDs is the "nonparametric approach," in which one treats all NDs as if they were tied at some value just below the LOD. Thus, if one wished to correlate two biomarkers X and Y, at least one of which was undetectable in some samples, one could calculate Spearman's r_S using the ranks of the X and Y values based on the entire data set, where all NDs for each variable have been assigned the smallest mid-rank. (See Section 4.5.1.1 for details on Spearman's r_S.) If one wished to compare two groups in terms of a biomarker for which NDs were present, one could apply the M-W-W or median test (Section 4.2.3.3) after computing the ranks on the combined sample of data from the two groups, again assigning the smallest mid-rank to each of the NDs. Atawodi et al. (1998) used this approach in their statistical evaluation of hemoglobin adducts as biomarkers of exposure to tobacco smoke, and found that the HPB-Hb adduct was significantly higher in smokers than in never smokers ($p = 0.02$).

4.8.1 Statistical Inference When NDs Are Present

Wang (2006) demonstrated via simulation that none of the "standard" methods described above for dealing with NDs when correlating two biomarkers that are both subject to left censoring are satisfactory, especially if the two biomarkers are strongly positively correlated ($\rho \geq 0.5$). An approach that is preferable when the biomarker concentrations for X and Y appear to follow a bivariate normal distribution is the maximum likelihood (ML) method developed by Lyles et al. (2001). Other more advanced methods, such as multiple imputation (Scheuren 2005), could be applied if the appropriate missing data mechanism is present. However, these methods are beyond the scope of this textbook.

An approach similar to the ML-based method of Lyles et al. (2001) was proposed by Taylor et al. (2001) for comparing two groups in terms of the mean of a variable that is subject to NDs. It is likely that this method is preferable to the simple imputation methods and the nonparametric approaches described above for dealing with NDs in the two-group problem, although a comprehensive comparison has yet to be performed.

Helsel (2012) provides a very comprehensive discussion of statistical methods that can be used for estimation and hypothesis testing in the presence of censored environmental data. Many of these methods are directly relevant to the analyses of biomarker data subject to NDs in the published studies mentioned above. Helsel also shows how to use either Minitab® or R to perform many of the statistical methods that he describes. However, in his book, Helsel does not discuss the estimation of the correlation between two variables that are both subject to an LOD. Thus, that is the focus of our discussion of the analysis of left-censored biomarker data.

4.8.2 Maximum Likelihood Estimation of a Correlation Coefficient When Both *X* and *Y* Are Subject to Non-Detects

In this section, we briefly describe the statistical theory behind the ML method proposed by Lyles et al. (2001) for estimating the PCC when X and Y have known limits of detection. This section may be omitted without loss of continuity with the discussion that follows.

*Technical Details of the Maximum Likelihood Method** Let X and Y denote the two biomarkers to be correlated and denote their known detection limits by L_x and L_y, respectively. Assuming that the non-censored values of X and Y follow a bivariate normal distribution, Lyles et al. proposed that one estimate the population parameter vector $\theta = [\mu_x, \mu_y, \sigma_x^2, \sigma_y^2, \rho]$ using MLE applied to a random sample of (x, y) values: $\{(x_1, y_1), (x_2, y_2), \ldots, (x_n, y_n)\}$. They noted that there are four types of observed pairs of (x, y) values: (1) pairs with both x and y observed, (2) pairs with x observed and $y < L_y$, (3) pairs with y observed and $x < L_x$, and (4) pairs with $x < L_x$ and $y < L_y$. Following the notation in Lyles et al. (2001), the contribution of each (x, y) pair of type 1 to the likelihood function is given by

$$t_{i1} = \left(2\pi\sigma_x\sigma_{y|x}\right)^{-1} \exp\left\{-0.5\left[\frac{(y_i - \mu_{y|x_i})^2}{\sigma_{y|x}^2} + \frac{(x_i - \mu_x)^2}{\sigma_x^2}\right]\right\}, \tag{4.99}$$

where $\mu_{y|x_i} = \mu_y + \rho\frac{\sigma_y}{\sigma_x}(x_i - \mu_x)$ and $\sigma_{y|x}^2 = \sigma_y^2(1 - \rho^2)$. The contribution of each pair of type 2 to the likelihood function is given by

$$t_{i2} = \left(2\pi\sigma_x^2\right)^{-1/2} \exp\left[-0.5\frac{(x_i - \mu_x)^2}{\sigma_x^2}\right] \times \Phi\left(\frac{L_y - \mu_{y|x_i}}{\sigma_{y|x}}\right), \tag{4.100}$$

where $\Phi(\cdot)$ denotes the standard normal distribution function. Similarly, the contribution of each pair of type 3 to the likelihood function is given by

$$t_{i3} = (2\pi\sigma_y^2)^{-1/2} \exp\left[-0.5\frac{(y_i - \mu_y)^2}{\sigma_y^2}\right] \times \Phi\left(\frac{L_x - \mu_{x|y_i}}{\sigma_{x|y}}\right), \tag{4.101}$$

where $\mu_{x|y_i} = \mu_x + \rho\frac{\sigma_x}{\sigma_y}(y_i - \mu_y)$ and $\sigma_{x|y}^2 = \sigma_x^2(1 - \rho^2)$.

Finally, the contribution of each pair of type 4 to the likelihood function is given by

$$t_4 = \int_{-\infty}^{L_y} \Phi\left\{\frac{L_x - \mu_{x|y}}{\sigma_{x|y}}\right\} \times \left(2\pi\sigma_y^2\right)^{-1/2} \exp\left[-0.5\frac{(y - \mu_y)^2}{\sigma_y^2}\right] dy. \tag{4.102}$$

Using the contributions of type 1, 2, 3, and 4 pairs, the total likelihood can be expressed as

$$L(\theta|\mathbf{x}, \mathbf{y}) = \prod_{i=1}^{n_1} t_{1i} \times \prod_{i=n_1+1}^{n_2} t_{2i} \times \prod_{i=n_2+1}^{n_3} t_{3i} \times \prod_{i=n_3+1}^{n_4} t_{4i}. \tag{4.103}$$

Once the ML estimates of the parameters $\mu_x, \mu_y, \sigma_x^2, \sigma_y^2, \rho$ have been found by maximizing the likelihood function in (4.103) and the corresponding estimated standard errors have been obtained, one can construct an approximate $100(1 - \alpha)\%$ Wald-type

CI) for ρ by using $\hat{\rho}_{\mathrm{ML}} \pm z_{\alpha/2}\widehat{\mathrm{SE}}(\hat{\rho}_{\mathrm{ML}})$, where $z_{\alpha/2}$ denotes the upper $\alpha/2$-percentage point of the standard normal distribution. Lyles et al. also considered profile likelihood (PL) CIs since Wald-type CIs are known to be potentially suspect when the sample size is small, and they found that the PL intervals generally performed better than the Wald-type intervals. However, the PL intervals are more difficult computationally, and generally do not have a closed-form expression. An alternative approach would be to use a CI based on an improved Fisher z-transformation, as will be discussed in the following section.

4.8.3 Comparison of Confidence Interval Methods for Correlation Coefficients When Both Variables Are Subject to Limits of Detection

McCracken (2013) performed a thorough comparison of eight methods of finding point and CI estimates of the correlation between X and Y when both X and Y are subject to LOD. These eight methods included several "standard methods," as well as the ML method developed by Lyles et al. (2001). The methods compared were as follows.

1. Maximum likelihood (Lyles et al. (2001))
2. Simple substitution: replace each ND by
   (a) LOD
   (b) LOD/2
   (c) $LOD/\sqrt{2}$.
3. Complex substitution (Lynn 2001, McCracken 2013): Replace each ND among the x-values by $E(X_i|X_i < LOD_x)$ and each ND among the y-values by $E(Y_i|Y_i < \mathrm{LOD}_y)$. In other words, each ND for each variable is replaced by the conditional mean of that variable, given that it is known that the value is less than the LOD for that variable. See Lynn (2001) for computational details.
4. Random imputation from a uniform distribution: Replace each ND among the x-values by a randomly selected value from the interval $[0, \mathrm{LOD}_x]$. Similarly, replace each ND among the y-values by a randomly selected value from the interval $[0, LOD_y]$.
5. Spearman's correlation r_S: Treat each ND among the x-values as tied at some value smaller than the smallest observed x-value. Similarly, treat each ND among the y-values as tied at some value smaller than the smallest observed y-value.

For estimation methods (1)–(4) above, a second-order Fisher z-transformation, which provides a more accurate estimate of the variance of $z(\hat{\rho})$, was used to find a 95% CI for the true value of the Pearson correlation between X and Y. CIs based on this method have improved coverage probabilities relative to those based on the usual Fisher z-transformation, and the improved transformation poses no computational difficulties. Details of this method are provided in Li et al. (2005) and McCracken (2013).

For estimation method (5), both the Jackknife and approximate bootstrap confidence interval (ABC) methods were used to find a 95% CI for the true value of the correlation. McCracken examined r_s both as a surrogate for r (to be used in place of r when there is evidence that the data do not follow a BVN distribution), as well as an estimate of the true population rank correlation ρ_s. Defining the true value of the Spearman coefficient is itself controversial (Gibbons and Chakraborti 2003); McCracken followed the approach of Newton and Rudel (2007) and used a simulation-based estimate. Namely, the true value, ρ_s, was defined to be the mean of the r_s values calculated from the Monte Carlo samples before the censoring schemes were applied.

An extensive Monte Carlo simulation study was undertaken by McCracken to compare the various point estimates and 95% CI procedures. This Monte Carlo study examined various settings of several simulation parameters: (1) sample size ($n = 20$, 30, 50, 75, 100, 200, 500); (2) true correlation between X and Y prior to censoring ($\rho = -0.9$, -0.6, -0.5, -0.25, 0.0, 0.1, 0.2, 0.25, 0.3, 0.4, 0.5, 0.6, 0.7, 0.75, 0.8 and 0.9); (3) true bivariate distribution of X and Y (bivariate normal, bivariate gamma, bivariate beta); and (4) censoring proportions on X (p_1) and Y (p_2). A total of 55 combinations of censoring proportions were examined, including balanced and unbalanced combinations. Balanced combinations included $(p_1, p_2) = (0,0)$, (10, 10), (20, 20), (25, 25), (30, 30), (40, 40), (50, 50), (60, 60), (70, 70), (75, 75), (80, 80), and (90, 90). Examples of unbalanced combinations included (10, 0), (10, 5), (10, 50), (10, 75), (20, 50), (25, 75), (30, 75), (90, 45), and (90, 0). All together, 18,480 different combinations of simulation parameter settings were considered. A Monte Carlo simulation size (MCSS) of 5000 was used.

Each of the point estimates and corresponding 95% CI procedure described above were evaluated in terms of the following criteria: (1) bias (and absolute bias), (2) median absolute deviation, (3) CI width, (4) CI coverage probability (CP). Our discussion of the comparisons of the various methods will focus on the CP of the 95% CIs.

The findings of such an extensive simulation study can only be summarized here. The MLE had the best overall performance in terms of all of the criteria that were examined and, somewhat surprisingly, it can be recommended for estimating ρ even when the assumption of bivariate normality is suspect. However, for extreme negative values of ρ, small sample sizes and/or extremely heavy or imbalanced censoring, the ML method may not be able to produce a point estimate (due to failure of the optimization routine to converge) or the resulting ML estimate may be unreliable. This is especially true when the true joint distribution of X and Y differs substantially from the BVN. In McCracken's simulation study, the non-BVN distributions were chosen to represent substantial departures from the BVN, as measured by Mardia's measures of multivariate skewness and kurtosis, denoted by $\beta_{1,p}$ and $\beta_{2,p}$, respectively. For the bivariate normal, $\beta_{1,2} = 0$ and $\beta_{2,2} = 8$. For the bivariate gamma used in the simulation study, $\beta_{1,2} = 3.5$ and $\beta_{2,2} = 12$ and, for the bivariate beta, $\beta_{1,2} = 3$ and $\beta_{2,2} = 10$. Somewhat unexpectedly, the ML method performed quite well under most simulation scenarios when the simulated data were generated from these non-BVN distributions, even though the MLEs were derived under the assumption of BVN.

TABLE 4.37 Comparison of Median Coverage Probability of Three CI Methods, by Censoring Proportions

		Method		
Distribution	Censoring Proportions (p_1, p_2)	Maximum Likelihood	Complex Substitution	Spearman's r_s (Jackknife Interval)
Normal	(0, 0)	94.8	94.8	93.8
Normal	(0.1, 0.7)	94.8	**81.0**	**91.5**
Normal	(0.25, 0.25)	94.8	**92.2**	94.1
Normal	(0.25, 0.75)	94.8	**76.2**	**89.9**
Normal	(0.5, 0.5)	94.7	**84.3**	92.5
Normal	(0.75, 0.375)	94.9	**75.7**	**88.4**
Normal	(0.9, 0)	94.9	**26.5**	**33.8**
Normal	(0.9, 0.9)	**90.0**	**27.2**	**61.8**
Non-normal	(0, 0)	**91.0**	**90.7**	93.9
Non-normal	(0.1, 0.7)	93.9	**81.4**	92.9
Non-normal	(0.25, 0.25)	93.4	**89.3**	94.1
Non-normal	(0.25, 0.75)	94.0	**76.6**	**91.8**
Non-normal	(0.5, 0.5)	93.8	**85.5**	93.7
Non-normal	(0.75, 0.375)	94.0	**80.0**	92.5
Non-normal	(0.9, 0)	93.2	**60.0**	**69.7**
Non-normal	(0.9, 0.9)	**85.8**	**38.6**	**74.3**

McCracken's simulated CP results are summarized very briefly in Tables 4.37, 4.38, and 4.39 for the ML method, complex substitution (CS), and Spearman's coefficient (with Jackknife-based CI) considered as an estimate of ρ_S. Table 4.37 examines the effect of the censoring proportions for X and Y on CP. Summary simulation results for a subset of the censoring proportions considered by McCracken {(0, 0) (0.1, 0.7) (0.25, 0.25) (0.25, 0.75) (0.5, 0.5) (0.75, 0.375) (0.9, 0) (0.9, 0.9)} were obtained by calculating the median CP over all settings of the other simulation parameters (namely, the true value of ρ or ρ_S, and sample size). The results for the "non-normal" simulated data presented in the bottom half of the table were obtained by averaging the CP results for the simulated bivariate gamma and bivariate beta data. For example, for censoring proportions $p_1 = 0.1$ and $p_2 = 0.7$, the median CP over all other simulation parameter settings was 94.8% for the ML method, 81.0% for CS, and 91.5% for Spearman's coefficient when data were generated from the bivariate normal. When data were generated from the non-BVN distributions, the median CPs for the ML and CS methods and Spearman's coefficient were 93.9%, 81.4%, and 92.9%, respectively.

In order to determine if the coverage probabilities of the various methods differed in any meaningful way from the nominal 95% confidence level, McCracken (2013) adopted the "liberal" guideline proposed by Bradley (1978) for evaluating the robustness of a statistical test: if the true significance level differs from the nominal level

TABLE 4.38 Comparison of Median Coverage Probability of Three CI Methods, by True Parameter Value

		Method		
Distribution	True Value of ξ^a	Maximum Likelihood	Complex Substitution	Spearman's r_s (Jackknife Interval)
Normal	−0.9	**90.8**	**0.0**	**15.8**
Normal	−0.5	94.6	**82.5**	**91.6**
Normal	−0.25	94.9	93.6	93.3
Normal	0.0	95.0	94.9	94.4
Normal	0.25	95.0	**91.8**	93.0
Normal	0.5	94.9	**86.0**	**91.9**
Normal	0.75	94.7	**70.4**	**89.0**
Normal	0.9	94.4	**24.9**	**76.7**
Non-normal	−0.9	**87.6**	**2.9**	**15.4**
Non-normal	−0.5	**91.7**	**75.1**	**92.0**
Non-normal	−0.25	92.9	**89.5**	93.3
Non-normal	0.0	**89.3**	95.0	94.2
Non-normal	0.25	94.0	**91.6**	94.2
Non-normal	0.5	93.5	**85.8**	93.4
Non-normal	0.75	93.4	**72.8**	**91.1**
Non-normal	0.9	**91.4**	**31.7**	**79.8**

[a] $\xi = \rho$ for Pearson correlation, $\xi = \rho_S$ for Spearman's coefficient.

by no more than $\alpha/2$, one can conclude that the test is robust. If the true significance level differs by more than $\alpha/2$ from the nominal level (either above or below), one can conclude that the test is not robust. In the present study, McCracken applied the Bradley criterion as follows: if CP differed from the 0.95 nominal confidence level by no more than 0.025, the CP produced by the CI method was deemed to be within acceptable limits. If the CP differed by more than 0.025 from the nominal confidence level (either above or below), the CP for that method was deemed to be unacceptable. Thus, for a 95% CI, the CP had to be between 92.5% and 97.5% for a CI procedure to be classified as "acceptable."

In Table 4.37, the values in boldface indicate median CPs that were less than the lower acceptability criterion of 92.5%. Note that the ML method maintained an acceptable value of CP for all censoring proportions except (0.9, 0.9) with BVN data and (0, 0) and (0.9, 0.9) for non-BVN data. Spearman's performed as well as the ML method for many of the censoring proportions, but failed to maintain the 92.5% level for several censoring proportions, especially when the data were generated from a BVN distribution. The CIs based on CS maintained the 92.5% level for very few of the censoring proportions. However, the results were generally comparable to those obtained when r_S was treated as an estimate of ρ, rather than as a estimate of ρ_S (results not shown).

TABLE 4.39 Comparison of Median Coverage Probability of Three CI Methods, by Sample Size

		Method		
Distribution	Sample Size	Maximum Likelihood	Complex Substitution	Spearman's r_s (Jackknife Interval)
Normal	20	94.1	**92.3**	**92.3**
Normal	30	94.4	**92.2**	93.3
Normal	50	94.5	**89.3**	93.0
Normal	75	95.2	**88.2**	93.1
Normal	100	95.0	**86.1**	**92.2**
Normal	200	94.8	**78.3**	**88.0**
Normal	500	95.2	**56.6**	**73.3**
Non-normal	20	93.3	**91.8**	**92.4**
Non-normal	30	93.7	**91.4**	93.4
Non-normal	50	93.8	**88.6**	93.7
Non-normal	75	93.8	**87.0**	93.8
Non-normal	100	93.7	**85.1**	93.9
Non-normal	200	93.2	**78.7**	93.7
Non-normal	500	**91.7**	**59.7**	**90.6**

Table 4.38 examines the relationship between the true value of the correlation parameter (either Pearson's correlation or Spearman's coefficient) and median CP of the CIs based on the MLE, CS, and Spearman's r_S. As in Table 4.37, the values in boldface indicate median CPs that did not exceed the lower acceptability criterion of 92.5%. Note that the ML method maintained an acceptable value of CP for all values of ρ except -0.9 with BVN data; however, it did not perform as well with non-BVN data. Spearman's coefficient generally performed as well as the ML method with non-BVN data, but failed to maintain the 92.5% level for several values of the true correlation when the data were generated from a BVN distribution. The CIs based on CS maintained the 92.5% level for very few of the true values of ρ.

Table 4.39 examines the effect of sample size (n) on the median CP of the CIs based on the ML and CS methods and Spearman's r_S. As in Tables 4.37 and 4.38, the values in boldface indicate median CPs that did not exceed the lower acceptability criterion of 92.5%. Note that the ML method maintained an acceptable value of CP for all sample sizes except $n = 500$ when the data were non-BVN. Spearman's performed almost as well as the ML method with the non-BVN data, but failed to maintain the 92.5% level for several sample sizes when the data were generated from a BVN distribution. The CIs based on CS failed to maintain the 92.5% level for any of the sample sizes in Table 4.39.

In summary, McCracken's results showed that when the data were generated from a BVN distribution, the ML method was superior to all other estimation methods under all conditions considered and had median CP above 92.5% except when

$p_1 = p_2 = 0.9$. When the data were generated from the non-BVN distributions, the performance of the ML method was still superior to the other estimation methods except under some scenarios involving moderate to large n, small $|\rho|$, and very light censoring combinations. Methods based on Spearman's r_s (as an estimate of ρ_s) performed acceptably as long as $|\rho_s|$ was small or moderate, the sample size was not too large (i.e., less than 500), and the proportion of censoring on X was small to moderate and there was little or no censoring on Y. The CIs based on r_s generally performed better for non-BVN data than for BVN data.

The CS method, proposed by Lynn (2001) when only one of the variables is subject to NDs and extended to the situation when both variables are subject to NDs by McCracken (2013), performed acceptably for some settings of the simulation parameters, primarily when $|\rho| < 0.25$, $n \leq 100$, and when the censoring proportions were both 50% or less and not too dissimilar. Its performance was generally greatly superior to that of any of the simple substitution or random substitution methods, and was generally comparable to that of Spearman's r_s when thought of as an estimate of ρ. However, CIs based on the CS method were generally greatly inferior to those based on either the MLE or on r_s when treated as an estimate of ρ_s. The true distribution of the data (either BVN or non-BVN) had only minimal impact on the performance of the CS method.

If the ML method fails to produce an estimate of ρ due to failure of the optimization routine to converge, we recommend that Spearman's r_s be used if one is interested only in measuring the strength of association between X and Y, and not in measuring linear association between X and Y. If estimation of ρ (as a measure of linear association) is the primary aim of the analysis, and the MLE does not exist or cannot be found, then we recommend that the CS method be used to estimate ρ. However, for some combinations of the simulation parameters considered here (heavy or imbalanced censoring proportions, moderate to large values of ρ, and large sample size), the CS method performed extremely poorly, so the CI based on the CS method should be considered to be only a rough approximation under those conditions.

Each of the CI methods considered by McCracken (2013) are illustrated in Example 4.31, and R code for finding each of the point estimates and corresponding CIs is provided on the companion website.

Example 4.31 Estimating the Correlation Coefficient in the Presence of Non-Detects

Consider once again the study by Amorim and Alvarez-Leite (1997), who examined the concurrent validity of urinary *o*-cresol as a biomarker of exposure to toluene by correlating the urinary concentrations of *o*-cresol with urinary concentrations of hippuric acid. They obtained data on the concentrations of these analytes in urine samples of individuals exposed to toluene in shoe factories, painting sectors of metal industries, and printing shops. Table 4.40 contains the data provided in their article, after combining the data from the three industries. These data are plotted in Figure 4.13, with a value of zero used to indicate the NDs. There is strong evidence against the bivariate normality assumption for these data (S-W $p < 0.0001$ for both the 15 *o*-cresol values and the 50 hippuric acid values). Applying the ML method

TABLE 4.40 Data on *o*-Cresol and Hippuric Acid

Specimen	o-Cresol	Hippuric Acid
1	0.92	ND
2	0.76	ND
3	0.40	ND
4	0.27	ND
5	0.68	ND
6	0.48	ND
7	0.22	ND
8	1.19	0.34
9	0.68	ND
10	0.70	ND
11	0.57	ND
12	0.73	ND
13	0.32	ND
14	0.27	ND
15	0.21	ND
16	0.36	ND
17	0.40	ND
18	0.24	ND
19	3.02	2.80
20	1.33	0.76
21	0.67	ND
22	0.44	ND
23	1.08	0.44
24	0.80	ND
25	1.20	0.59
26	0.67	ND
27	0.70	ND
28	2.10	1.36
29	ND	ND
30	1.30	0.41
31	1.10	0.32
32	1.10	0.44
33	0.40	0.25
34	0.20	1.25
35	0.20	ND
36	0.20	ND
37	0.30	ND
38	ND	ND
39	0.20	ND
40	1.20	0.51
41	0.30	ND
42	ND	ND
43	0.20	ND

TABLE 4.40 (*Continued*)

Specimen	o-Cresol	Hippuric Acid
44	0.60	ND
45	0.30	0.21
46	0.50	ND
47	0.20	ND
48	0.20	ND
49	0.50	0.28
50	ND	ND
51	0.40	ND
52	0.10	ND
53	0.10	ND
54	0.80	0.21

Source: Adapted, with permission, from Tables 1–3 of Amorim and Alvarez-Leite (1997) reprinted with permission of the publisher Taylor & Francis Ltd.

for estimating the correlation in the presence of non-detects yields $\hat{\rho}_{\text{ML}} = 0.79$, with a 95% modified Fisher z CI(ρ) of (0.66, 0.87). Analyzing only the 15 cases with complete data yields $r = 0.76$ with a 95% CI(ρ) of (0.40, 0.92), using the standard approach for Pearson's correlation based on the Fisher z-transform. (See Section 4.5.2.) Imputing LOD/2, as was done by Amorim and Alvarez-Leite yields $\hat{\rho}_{\text{LOD}/2} = 0.79$,with a 95% modified Fisher z CI(ρ) of (0.65, 0.87).

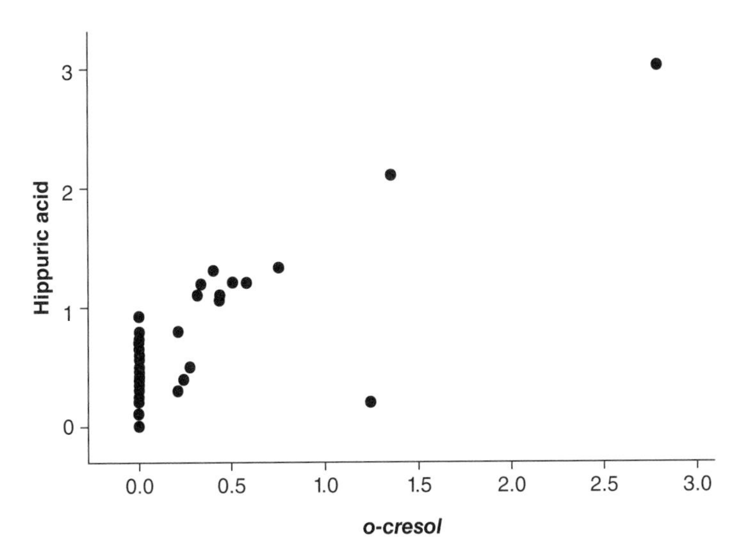

FIGURE 4.13 Scatterplot of *o*-cresol vs. hippuric acid concentrations in urine samples of 54 individuals exposed to toluene in shoe factories, painting sectors of metal industries, and printing shops. Observations below the detectable limit of either assay are plotted as zero for purposes of illustration only.

TABLE 4.41 Summary of Results for Data from Amorim and Alvarez-Leite (1997)

Method	n	Estimate	p-value	95% CI (ρ)
Complete cases	15	0.76	<0.001	(0.40, 0.92)
Substitute zero	54	0.79	<0.001	(0.67,0.88)
Substitute LOD	54	0.77	<0.001	(0.63, 0.85)
Substitute LOD/2	54	0.79	<0.001	(0.65, 0.87)
Substitute LOD/$\sqrt{2}$	54	0.78	<0.001	(0.64, 0.86)
Random substitution	54	0.63	<0.001	(0.43, 0.76)
Complex substitution	54	0.78	<0.001	(0.65, 0.86)
Spearman	54	0.58	<0.001	(0.34, 0.82)
Kendall	54	0.49	<0.001	(0.12, 0.74)
Maximum likelihood	54	0.79	<0.001	(0.66, 0.87)

The R code used to produce the above results for all of the methods except "substitute zero" and Kendall's coefficient is provided on the companion website. These results for "substitute zero" and Kendall's coefficient were obtained using SAS (see Example 4.20). Note that the results obtained for the random substitution method will vary from one run to the next, as randomly generated values are imputed for the NDs.

Table 4.41 provides a summary of the results obtained using all of the methods examined by McCracken (2013). Results are also provided for two methods not examined in the simulation study; namely, Kendall's coefficient and substituting 0 for all of the NDs, both of which have been used in biomarker studies in which NDs were present. As can be seen from the table, the results for the ML approach differ very little from those produced by the substitution methods, with the exception of random substitution. However, there is quite a discrepancy between the results obtained using the ML method and those based on either Spearman's or Kendall's coefficients. Note that the censoring proportions in this example are $p_1 = 7\%$ (4/54) for hippuric acid and $p_2 = 72\%$ (39/54) for o-cresol. If we consider the summary results presented in Table 4.37, the closest censoring proportions in the table are (0.1, 0.7). For data that do not appear to follow a BVN distribution (as is apparently the case in this example), we see that CIs based on either the MLE or Spearman's r_s maintain acceptable CP under these censoring proportions (93.9% for ML and 92.9% for r_s). If we consider the summary results presented in Table 4.38 for non-BVN data, we see that CIs based on the MLE maintain acceptable CP (93.4%) when the true value of ρ is approximately 0.75, which seems to be a reasonable assumption based on the results in Table 4.41 ($\hat{\rho}_{ML} = 0.79$). Similarly, CIs based on Spearman's r_s maintain acceptable CP (93.4%) when the true value of ρ_s is approximately 0.5, which appears to be a reasonable assumption based on the results in Table 4.41 ($r_s = 0.58$). Finally, from the results for non-BVN data in Table 4.39, we see that CIs based on either the MLE (93.8%) or Spearman's r_s (93.7%) maintain acceptable CP when n is approximately 50, which it is in this example ($n = 54$). Thus, based on McCracken's simulation results (summarized in Tables 4.37–4.39), we have no reason to doubt the validity of either the ML-based CI or the r_s-based CI (r_s considered as an estimate of ρ_s). Given the strong departure from normality for these data, and that the authors were evaluating the concurrent validity of o-cresol by examining its association with hippuric acid (not necessarily its linear association), we recommend that the results for Spearman's coefficient be used: $\hat{\rho}_S = 0.58$ with a 95% Jackknife CI(ρ_S) of (0.34, 0.82). Thus, the association between *o*-cresol and hippuric acid appears to be quite a bit weaker than that claimed by Amorim and Alvarez-Leite ($r = 0.777$).

The use of Spearman's coefficient with these data is consistent with Amorim and Alvarez-Leite's use of the nonparametric K-W test to compare the *o*-cresol concentrations among the three groups of individuals exposed to toluene that they studied: workers in shoe factories, painting sectors of metal industries, and printing shops If the authors had been primarily interested in the linear association between the hippuric acid and *o*-cresol concentrations, then we would recommend that the ML method be used instead of r_S. Even though there is very strong evidence that the data in this study do not follow a bivariate normal distribution, McCracken's simulation results show that the ML-based method is still preferable to any of the other methods of estimating the PCC when LODs are present in both variables, regardless of the bivariate distribution of X and Y. Thus, we feel it would be safe to use the PCC if estimating the degree of linear relationship between the two biomarkers was the primary goal of the analysis.

4.9 THE ANALYSIS OF CROSS-CLASSIFIED CATEGORICAL DATA

4.9.1 Choosing the Appropriate Measure of Association

In Chapter 2, we discussed several of the issues related to the design of research studies involving biomarkers. In particular, we addressed the issue of choosing the appropriate measure of association when analyzing cross-classified categorical data. Table 2.1 can provide assistance in selecting the appropriate measure of association between exposure and outcome to use in a research study when both the predictor and the outcome are categorical.

4.9.1.1 The Odds Ratio It is often the case in research studies involving biomarkers that both the predictor and the outcome are dichotomous. The predictor might be exposure to a hazardous substance, classified as "high" or "low" according to the observed value of a particular biomarker, and the outcome might be the presence or absence of a disease or condition. For example, Tunstall-Pedoe et al. (1995) examined the association between the level of serum cotinine (a biomarker for passive smoking) and the presence or absence of several adverse health outcomes (chronic cough, CHD, etc.). Serum cotinine level was grouped into four ordinal categories: "non-detectable," 0.01–1.05 ng/mL, 1.06–3.97 ng/mL, and 3.98–17.49 ng/mL. The authors correctly used the OR (Section 3.10.2) in their comparisons of each serum cotinine category vs. the referent category of "non-detectable" in terms of the adverse health outcomes they considered. Table 4.42 contains an excerpt from their Table 3 for the outcome of diagnosed CHD.

TABLE 4.42 Adjusted Odds Ratios for Diagnosed CHD with Level of Serum Cotinine as the Risk Factor

	Serum Cotinine Group			
	Non-detectable	0.01–1.05 ng/mL	1.06–3.97 ng/mL	3.98–17.49 ng/mL
Odds Ratio	1.0	1.5	1.7	2.7
95% CI	—	(0.8, 3.0)	(0.8, 3.3)	(1.3, 5.6)

Source: Adapted from Table 3 of Tunstall-Pedoe et al. (1995), with permission from BMJ Publishing Group Ltd.

The OR is the most commonly used measure of association in epidemiological research studies. It is appropriate for a wide variety of research scenarios. Following the generic terminology typically used when describing epidemiological research, the predictor variable is referred to as the "exposure," and the outcome variable is referred to as the "disease." This nomenclature leads to the general term "E-D association," which is used to describe whatever association between the exposure (E) and disease (D) is currently being examined. For example, according to Table 4.42, Tunstall-Pedoe et al. (1995) found an OR of 1.7 for the E-D association between "exposure" to 1.06–3.97 ng/mL of serum cotinine and the "outcome" of diagnosed CHD.

As discussed in Section 3.10.2, the OR is given by the ratio of the odds of disease for the exposed study subjects, divided by the odds of disease for the unexposed subjects. (If π represents the probability that an event will occur, the *odds* that the event will occur is defined to be $\pi / (1 - \pi)$.) Thus, using the proportions of disease among the exposed (p_1) and unexposed (p_2) in the sample, an estimate of the true OR can be calculated as follows (Equation 3.36):

$$\widehat{\text{OR}} = \frac{p_1/(1-p_1)}{p_2/(1-p_2)}. \tag{4.104}$$

Example 4.32 Estimating the Odds Ratio

To illustrate the use of the OR in a study involving biomarker data, consider the study by Hobbs et al. (2005). In their case–control study, the authors examined the association of low plasma methionine level (<24.17 μmol/L) in pregnant women with presence of congenital heart defects in their offspring. Out of the 130 mothers with a low plasma methionine level, 103 (79.2%) of their infants had a congenital heart defect; of the 183 mothers who had a normal plasma methionine level, 120 (65.6%) of their infants had a heart defect, yielding an OR of 2.00:

$$\widehat{\text{OR}} = \frac{p_1/(1-p_1)}{p_2/(1-p_2)} = \frac{0.792/(1-0.792)}{0.656/(1-0.344)} = 2.00.$$

Note that an equivalent way to calculate the OR would be to consider the proportion of cases (infants with a heart defect) whose mother had the exposure (low plasma methionine level) with the proportion of the controls (infants without a heart defect) whose mother had the exposure. Of the 223 mothers whose infants had a congenital heart defect, 103 (46.2%) had a low plasma methionine level; of the 90 mothers whose infants did not have a heart defect, 27 (30.0%) had a low level, yielding the same OR of 2.00:

$$\widehat{\text{OR}} = \frac{0.462/(1 - 0.462)}{0.300/(1 - 0.300)} = 2.00.$$

4.9.1.2 Risk Ratio Another measure of association that one should consider when designing a research study involving biomarkers is the *risk ratio* (RR), also known as the *relative risk* (Section 3.10.2). It is given by

$$\widehat{\text{RR}} = \frac{p_1}{p_2}.$$

The RR is an appropriate measure of the E-D association only if the study participants can be considered to consist of representative samples from the populations of exposed and unexposed subjects. In a case–control study (Section 2.2.3), subjects with disease (cases) are often matched with subjects without disease (controls). The matching criteria are usually patient characteristics thought to be associated with increased (or decreased) risk of the disease (e.g., age, race, gender) and/or known risk factors for the disease other than the risk factor of interest. Matching is commonly used in an attempt to ensure that the cases and controls are as alike as possible in terms of possible confounders of the E-D association, so that attention can be focused on the primary risk factor of interest. If 1:1 matching is used, the estimated prevalence of disease based on the sample of cases and controls is 50%, which in general will not be a valid estimate of the true prevalence of the disease in the population. Therefore, using estimates of the prevalence of disease for exposed (p_1) and unexposed (p_2) subjects based on case–control study data is not valid, so a measure of association other than the RR is needed. The OR is the preferred measure of association in a case–control study, unless the sample prevalence of the disease is a valid estimate of the population prevalence. The OR and the RR are similar for rare diseases, but become more dissimilar as the disease prevalence increases (see Agresti 2007, p. 32).

Referring to the study by Hobbs et al. (2005) mentioned earlier, the (invalid) estimated RR based on their study data would be

$$\widehat{\text{RR}} = \frac{103/130}{120/183} = \frac{0.792}{0.656} = 1.21,$$

giving the impression of a much weaker association between having a low plasma methionine level during pregnancy and giving birth to a baby with a congenital heart defect than would be obtained using the OR ($\widehat{\mathrm{OR}} = 2.00$). This study illustrates why the RR is not a valid measure of association for a case–control study: the proportion of babies born with a congenital heart defect in the general population is much lower than the estimated prevalence of 223/(223 + 90) = 71.2% in the study data. Thus, whatever the value of the RR might be for these data, it would not be a valid estimate of the true E-D association.

As we pointed out earlier, a convenient feature of the OR is that the estimated OR will be the same even if the roles of "exposure" and "disease" in the study are reversed. For example, in the study by Hobbs et al., if we define "exposure" to be giving birth to an infant with a congenital heart defect and define "disease" to be low plasma methionine level, we still obtain $\widehat{\mathrm{OR}} = 2.00$, but the estimated relative risk is now $\widehat{\mathrm{RR}} = 1.54$. In other words, the OR is the same regardless of whether we compute the odds of disease conditional on exposure status or the odds of exposure conditional on disease status. This feature is particularly useful when it is difficult to establish a temporal relationship between exposure and disease (i.e., to establish which one came first), as is the case in many case–control studies.

4.9.1.3 Risk Difference The difference in disease risk for populations that are "exposed" vs. "unexposed" to a risk factor can be a useful measure of the absolute change in disease risk due to the exposure. The difference between the estimated disease *incidence* (proportion of the at-risk population who develop a new case of the disease during a specified time period) between the exposed and unexposed groups can be used to compute the *risk difference* (sometimes called the "attributable risk"). Alternatively, the risk difference can be computed as the difference in the estimated disease *prevalence* (proportion of the population with the disease at a specified point in time) between the exposed and unexposed groups. Either way, the risk difference is merely the difference between two binomial proportions and, thus, the formula given in (3.32) can be used to compute approximate $100(1 - \alpha)\%$ CI for the true difference between the risk of disease for exposed and unexposed populations.

For example, Cummings et al. (2002) found that the incidence of breast cancer in post-menopausal women with a baseline serum estradiol concentration exceeding 10 pmol/L was 13/1771 = 0.7% for women taking the drug Raloxifene compared to 26/879 = 3.0% for women taking placebo. They report a risk difference of 2.2%, 95% CI (1.0%, 3.5%) for these women. On the other hand, for women with undetectable levels of serum estradiol at baseline, Cummings et al. report incidences of 11/1710 = 0.64% for women taking Raloxifene compared to 4/716 = 0.56% for women taking placebo, and a risk difference of −0.1%, 95% CI (−0.8%, 0.6%). Note that their calculation of the risk difference treats the placebo as the "exposure," but one could reverse the signs to arrive at a risk difference of −2.2% for women with a baseline serum estradiol concentration over 10 pmol/L, and a risk difference of 0.1% for women with undetectable levels of serum estradiol, when Raloxifene is considered to be the exposure.

Although the risk difference represents an estimate of the absolute difference in disease risk for exposed and unexposed populations, dividing the risk difference by the disease risk in the exposed group yields the *etiologic fraction,* which is interpreted as the proportion of the risk in the exposed population that is attributable to the exposure. For example, considering Raloxifene as the exposure, the etiologic fraction is −2.2%/3.0% = −73%. Since the etiologic fraction is a negative value in this example, it can be interpreted to mean that, among post-menopausal women with a baseline serum estradiol concentration over 10 pmol/L who are taking Raloxifene, a 73% *reduction* in breast cancer incidence can be attributed to taking Raloxifene.

4.9.1.4 Odds Ratio for Paired Data Just as dependent data can cause complications in the comparison of means (Section 4.4.2) or proportions (Section 4.4.3) between groups, so too can the use of matched pairs (as in a matched case–control study) cause complications in the use of the OR. In many case–control studies, cases and controls are "matched" based on some criteria that are thought to be confounders of the true E-D association. The "Big 3" of these are age, race, and gender. While this matching may successfully control for the confounding effects of the matching criteria, it also introduces a dependence between the cases and controls that requires an alternative analysis of the OR. In fact, the OR is calculated differently for paired data (see Section 4.9.4.4). We follow the convention of Agresti (2007) and use the term "paired data" any time there is a dependence in the two groups being compared using the OR. In other words, by nature of the design of the study, there may be a dependence between the "exposed" and "unexposed" groups (e.g., before and after some treatment is applied to all study subjects) or a dependence between the cases and controls (e.g., because of matching).

As an example of a matched case–control study that utilized biomarker data, consider Wang et al. (2008), in which the investigators examined the association between attention deficit/hyperactivity disorder (ADHD) and blood lead levels in Chinese children. Cases (children with ADHD) and controls (children without ADHD) were matched on the basis of age, sex, and socio-economic status. However, the authors did not account for the paired nature of the data that results from matching when they examined the associations between ADHD status and various risk factors (maternal smoking, maternal drinking, etc.) As we discussed in Sections 4.4.2 and 4.4.3, the dependence that is present any time the data are "paired" must be accounted for in any valid statistical analysis. Preferred methods for statistical inference for the OR in the presence of paired data are covered in Section 4.9.4.4.

4.9.2 Choosing the Appropriate Statistical Analysis

Once one has selected the appropriate measure of association for cross-classified data, one must then use the appropriate statistical method(s) to determine if the study result is statistically significant. (See Section 2.3.2.) For example, in the study by Tunstall-Pedoe et al. (1995), the authors correctly used logistic regression to find CIs for the ORs in their study (see Table 4.42). (However, as we have discussed elsewhere (Section 2.4), it would have been preferable for the authors to also include p-values for the test of the null hypothesis H_0: $OR = 1$ in addition to their confidence limits.) An advantage of using logistic regression to analyze the data when the OR has been chosen as the measure of association is that adjustment for the effects of confounding variables is straightforward (Kleinbaum, Kupper, and Morgenstern 1982), thus making it rather easy to determine if there is an "independent effect" of the main predictor of interest. For example, the ORs extracted from Table 3 of Tunstall-Pedoe et al. (1995) and presented in Table 4.42 were adjusted for the effects of age, housing tenure, cholesterol, and diastolic blood pressure.

4.9.3 Choosing the Appropriate Sample Size

As discussed in Section 2.3.3, once one has designed the statistical analysis for a study, the next step is to determine the appropriate sample size to be used. *Both of these steps should be performed prior to beginning data collection.* Sample size determination is specific to the statistical method that is to be used to analyze the study data once they have been collected. For example, the sample size methods described in Fleiss et al. (2003), which have been implemented in the freely available Epi Info software http://wwwn.cdc.gov/epiinfo/7/ and many other statistical software packages, could have been used to determine the appropriate sample size for the study by Tunstall-Pedoe et al. (1995). (Note that the authors provided no justification at all for their sample size.) StatXact also has extensive capabilities for determining the appropriate sample size to use when planning a study that will require analysis of categorical data, and it is especially helpful when it is anticipated that the sample size will have to be small because of budget or time constraints; availability of resources, including specimens for biomarker determinations; etc. With regard to SAS, sample size and power calculations for more and more statistical methods are added to the POWER procedure with each new release. From a more general perspective, Goldsmith (2001) provides very useful practical advice on determining the appropriate statistical package(s) to use for sample size calculations for many of the statistical procedures described in this book.

4.9.4 Choosing a Statistical Method When Both the Predictor and the Outcome Are Dichotomous

4.9.4.1 Comparing Two Independent Groups in Terms of a Binomial Proportion

In research studies involving biomarkers, it is often of interest to compare two independent groups in terms of a binomial proportion (or a percentage) by focusing on the *risk difference* (i.e., the difference in estimated prevalence of the disease between the exposed and unexposed groups), rather than the RR. For example, Pérez-Stable et al. (1995) compared smokers and non-smokers in terms of the proportion diagnosed with depression using the Diagnostic Interview Schedule (DIS) (Table 4.43). Pérez-Stable et al. (1995) performed their comparison of smokers and non-smokers using the most commonly used method for this type of data, the χ^2 (chi-squared) test (Section 3.10.2). However, this test is known to have very poor statistical properties when comparing two independent proportions, especially if the number of subjects in either group is small (Mehrotra et al., 2003), and we do not recommend it for general use. A preferred method is Fisher's exact test (Agresti 2007, pp. 45–48), as

TABLE 4.43 Association Between Dichotomized Cotinine Level and Diagnosis of Depression Using the Diagnostic Interview Survey (DIS), Female Subjects Only

	DIS Diagnosis		
Cotinine ≥15 ng/mL	Positive	Negative	Total
Yes	27(11.8%)	202(88.2%)	229
No	7(5.5%)	121(94.5%)	128
Total	34(9.5%)	323(90.5%)	357

Source: Adapted from Table 4 of Pérez-Stable et al. (1995) with permission from Elsevier.

implemented in StatXact or in the FREQ procedure in SAS. This test is described below.

*Theoretical Details of Fisher's Exact Test** Suppose that it is desired to perform an exact test of the null hypothesis H_0: $\pi_1 = \pi_2$ vs. the alternative H_0: $\pi_1 \neq \pi_2$. (In this context, "exact" means that no approximation will be used for the null distribution of the test statistic.) Following the argument in Mehta and Patel (2010, pp. 393–397), let the common probability of success for the two populations be denoted by $\pi = \pi_1 = \pi_2$. The canonical 2 × 2 table for comparing the proportions in two independent groups is given in Table 4.44. Under the null hypothesis H_0: $\pi_1 = \pi_2$, the probability of observing the data in Table 4.44 is given by

$$f_0(x_{11}, x_{12}, x_{21}, x_{22}) = \binom{n_{1\bullet}}{x_{11}} \binom{n_{2\bullet}}{x_{21}} \pi^{x_{11}+x_{21}} (1 - \pi)^{x_{12}+x_{22}}, \qquad (4.105)$$

where x_{ij} denotes the count in cell (i, j) of the 2 × 2 table, and $n_{1\bullet}$ and $n_{2\bullet}$ denote the sample sizes for the two groups being compared.

For the upper-tailed alternative H_a: $\pi_1 > \pi_2$, any 2 × 2 table with the same marginal row and column totals as the observed table that has a count in the (1,1) cell that is greater than or equal to x_{11} in the observed table is considered to be "favorable" to H_a. The hypergeometric probability for each of these tables is accumulated in order to calculate the upper-tailed p-value for the test of H_0: $\pi_1 \leq \pi_2$ vs. H_a: $\pi_1 > \pi_2$. The

TABLE 4.44 Canonical form of a 2 × 2 Table for Comparing the Proportions in Two Independent Groups

	Response		
Group	Success	Failure	Total
1	x_{11}	x_{12}	$n_{1\bullet}$
2	x_{21}	x_{22}	$n_{2\bullet}$
Total	$n_{\bullet 1}$	$n_{\bullet 2}$	n

"reference set" under this conditional approach is defined to consist of all 2×2 tables with the same marginal row and column totals as the observed table.

In order to calculate the p-value for exact test of H_0, one must calculate the probability of obtaining a 2×2 table at least as extreme as the observed table. The probability of obtaining any such table will depend on the parameter π, as indicated in Equation (4.105). The "conditional" approach to exact inference for 2×2 tables is equivalent to eliminating π from the probability calculations by conditioning on its sufficient statistic (Cox and Hinkley, 1974, Chapter 2). This conditional approach is implemented in many of the statistical procedures in StatXact and in SAS, and we recommend it for general use.

After conditioning on the sufficient statistic for π (which is equal to the total number of successes in the two samples, $n_1 = x_{11} + x_{21}$, we find that the exact probability under the null hypothesis of observing the data in Table 4.44 is given by the hypergeometric. In particular,

$$p(\mathbf{x}) = \frac{\binom{n_{1\bullet}}{x_{11}}\binom{n_{2\bullet}}{x_{21}}}{\binom{n}{n_{\bullet 1}}}, \tag{4.106}$$

where $\mathbf{x}$ denotes the vector of cell counts $\{x_{11}, x_{12}, x_{21}, x_{22}\}$. Let $\mathbf{y}$ denote any table that is in the reference set; that is, any 2×2 table with the same marginal row and column totals as the observed table (Table 4.44). Let y_{11} denote the entry in the (1,1) position in $\mathbf{y}$. Then y_{11} ranges from a minimum of $y_{\min} = \max(0, n_{1\bullet} - n_{\bullet 2})$ to a maximum of $y_{\max} = \min(0, n_{1\bullet}, n_{\bullet 1})$. Thus, the exact upper-tailed p-value for the test of H_0: $\pi_1 \le \pi_2$ vs. H_a: $\pi_1 > \pi_2$ is given by

$$p_{\mathrm{U}} = \sum_{y_{11}=y_{\min}}^{x_{11}} p(\mathbf{y}), \tag{4.107}$$

where $p(\mathbf{y})$ is calculated using (4.106).

For the lower-tailed alternative H_a: $\pi_1 < \pi_2$, a similar argument shows that the exact lower-tailed p-value is given by

$$p_{\mathrm{L}} = \sum_{y_{11}=x_{11}}^{y_{\max}} p(\mathbf{y}). \tag{4.108}$$

The exact two-tailed p-value is given by

$$p_2 = \left\{ \begin{array}{l} 2p_{\mathrm{U}} \text{ if } x_{11} > n_{1\bullet}n_{\bullet 1}/n \\ 2p_{\mathrm{L}} \text{ if } x_{11} < n_{1\bullet}n_{\bullet 1}/n \end{array} \right\}, \tag{4.109}$$

using the same notation as in Table 4.44.

Example 4.33 Fisher's Exact Test for Comparing Two Proportions

Based on the data in Table 4.43, the test statistic for Fisher's exact test is $x_{11} = 27$, which is greater than $n_{1\bullet}n_{\bullet 1}/n = (229)(34)/357$. Thus, we first calculate the exact upper-tailed p-value by accumulating the hypergeometric probabilities for all possible tables in which the value in the (1, 1) position is greater than 27, assuming that the row and column totals are the same as in Table 4.43. Using Equation (4.107), this yields an exact upper-tail p-value of 0.0355, and an exact two-tailed p-value of 0.0710, indicating a non-significant result. Using the chi-squared test, $\chi_0^2 = 3.81$, $df = 1$, p-value $= 0.0510$, which is also non-significant.

The exact version of Fisher's exact test as we have described it is known to be conservative, especially if any of the cell counts are small (Agresti 2007, pp. 47–48). In other words, the true significance level of the test can be quite a bit lower than the desired significance level 0.05 (also called the "nominal" significance level). This is because the hypergeometric distribution used to calculate the exact p-value is highly discrete, especially when one or more of the cell sizes in Table 4.44 are small. This means that there will be only a small number of possible values that the test statistic x_{11} can assume, leading to a small number of possible p-values, and hence a small number of possible significance levels, none of which may be close to 0.05. By convention, we choose the appropriate one-tailed significance level that is closest to, but less than or equal to 0.025. For example, for the data in Table 4.43, examination of the exact conditional null distribution of x_{11} based on the hypergeometric distribution indicates that the upper-tailed significance level closest to, but less than, 0.025 is 0.013 (obtained using a critical value of $n_{11} = 28$). This means that the true significance level of the two-tailed test of H_0: $\pi_1 = \pi_2$ vs. H_a: $\pi_1 \neq \pi_2$ would be $2(0.013) = 0.026$, rather than the desired significance level of 0.05.

Mid-P value To help diminish the adverse effects of the conservativeness of Fisher's exact test (namely, loss of power) we follow the recommendation of Agresti (2007, p. 48) and recommend that one routinely use the *mid-P value*. For a one-tailed test, this is equal to the exact p-value minus half the exact point probability of the observed value of the test statistic. This approach has been shown to have extremely favorable properties relative to using chi-square or other approximate approaches to test the null hypothesis H_0: $\pi_1 = \pi_2$ (Hirji et al. 1991). The upper-tailed mid-P value for Fisher's exact test is given by $p_{\text{U}} - \frac{1}{2}p(\mathbf{x})$, the lower-tailed mid-$P$ value is given by $p_{\text{L}} - {}^1\!/_2 p(\mathbf{x})$, and the two-tailed mid-P value is given by $p_2 - p(\mathbf{x})$, where $p(\mathbf{x})$ is given by (4.106), p_{U} is given by (4.107), p_{L} is given by (4.108), and p_2 is given by (4.109).

For the data in Table 4.43, the exact point probability for the test statistic $n_{11} = 27$ is found using Equation (4.106):

$$p(\mathbf{x}) = \frac{\binom{n_{1\bullet}}{x_{11}}\binom{n_{2\bullet}}{x_{21}}}{\binom{n}{n_{\bullet 1}}} = \frac{\binom{229}{27}\binom{128}{7}}{\binom{357}{34}} = 0.0222.$$

This yields an upper-tailed mid-P value of $0.0355 - \frac{1}{2}(0.0222) = 0.0244$. Thus, the two-tailed mid-P value is $2(0.0244) = 0.0488$, which does meet the usual 0.05 criterion for statistical significance. As mentioned previously, if one uses the "usual" chi-squared test, the p-value is 0.0510, a non-significant result (although, admittedly, there is very little difference between the results for the two tests).

The mid-P value can be used with many exact tests for categorical data; it requires only the exact p-value and the exact point probability (p-prob) for the observed value of the test statistic. Then, as described above for Fisher's exact test, the mid-P value is calculated using (exact p-value $- \frac{1}{2}$ p-prob). We recommend using the mid-P value whenever it can be calculated using available software.

Note that there are also approximate versions of Fisher's exact test; for example, the method described by Ahlbom (1993), in which the null distribution of Fisher's exact test is approximated using the normal approximation to the hypergeometric. With the advent of modern computers and readily available software such as StatXact and SAS, there is no longer any need to resort to any approximate method for calculating p-values for Fisher's exact test. The only exception is when one or more of the cells (or marginal totals) in the 2×2 table are unusually large, in which case the computation of the exact p-value for Fisher's exact test may exceed the memory capabilities of the computer. In this case, approximate methods can be used, as it is precisely this situation in which the approximate methods are expected to be highly accurate (i.e., close enough to the exact value to be considered equivalent).

The following SAS code can be used to perform Fisher's exact test for the data in Table 4.43:

```
data DIS;
input cotinine DIS_DX count @@;
cards;
1 1 27   1 2 202
2 1  7   2 2 121
;

proc freq data=DIS order=data; weight count;
       tables cotinine * DIS_DX / fisher;
       title 'Fishers Exact Test';
       run;
```

4.9.4.2 Exact Test for Independence of Rows and Columns in a 2×2 Table It is a common misconception that there is a natural way to distinguish between "tests of independence" for a 2×2 table (i.e., testing that the row and column variables are independent of each other) and tests of equal proportions between two groups. In fact, the row and column variables in Table 4.44 are independent if and only if the true proportions of "success" in the two groups are equal if and only if the true OR is equal to 1 (Agresti 2007, pp. 45-46). Consistent with our earlier notation, let $\pi_1 =$ true proportion of "success" in the population defined by the first row and

$\pi_2 =$ true proportion of "success" in the population defined by the second row. Then $\mathrm{OR} = \frac{\pi_1/(1-\pi_1)}{\pi_2/(1-\pi_2)}$ is the ratio of the odds of "success" in the population defined by the first row variable divided by the odds of "success" in the population defined by the second row. Using this notation, all three of the following null hypotheses for a 2×2 table are equivalent, and rejecting any one of them means that the other two must be rejected. Similarly, failing to reject any one of them means that neither of the other two can be rejected.

H_{01}: The row classification variable and the column classification variable are independent,

$$H_{02} : \pi_1 = \pi_2, \tag{4.110}$$

$$H_{03} : \mathrm{OR} = 1$$

For example, in the study by Pérez-Stable et al. (1995) (Example 4.33), in which the investigators compared smokers and non-smokers in terms of the proportion diagnosed with depression, the row variable, as depicted in Table 4.43 is "Cotinine status" defined by the two categories "Cotinine ≥ 15 ng/mL" and "Cotinine <15 ng/mL." The column variable is DIS diagnosis of depression, either positive (depressed) or negative (not depressed). Thus, H_{01} in (4.110) can be restated as "Cotinine category is independent of depression status." The hypothesis H_{02} in (4.110) can be restated as "The true prevalence (proportion) of depression, as diagnosed using the DIS, is the same in the Cotinine ≥ 15 ng/mL population as in the Cotinine <15 ng/mL population." Finally, H_{03} in (4.110) can be restated as "The true odds ratio for depression (as diagnosed using DIS) in the Cotinine ≥ 15 ng/mL group relative to the Cotinine <15 ng/mL group is equal to 1.0."

Thus, in addition to being the generally recommended method for comparing two population proportions, Fisher's exact test with mid-*P* adjustment is also the recommended method for testing independence of rows and columns in a 2×2 table, and for testing the null hypothesis that the OR is equal to 1. Note that there is a similar equivalence in terms of the chi-square test: the traditional chi-square test for independence (Section 3.10.1) is equivalent to the "usual" method for comparing two population proportions (also called the "score test") that makes use of the following test statistic:

$$z_0 = \frac{\widehat{p_1} - \widehat{p_2}}{\mathrm{SE}\left(\widehat{p_1} - \widehat{p_2}\right)}, \tag{4.111}$$

where

$$\mathrm{SE}\left(\widehat{p_1} - \widehat{p_2}\right) = \sqrt{\bar{p}(1-\bar{p})\left(\frac{1}{n_1} + \frac{1}{n_2}\right)},$$

and

$$\bar{p} = \frac{\left(n_1\widehat{p_1} + n_2\widehat{p_2}\right)}{n_1 + n_2}$$

is the "pooled" proportion of "success" in the two samples. After squaring the test statistic in (4.111) and doing some rather tedious algebra, one obtains the test statistic for the traditional chi-square test for independence (Equation 3.31).

4.9.4.3 Exact Inference for Odds Ratios We have already discussed the "standard" statistical analysis of ORs in Section 3.10.2. However, under certain conditions, CIs and hypothesis tests for the true OR based on the normal approximation for the distribution of log(OR) may not perform adequately. For example, approximate methods for 2×2 tables generally perform well as long as all four of the expected cell counts are 5 or greater (Agresti 2007, p. 40); for smaller cell expected cell counts, the results can be quite misleading. With the advent of modern computing, there is very little need to use approximate methods for finding CIs and performing hypothesis tests for the OR. The only exception is when one or more of the four cell sizes in the 2×2 table (or the total sample size) is so large that performing the exact methods exceeds the memory capacity of the computer. It is precisely these conditions under which the methods based on the normal approximation perform best, and there will be very little meaningful difference between the results obtained using the normal approximation and those obtained using the exact method. Hence, there will be little or no harm in using the approximate methods when n is large. Our advice is to always use the exact method (with mid-P adjustment, if available) whenever possible, and resort to the approximate methods only if the available software cannot provide these analyses due to memory overflow.

*Theoretical Details of Exact Confidence Intervals for the Odds Ratio** In Section 4.9.4.1, we pointed out that the exact conditional null distribution of the test statistic for Fisher's exact test is hypergeometric. To derive an exact CI for the true OR, we must again consider the risk set, $\mathfrak{R}$, defined to consist of all 2×2 tables that have the same row and column totals as the observed table $\mathbf{x}$. Following the argument in Mehta et al. (1985), and using the same notation as in Table 4.44, the risk set is given by

$$\mathfrak{R} = \left\{ \mathbf{y} : \mathbf{y} \text{ is } 2 \times 2; \sum_{j=1}^{2} y_{ij} = n_{i\cdot}; \sum_{i=1}^{2} y_{ij} = n_{\bullet j}; \text{ for } i = 1,2; j = 1,2 \right\}.$$

Let y_{11} denote the cell count in the (1,1) position of any $\mathbf{y} \in \mathfrak{R}$. Then the exact probability of observing $\mathbf{y}$ depends on π_1 and π_2 only through the true OR. It can be shown that the exact probability of observing $\mathbf{y}$ is given by

$$p(\mathbf{y}) = \frac{\binom{n_{1\bullet}}{y_{11}} \binom{n_{2\bullet}}{y_{21}} \mathrm{OR}^{y_{11}}}{\sum_{y \in \mathfrak{R}} \binom{n_{1\bullet}}{y_{11}} \binom{n_{2\bullet}}{y_{21}} \mathrm{OR}^{y_{11}}} \tag{4.112}$$

(Ahlbom 1993, p. 80). Under the null hypothesis H_0 : OR = 1, Equation (4.112) reduces to the hypergeometric probability that was used in calculating the exact probability for Fisher's exact test (Equation 4.106):

$$p(y) = \frac{\binom{n_{1\bullet}}{y_{11}}\binom{n_{2\bullet}}{y_{21}}}{\binom{n}{n_{\bullet 1}}},$$

since

$$\sum_{y \in \Re} \binom{n_{1\bullet}}{y_{11}}\binom{n_{2\bullet}}{y_{21}} = \binom{n}{n_{\bullet 1}}.$$

The exact test of H_0 : OR = OR$_0$, where OR$_0$ is a null value different from 1, is based on using (4.112) to calculate the exact p-value, similar to the approach described in Section 4.9.4.1 for calculating the exact p-value for Fisher's exact test. An exact CI for the true value of the OR is then obtained by inverting this exact test; in other words, the exact CI based on a particular 2×2 table is defined to consist of exactly those null values not rejected when applying the exact test to that table. For more details, see Mehta et al. (1985), or the documentation in the StatXact manual.

Example 4.34 Exact Inference for the Odds Ratio

Although not considered by Pérez-Stable et al. (1995), one is usually interested in measuring the "E-D association" in a study such as theirs. In other words, we are usually interested not only in determining that there is a significant relationship between smoking and depression, but we also usually want to describe the strength of this relationship using a measure of association. Since the sample in Pérez-Stable et al. (1995) was cross-sectional in nature, the OR would be the appropriate measure of association (Table 2.1). Based on the data in Table 4.43, we obtain $\widehat{\text{OR}} = \frac{ad}{bc} = \frac{(27)(121)}{(7)(202)} = 2.31$, using the standard notation for a 2×2 table. Applying the methods described in Section 3.10.2 (see Equation 3.37), we obtain an approximate 95% CI of (0.98, 5.47). Applying the methods described above for exact inference for the OR, we obtain an exact 95% CI of (0.94, 6.47). As expected, the exact 95% CI is somewhat wider than the approximate interval. Note that the p-value for the test of H_0 : OR = 1 that corresponds to the approximate CI for the OR is the same as the p-value for the usual chi-square test of independence ($p = 0.0510$). Similarly, the p-value for the exact test of H_0 : OR = 1 that corresponds to the exact CI for the OR is the same as the p-value for Fisher's exact test ($p = 0.071$). As we saw in Example 4.33, the two-tailed mid-P value is 0.0488, which does meet the usual 0.05 criterion for statistical significance. The 95% mid-P CI (available in StatXact) is (1.004, 5.868). These results are consistent with the findings by Hirji et al. (1991) that the mid-P approach can be more powerful than chi-square under some circumstances.

The following SAS code can be used to find approximate and exact CIs for the OR for the data in Table 4.43.

```
data DIS;
input cotinine DIS_DX count @@;
cards;
1 1 27  1 2 202
2 1  7  2 2 121
;

proc freq data=DIS order=data; weight count;
      tables cotinine * DIS_DX / fisher;
      exact OR;
      title1 'Exact Inference for Odds Ratios';
      run;
```

4.9.4.4 Inference for the Odds Ratio for Paired Data Consider again the study by Wang et al. (2008), who used a matched case–control study design to examine the association between ADHD and blood lead in Chinese children. One of the potential confounders of the E-D association that the authors considered was maternal smoking during pregnancy (coded as yes/no). In their Table 2, the authors report that mothers of 6 of the 630 children (0.95%) with ADHD smoked, whereas mothers of 9 of the 630 children (1.43%) without ADHD smoked. They claim that this yields an OR of 4.04 for the association between maternal smoking and ADHD. This is an obvious typo, as the rate of maternal smoking among the cases is actually lower than that among the controls, which cannot possibly yield an OR greater than 1. Even if one assumes that the frequencies of 6 and 9 were inadvertently reversed in the table, this yields an OR of only $\widehat{\text{OR}} = \frac{ad}{bc} = \frac{(9)(624)}{(6)(621)} = 1.51$. However, this is not the correct way to calculate the OR for matched data, as we discuss below.

Wang et al. did not provide sufficient data for a matched pair analysis of the E-D associations that they considered. In order to properly account for the dependence among case–control pairs that results from the matching, one must first put the cross-classified data into what is called the "canonical form" for matched pair data. (A similar structure for cross-classified data was used in our discussion of the comparison of two dependent proportions in Section 4.4.3.1.) In Table 4.45, we present hypothetical matched pair data that would yield an OR of 4.0 for the association between maternal smoking and ADHD status of the child. We assume that, among the 630 cases of ADHD, 12 had mothers who smoked during pregnancy. Similarly, among the 630 controls, we assume that 6 had mothers who smoked. It is important to note the special structure of Table 4.45. The rows and columns are each labeled "case" and "control." Each cell entry in the 2×2 table represents the number of matched case–control pairs that satisfied the particular combination of exposure status (in this case, presence or absence of maternal smoking). For example, for only four of the case–control pairs did the mother of the case and the mother of

TABLE 4.45 Canonical Form for Hypothetical Matched Case–Control Data

	ADHD Control		
ADHD Case	Smoker	Non-Smoker	Total
Smoker	4	8	12
Non-Smoker	2	616	618
Total	6	624	630

the matching control both smoke. For 616 of the case–control pairs, neither mother smoked. These 620 "concordant" case–control pairs are irrelevant as far as the statistical analysis for matched pairs is concerned. Instead, only the "discordant pairs" are included in the statistical analysis. These consist of the eight case–control pairs for which the mother of the ADHD case smoked during pregnancy, but the mother of the matched control did not smoke, together with the two case–control pairs for which the mother of the ADHD case did not smoke, but the mother of the matched control did smoke. The estimated OR for such matched case–control studies is given by $\widehat{\mathrm{OR}}_{\mathrm{m}} = b/c = 8/2 = 4.0$, where the cells in Table 4.45 are labeled in the usual "*a, b, c, d*" format used in 2 × 2 contingency tables (see Table 3.9). In Section 3.10.2, we saw that the sampling distribution of $\widehat{\mathrm{OR}}$ tends to be highly skewed, so a log transformation is applied for the purposes of deriving CIs and hypothesis tests for the true OR. The sampling distribution of $\widehat{\mathrm{OR}}_{\mathrm{m}}$ also tends to be highly skewed, and applying the log transformation to $\widehat{\mathrm{OR}}_{\mathrm{m}}$ also yields a random variable that is approximately normally distributed. This log-transformed $\widehat{\mathrm{OR}}_{\mathrm{m}}$ is then used to derive an approximate CI for the true OR. An approximate $100(1-\alpha)\%$ CI for the true OR when the data are matched is given by

$$\exp\left[\log(\widehat{\mathrm{OR}}_{\mathrm{m}}) \pm z_{\alpha/2}\sqrt{\frac{1}{b}+\frac{1}{c}}\right]. \tag{4.113}$$

An approximate test of the null hypothesis H_0: $\mathrm{OR}_{\mathrm{m}} = 1$ can be performed by calculating the following test statistic and comparing it with the standard normal distribution:

$$z_0 = \frac{\log(\widehat{\mathrm{OR}}_{\mathrm{m}})}{\sqrt{\frac{1}{b}+\frac{1}{c}}}, \tag{4.114}$$

where $\sqrt{\frac{1}{b}+\frac{1}{c}}$ is the estimated standard error of $\log(\widehat{\mathrm{OR}}_{\mathrm{m}})$.

Exact methods of statistical inference for the OR when the data are paired are also available (Newcombe 1998). The exact version of McNemar's test is used to test the null hypothesis H_0: $\mathrm{OR}_{\mathrm{m}} = 1$, and an exact conditional approach similar to the one

TABLE 4.46 2 × 2 Table for Association Between Blood Lead and ADHD Ignoring Matching (Hypothetical Data)

ADHD Status	Smoker	Non-smoker	Total
Case	12(1.90%)	618(98.1%)	630
Control	6(0.95%)	624(99.05%)	630
Total	18(1.43%)	1242(98.57%)	1260

used to find an exact CI for the OR when there is no pairing (Section 4.9.4.3) is also available. StatXact can be used to obtain these exact results.

Although the approximate methods based on $\log(\widehat{\mathrm{OR}}_{\mathrm{m}})$for dealing with the OR when the data are paired are not directly available in SAS, the LOGISTIC procedure can be "tricked" into providing them (Agresti 2007, p. 275). SAS code for analyzing the data in Table 4.45 is given following Example 4.35.

Example 4.35 Inference for the Odds Ratio When the Data Are Paired

As mentioned previously, for the data in Table 4.45, $\widehat{\mathrm{OR}}_{\mathrm{m}} = b/c = 8/2 = 4.0$. Applying Equation (4.113), we obtain an approximate 95% CI for OR_{m} of (0.85, 18.84). We have $\log(\widehat{\mathrm{OR}}_{\mathrm{m}}) = \log(4.00) = 1.39$ and $\mathrm{SE}[\log(\widehat{\mathrm{OR}}_{\mathrm{m}})] = \sqrt{\frac{1}{b} + \frac{1}{c}} = \sqrt{\frac{1}{8} + \frac{1}{2}} = 0.79$. Equation (4.114) yields a test statistic of $z_0 = 1.75$, with an approximate p-value of 0.080. Using StatXact, the exact p-value is 0.109 (mid-P value = 0.066), with an exact 95% CI of (0.80, 26.20).

If one ignores the fact that the ADHD cases and controls were matched in Wang et al. (2008), then one obtains the 2 × 2 table given in Table 4.46.

Applying the "usual" analysis for the OR (ignoring the fact that cases and controls were matched) yields $\widehat{\mathrm{OR}} = \frac{ad}{bc} = \frac{(12)(624)}{(6)(618)} = 2.11$, chi-square p-value = 0.155, approximate 95% CI (0.75, 5.42). Note that the estimated OR is almost twice as large if the matching is taken into account (4.0 vs. 2.1), and the p-value is almost half as large (0.080 vs. 0.155). While neither analysis indicates statistical significance for these data, it is obvious that appropriately taking the matching into account could yield entirely different conclusions.

The following SAS code can be used to obtain the approximate results for $\widehat{\mathrm{OR}}_{\mathrm{m}}$ presented in Example 4.35.

```
data ADHD;
input case_exp cont_exp count @@;
cards;
1  1  4
1  0  8
0  1  2
0  0  616
;
```

```
data ADHD;
    set ADHD;
    y_star=1;
    if case_exp=cont_exp then x_star=0;
    if case_exp=1 and cont_exp=0 then x_star= 1;
    if case_exp=0 and cont_exp=1 then x_star=-1;

proc logistic desc data=ADHD;
     weight count;
     model y_star=x_star / noint ;
     title1 'OR Inference for Matched Pair Data';
     run;
```

4.9.5 Choice of a Statistical Method When the Predictor Is Ordinal and the Outcome is Dichotomous

4.9.5.1 Tests for a Significant Trend in Proportions As described previously, Tunstall-Pedoe et al. (1995) examined the association between level of serum cotinine (as a biomarker of passive smoking) and the presence or absence of several adverse health outcomes. They classified serum cotinine level into four ordinal categories and calculated ORs and associated 95% CIs for the comparison of each of their three ordinal categories vs. the referent category of "non-detectable" in terms of the prevalence of CHD (Table 4.42). The observed frequency and estimated prevalence of CHD in each cotinine category are provided in Table 4.47.

As can be seen from an examination of this table (or Table 4.42), there appears to be an increasing trend in risk of CHD across the serum cotinine categories. In fact, in their discussion, Tunstall-Pedoe et al. spoke in terms of a "gradient" of adverse health outcomes across the passive smoking categories, but performed no statistical test to determine if, in fact, their data supported the existence of such a gradient.

An additional analysis that would support the claims of a gradient for CHD that we recommend for data of this type (in which the predictor is ordinal and the outcome is binary) is a test for trend across the serum cotinine categories in terms of the estimated

TABLE 4.47 Frequency and Estimated Prevalence of Diagnosed CHD with Level of Serum Cotinine as the Risk Factor

	Serum Cotinine Group			
	Non-detectable	0.01–1.05 ng/mL	1.06–3.97 ng/mL	3.98–17.49 ng/mL
Sample Size	756	674	553	295
Frequency	15	20	19	16
Prevalence	0.020	0.030	0.034	0.054

prevalence of CHD. Such an analysis would be especially helpful in identifying any dose–response relationships that might be present between passive smoking and the adverse health outcomes considered in the Tunstall et al. study.

Recommended procedures for performing the test for trend include the permutation test (Gibbons and Chakraborti 2003, Chapter 8) and the Cochran–Armitage (C-A) test (Cochran 1954; Armitage 1955). Both of these methods require assigning a numerical "score" to each of the ordinal categories of the predictor variable.

To perform the C-A test for data in which the predictor is a biomarker whose levels have been grouped into ordinal categories, let c denote the number of ordinal categories, and let s_i denote the score that has been assigned to the ith category ($i = 1, 2, \ldots, c$). For the most commonly used version of the C-A test (e.g., the one that is available in StatXact and SAS), equally spaced scores $s_i = i - 1$ are used. Thus, for the data in Table 4.47, the scores 0, 1, 2, 3 would be assigned. (Note that any set of equally spaced scores will yield identical results for the C-A test.) Within the ith category, assume that y_i specimens out of a total of n_i have been classified as "positive" using the biomarker. Then the total sample size is $n = \sum_{i=1}^{c} n_i$. Let $y = \sum_{i=1}^{c} y_i$ denote the total number of positive specimens in the sample of size n, and let $\bar{s} = \left(\sum_{i=1}^{s} n_i s_i\right)/n$ denote the weighted average of the scores (the s-values) assigned to the categories. Then the test statistic for the C-A test for trend is given by

$$\chi_o^2 = \frac{\left(\sum_{i=1}^{k} s_i y_i - \bar{s}y\right)^2}{p(1-p)\left(\sum_{i=1}^{k} n_i s_i^2 - n\bar{s}^2\right)}, \tag{4.115}$$

where $p = y/n$ denotes the overall proportion of "positive" specimens. To perform the approximate version of the C-A test, the test statistic in Equation (4.115) is compared with a χ^2 distribution with one degree of freedom (upper-tailed test only). An exact test for trend based on the test statistic in (4.115) can be performed by using the same conditioning argument as that used in our description of Fisher's exact test in Section 4.9.4.1.

The test statistic for the general permutation test for trend is obtained by applying the formula in Equation (4.115) using whatever scores were assigned to the ordinal categories. (These scores need not be equally spaced.) The general permutation test approach (Gibbons and Chakraborti 2003, Chapter 8) is then used to calculate the exact p-value.

The exact and approximate versions of both the permutation test for trend and the C-A test are available in StatXact, which can also be used to determine the appropriate sample size to use when planning a study that will require either of these tests. The asymptotic and exact versions of the C-A and permutation tests are also available in the FREQ procedure in SAS. SAS code that can be used to perform the C-A and permutation tests for the data in Table 4.47 is provided following Example 4.36.

Example 4.36 Cochran–Armitage and Permutation Tests for Trend

In the Tunstall-Pedoe study, we assigned scores corresponding to the midpoint of each of the four serum cotinine categories (0.00, 0.53, 2.52, and 10.74 ng/mL) and then performed the exact permutation test for trend and the exact C-A test using the FREQ procedure in SAS. For the data in Table 4.47 with midpoint scores, Equation (4.115) yields $\chi_o^2 = 7.76$. The approximate chi-squared test ($df = 1$) yields a p-value of 0.0053, a strongly significant result. The exact upper-tailed p-value for the test statistic in (4.115) is 0.0094, with point probability 0.0001. Putting these results together yields a mid-P value of $0.0094 - {}^1\!/_2(0.0001) = 0.0093$. For the data in Table 4.47 with equally spaced scores, Equation (4.115) yields $\chi_o^2 = 8.05$. The chi-squared test ($df = 1$) yields an approximate p-value of 0.0046 for the C-A test. The exact upper-tailed p-value for the C-A test is 0.0060, with point probability 0.0009. Putting these results together yields a mid-P value of $0.00600 - {}^1\!/_2(0.0009) = 0.0051$. Both tests indicate a strongly significant increasing trend in the prevalence of diagnosed CHD as serum cotinine level increases. This finding, not reported by the authors, would have provided justification for their claim of a gradient of adverse health outcomes across the passive smoking categories. Note that, for both exact tests, the mid-P adjustment had only minimal effect. This is due to the large sample size in this study ($n = 2278$) and the fact that the numbers in each ordinal category did not vary greatly (Table 4.47).

The following SAS code can be used to perform the exact and approximate versions of the C-A and permutation tests for the data in Table 4.47.

```
data tunstall;
input cotinine chd count @@;
datalines;
0.00 0 741   0.53 0 654   2.52 0 534   10.74 0 279
0.00 1  15   0.53 1  20   2.52 1  19   10.74 1  16
;

proc freq data=tunstall order=data; weight count;
     tables cotinine * chd / nocol nopct trend;
     exact trend;
     title1 'Exact Permutation Test for Trend';
     title2 'Using Midpoints of Exposure Categories';
     run;

data tunstall_2;
input cotinine chd count @@;
datalines;
0.00 0 741   1.00 0 654   2.00 0 534   3.00  0 279
0.00 1  15   1.00 1  20   2.00 1  19   3.00  1  16
;
```

```
proc freq data=tunstall_2 order=data; weight count;
     tables cotinine * chd  / nocol nopct trend;
     exact trend;
     title1 'Exact Cochran-Armitage Test for Trend';
     run;
```

One difficulty with the C-A test is that it requires preassigned fixed scores for each level of the ordinal predictor variable. While it was not the case in Example 4.36, the choice of scores can make quite a difference in the value of the test statistic, as well as the approximate and exact p-values (Agresti 2007, pp. 43–44); however, the choice of scores is usually arbitrary and, in some cases, there may be no reasonable way to select appropriate scores. If there is no reasonable justification for the choice of scores, one should simply use scores that are equally spaced. Any choice of equally spaced scores will yield identical results for the C-A and permutation tests. One may also wish to perform a sensitivity analysis to examine the effects that different choices of scores have on the statistical results.

It is known that the C-A test is more powerful when the scores and the observed binomial proportions in the ordinal categories follow a similar observed trend; for example, when both the scores and the proportions follow a linear trend (Neuhäuser and Hothorn 1999). Neuhäuser and Hothorn proposed alternative methods for testing for trend that do not require specifying scores for the categories and are robust with respect to the shape of the dose–response curve. However, to the best of our knowledge, software for performing these methods is not yet available in any commonly used statistical package, so we are currently unable to recommend them for general use.

4.9.6 Choice of a Statistical Method When Both the Predictor and the Outcome are Ordinal

4.9.6.1 Test for Linear-by-Linear Association In their evaluation of salivary cotinine as a biomarker for passive smoking, Cook et al. (1993) considered the association between the number of smokers to whom children had been exposed and their salivary cotinine concentration, measured in ng/mL. They categorized "number of smokers" as 0, 1, 2, and ≥ 3, and salivary cotinine as "non-detectable," 0.1–0.2, 0.3–0.6, 0.7–1.7, 1.8–4.0, 4.1–14.7, and >14.7 ng/mL. The authors stated that "salivary cotinine concentration was strongly related to the number of smokers to whom the child was usually exposed" (p. 16). However, they provided no statistical test results to justify this assertion. Their data are presented in Table 4.48.

As indicated in Table 2.2, the appropriate statistical method for testing for significant association between these two variables would be the linear-by-linear association test (Agresti et al., 1990). In addition, as indicated in Table 2.1, Spearman's correlation (or Kendall's coefficient) could be used to produce a single numerical measure of this association, and a statistical test could be performed to determine if the population value of Spearman's correlation differs from zero (or some other hypothesized

TABLE 4.48 Contingency Table Showing Association Between Number of Smokers to Whom Exposed and Salivary Cotinine Category

	No. of Smokers to Whom Exposed				
Salivary Cotinine Category (ng/mL)	0	1	2	≥3	Total
ND	143	17	1	0	161
0.1–0.2	371	41	3	0	415
0.3–0.6	397	122	11	1	531
0.7–1.7	184	205	76	8	473
1.8–4.0	51	208	186	22	467
4.1–14.7	10	112	232	49	403
>14.7	1	0	29	5	35
Total	1157	705	538	85	2485

Source: Adapted from Table 1 of Cook et al. (1993), with permission from BMJ Publishing Group Ltd.

null value). We also recommend that a CI be reported any time correlation analysis is used. These methods are covered in Section 4.5.2.

In order to perform the linear-by-linear association test, we must first assume that the rows and columns of the $r \times c$ contingency table have been ordered according to some underlying variable. In the example taken from Cook et al. (1993), there is a natural ordering in both the rows (salivary cotinine levels) and columns ("number of smokers"). Following the approach of Mehta and Patel (2005), let x_{ij} denote the count in the (i, j) position of the "ordered" contingency table and consider the test statistic:

$$T_0 = \sum_{i=1}^{r} \sum_{j=1}^{c} u_i v_j x_{ij}, \tag{4.116}$$

where $\{u_1, u_2, \ldots, u_r\}$ are appropriately assigned row scores, and $\{v_1, v_2, \ldots, v_c\}$ are appropriately assigned column scores. Note that $u_1 \leq u_2 \leq \cdots \leq u_r$ and $v_1 \leq v_2 \leq \cdots \leq v_c$. Let $\{m_1, m_2, \ldots, m_r\}$ denote the row totals, and $\{n_1, n_2, \ldots, n_c\}$ denote the column totals of the $r \times c$ table. Under the null hypothesis of no association between the row and column variables, the test statistic given in Equation (4.116) has mean

$$E[T_0] = \frac{\sum_{i=1}^{r} u_i m_i \sum_{j=1}^{c} v_j n_j}{n}, \tag{4.117}$$

and variance

$$\mathrm{Var}[T_0] = \frac{1}{n-1} \left[\sum_{i=1}^{r} u_i^2 m_i - \frac{\left(\sum_{i=1}^{r} u_i m_i \right)^2}{n} \right] \left[\sum_{j=1}^{c} v_j^2 n_j - \frac{\left(\sum_{j=1}^{c} v_j n_j \right)^2}{n} \right], \tag{4.118}$$

where $n = \sum_{j=1}^{c} n_j = \sum_{i=1}^{r} m_i$ is the total sample size.

Since the test statistic given by

$$z_0 = \frac{T_0 - E(T_0)}{\sqrt{\mathrm{Var}(T_0)}} \tag{4.119}$$

is approximately distributed as standard normal under the null hypothesis, one can compare the value of z_0 calculated from the sample data with the standard normal to obtain an approximate p-value. Exact p-values can be obtained for the linear-by-linear association test by considering the conditional permutation distribution of the test statistic T_0 under the null hypothesis. As in our earlier discussion of exact distributions based on the conditional approach (Section 4.9.4.1), the reference set is defined to be the set of all $r \times c$ contingency tables with the same row and column totals as the observed table.

StatXact is capable of performing the exact and approximate versions of the linear-by-linear association test. The FREQ procedure in SAS can be used to perform the linear-by-linear association test, and to calculate the Spearman and Kendall coefficients. The SAS code provided following Example 4.20 can be used to perform inference for the Spearman and Kendall coefficients (see Section 4.5.2). Note that it would not be appropriate to use PCC to measure the association between the ordinal row and column scores in Table 4.48 since such ordinal scores cannot follow a bivariate normal distribution. (See Table 2.1.)

Example 4.37 Linear-By-Linear Association Test

For the data in Table 4.48, the formula in Equation (4.119) yields $z_0 = 37.45$ and $p = 0.0005$ for the normal approximation to the linear-by-linear association test, indicating a strongly significant association between "number of smokers" and salivary cotinine. The sample size in this problem was too large for either StatXact or SAS to perform the exact test. However, with such a large n, we have no reason to doubt the validity of the approximate test. Spearman's correlation also indicates a strongly significant association between the ordinal categories for number of smokers and salivary cotinine: $r_s = 0.72$; 95% Fisher-z CI, 0.70–0.74; $p < 0.001$), as does Kendall's coefficient: $t_b = 0.62$; 95% Fisher-z CI, 0.61–0.64; $p < 0.001$).

SAS code that can used to perform these analyses for the data in Table 4.48 is given below:

```
data cook;
input cotinine smokers count @@;
cards;
0.00 0 143    0.00 1 17     0.00 2 1      0.00 3 0
0.15 0 371    0.15 1 41     0.15 2 3      0.15 3 0
0.45 0 397    0.45 1 122    0.45 2 11     0.45 3 1
1.20 0 184    1.20 1 205    1.20 2 76     1.20 3 8
2.90 0 51     2.90 1 208    2.90 2 186    2.90 3 22
9.40 0 10     9.40 1 112    9.40 2 232    9.40 3 49
```

```
14.7 0 1     14.7 1 0     14.7 2 29    14.7 3 5
;

proc freq order=data; weight count;
      tables  smokers * cotinine / jt measures;
*     exact jt;
      title 'Linear-by-Linear Association Test';
      title2 'Spearman and Kendall Coefficients';
      run;
```

Note that the hypothesis testing and CI results for the SCC and KCC were obtained using the SAS code provided following Example 4.20.

4.9.7 Choice of a Statistical Method When Both the Predictor and the Outcome are Nominal

4.9.7.1 Fisher–Freeman–Halton Test The most commonly used statistical method for examining the association between two nominal variables, regardless of the number of rows and columns, is the chi-square test (Section 3.10.1). However, just as in the case of 2×2 tables, this test is known to have very poor statistical properties, especially if the expected frequencies in any of the cells of the contingency table are too small (Mehrotra et al. 2003), and we do not recommend it for general use.

Just as Fisher's exact test is generally preferable to the traditional chi-square test for 2×2 tables, there is a corresponding exact test that is generally preferable when the number of nominal rows (r) and/or the number of nominal columns (c) are greater than two. This is a generalization of Fisher's exact test known as the Fisher-Freeman-Halton (F-F-H) test (Freeman and Halton 1951). This test can be performed using StatXact or the FREQ procedure in SAS. The F-F-H test is described below.

Example 4.38 Testing Independence in an $r \times c$ Contingency Table

Consider the data in Table 4.49 showing the association of a particular genetic variant of methionine metabolism (CBS c.844_855ins68) in 290 patients with WHO Grade I–III meningioma and 287 controls without the disease (Semmler et al. 2008).

TABLE 4.49 Association Between Allelotype of CBS c.844_855ins68 and Presence of WHO Grade I–III Meningioma

	Number with Variant		
Allelotype	Controls	Patients	Total
dd	253	235	488
id	34	52	86
ii	0	3	3
Total	287	290	577

Source: Adapted from Table 1 of Semmler et al. (2008, p. 101), with permission from the American Association of Neurological Surgeons (http://www.aans.org/).

Semmler et al. wished to examine the utility of CBS c.844_855ins68 and other genetic variants as potential markers for susceptibility to meningioma formation. Their statistical analyses included use of the chi-squared test to test for independence between presence of the genetic variants and presence of meningioma.

In general, for an $r \times c$ contingency table, we wish to test the following hypotheses:

H_0: The row classification variable and the column classification variable are independent.

vs. (4.120)

H_a: The row classification variable and the column classification variable are not independent.

The null hypothesis H_0 in (4.120) can be restated in terms of the marginal probabilities in the population in a manner similar to our description of the chi-square test (Section 3.10.1). To be more specific, let π_{ij} denote the probability that a study subject will be classified as belonging to row i and column j in the $r \times c$ table. Thus, $i = 1, 2, \ldots, r$ and $j = 1, 2, \ldots, c$. Then the marginal probabilities for row i and column j, respectively, are defined by

$$\pi_{i+} = \sum_{j=1}^{c} \pi_{ij}, \quad i = 1, 2, \ldots, r,$$

$$\pi_{+j} = \sum_{i=1}^{r} \pi_{ij}, \quad j = 1, 2, \ldots, c.$$

Using this notation, the null hypothesis H_0 in (4.120) can be rewritten as

$$H_0 : \pi_{ij} = \pi_{i+}\pi_{+j} \text{ for all } (i,j) \text{ pairs.} \qquad (4.121)$$

Whereas the chi-squared test for an $r \times c$ is based on the normal approximation to the multinomial, exact tests such as F-F-H are based on the multiple hypergeometric distribution. Similar to the approach we described for Fisher's exact test (Section 4.9.4.1), Freeman and Halton (1951) considered the "reference set," which is the collection of all $r \times c$ tables with the same marginal totals as those observed in the sample data. For example, if we let m_i denote the total for row i, and n_j denote the total for column j, for the 3×2 data in Table 4.49, the marginal totals are $m_1 = 488$, $m_2 = 86$, $m_3 = 3$, $n_1 = 287$, and $n_2 = 290$. For these data, the exact p-value for the F-F-H test is given by the accumulated multiple hypergeometric probabilities for the set of all 3×2 tables with the same marginal totals that are no more likely to occur than Table 4.49.

*Technical Details of Fisher–Freeman–Halton Test** The main objective of the F-F-H test, as well as the traditional chi-square test, is to determine whether the observed contingency table **x** is consistent with the null hypothesis that the row and column classifications are independent. In order to calculate the exact p-value for the F-F-H test (or the chi-square test, for that matter), the following steps are required.

1. Define a "reference set," denoted by $\mathfrak{R}$, of all $r \times c$ tables in which each table has a known probability of occurring under the assumption that the row and column classifications are independent.
2. Order all of the tables in $\mathfrak{R}$ according to a *discrepancy measure* (i.e., a test statistic) that quantifies the degree to which each $r \times c$ table in $\mathfrak{R}$ deviates from the null hypothesis of independence.
3. Sum the probabilities of all tables in $\mathfrak{R}$ that are at least as discrepant as the observed $r \times c$ table.

Throughout this discussion, we will use $\mathbf{x}$ to denote the $r \times c$ table constructed from the sample data, and $\mathbf{y}$ to denote a typical $r \times c$ table in $\mathfrak{R}$. As discussed in Section 4.9.4.1 when describing Fisher's exact test, the key to exact inference for categorical data is to remove the effect of all nuisance parameters from the distribution of $\mathbf{y}$. For the analysis of $r \times c$ contingency tables, this is accomplished by restricting the sample space to the set of all $r \times c$ tables that have the same row and column totals as the observed table $\mathbf{x}$. Thus, for the F-F-H test, we define the reference set to be

$$\mathfrak{R} = \left\{ \mathbf{y} : \mathbf{y} \text{ is } r \times c;\ \sum_{j=1}^{c} y_{ij} = m_i;\ \sum_{i=1}^{r} y_{ij} = n_j;\ \text{for all } i, j \right\},$$

where y_{ij} is the count in cell (i, j); $i = 1, 2, \ldots, r$; $j = 1, 2, \ldots, c$. Then, under the null hypothesis that rows and columns are independent, the probability of observing any particular $\mathbf{y} \in \mathfrak{R}$ is given by

$$P(\mathbf{y}) = \frac{\prod_{j=1}^{c} n_j! \prod_{i=1}^{r} m_i!}{N! \prod_{j=1}^{c} \prod_{i=1}^{r} y_{ij}!}, . \tag{4.122}$$

where $N = \sum_{j=1}^{c} n_j = \sum_{i=1}^{r} m_i$ is the total sample size.

To perform the exact test of independence of row and column classifications, each $r \times c$ table $\mathbf{y} \in \mathfrak{R}$ is ordered according to its discrepancy measure (i.e., the value of the test statistic calculated from it). Denote this discrepancy measure by $D(\mathbf{y})$. Large absolute values of D provide evidence against the null hypothesis, whereas small absolute values are consistent with H_0. The discrepancy measure (i.e., test statistic) for the F-F-H test, denoted by $D_0(x)$ is given by

$$D_0(x) = -2\log(\gamma P(\mathbf{x})), \tag{4.123}$$

where

$$\gamma = (2\pi)^{(r-1)(c-1)/2}(N)^{-(rc-1)/2} \prod_{i=1}^{r} (m_i)^{(c-1)/2} \prod_{i=1}^{r} (n_j)^{(r-1)/2},$$

and $P(\mathbf{x})$ is calculated using (4.122).

The exact p-value for testing the null hypothesis H_0 in (4.120) using the F-F-H test is calculated by accumulating the null probabilities of all the $r \times c$ tables in $\mathfrak{R}$ that are at least as extreme as the observed table $\mathbf{x}$, as calculated using the F-F-H discrepancy measure. In particular, this p-value is given by

$$p_2 = \Pr[D(\mathbf{y}) \geq D_0(\mathbf{x})] = \sum_{\mathbf{y}:D(\mathbf{y}) \geq D_0(\mathbf{x})} P(\mathbf{y}), \tag{4.124}$$

where $D(\cdot)$ is calculated using Equation (4.123).

For the data in Table 4.49, the F-F-H test statistic, calculated using (4.123), is $D_0(\mathbf{x}) = 7.013$. The exact p-value based on (4.124) is $p_2 = 0.0176$, and the exact point probability of obtaining Table 4.49, as calculated using (4.122), is $P(\mathbf{x}) = 0.0026$. Thus, the mid-P value is given by $0.0176 - {}^1/_2(0.0026) = 0.016$. The p-value for the chi-square test, as reported by Semmler et al. (2008) was 0.039. While this difference in p-values between the chi-square and F-F-H tests does not lead to a different conclusion, a difference of this magnitude could result in different conclusions in other situations. In fact, in our experience, we have encountered examples in which the exact version of the F-F-H test without the mid-P adjustment yielded a lower p-value than the traditional χ^2 test, despite the widely held mistaken belief that the χ^2 test is always more powerful than the F-F-H test.

The F-F-H test can be performed using StatXact or the FREQ procedure in SAS. The following SAS code can be used to perform the F-F-H test for the data in Table 4.49.

```
data meningioma;
input CBS $ group $ count @@;
cards;
dd CONTROL 253   dd CASE 235
id CONTROL 34    id CASE 52
ii CONTROL 0     ii CASE 3
;

proc freq data=meningioma; weight count;
 tables CBS * group / Fisher;
 title 'Fisher-Freeman-Halton Test';
run;
```

PROBLEMS

4.1. The following table provides hypothetical preoperative hemoglobin A1c levels on 21 diabetes mellitus patients and 28 non-diabetic patients undergoing coronary artery bypass graft (CABG) surgery.

A. Use the data in the table to generate descriptive statistics (n, $\bar{x}$, and s) separately for diabetic and non-diabetic patients.

B. Generate side-by-side box plots of the hemoglobin A1c levels of diabetic and non-diabetic patients.

C. Compute 95% CIs on the true mean hemoglobin A1c level of diabetic and non-diabetic patients.

D. Use the appropriate statistical method to compare the hemoglobin A1c levels of diabetic and non-diabetic patients.

Hypothetical Preoperative Hemoglobin A1c Data on 21 Diabetic and 28 Non-Diabetic Patients Undergoing CABG Surgery

Diabetes Status	Hemoglobin A1c (%)					
Diabetic						
	7.4	6.7	8.2	7.2	9.5	
	11.1	8.0	7.2	7.6		
	8.5	6.5	10.1	5.9		
	6.9	9.5	4.3	11.4		
	9.6	10.5	6.7	7.1		
Non-diabetic	5.9	5.6	6.3	5.9	6.9	6.5
	7.6	6.2	5.8	6.0	6.9	5.9
	6.4	5.5	7.1	5.3	6.9	5.6
	5.7	6.9	4.5	7.7	5.3	
	6.9	7.4	5.6	5.8	6.1	

4.2. Seventeen adult subjects were randomly selected from the 2009–2010 National Health and Nutrition Examination Survey (NHANES) data (CDC, 2010). Data on the subjects' age and fasting blood glucose level (mg/dL) are given in the following table. Use the data in the table to determine if there is a significant association between age (years) and fasting blood glucose level (mg/dL).

Age and Fasting Blood Glucose Levels of 17 Randomly Selected Adult Subjects from 2009–2010 NHANES Data

Subject	Age (years)	Fasting Blood Glucose (mg/dL)
1	80	101
2	51	98
3	45	94
4	63	108
5	80	99
6	47	98
7	28	104
8	67	93
9	52	106
10	30	102
11	62	100

(continued)

Subject	Age (years)	Fasting Blood Glucose (mg/dL)
12	25	95
13	64	98
14	26	100
15	51	99
16	40	96
17	71	243

4.3. The serum HDL cholesterol levels (mg/dL) of 74 randomly selected subjects from the NHANES study (CDC 2010) are shown in the following table. Use the appropriate statistical method to compare HDL cholesterol levels across the three ethnic groups.

HDL Cholesterol Levels (mg/dL) of 74 Randomly Selected Subjects from the NHANES Study

Ethnic Group	HDL Cholesterol (mg/dL)				
White	76	40	48	43	48
	35	45	65	28	50
	28	59	55	15	34
	24	48	39	32	60
	44	74	39	90	48
	25	35	45	36	
Black	32	70	44	50	
	49	57	53	56	
	49	98	40	71	
	49	77	29		
	179	43	39		
	75	83	45		
Hispanic	39	62	32	69	
	47	37	28	38	
	59	31	31	32	
	33	48	74	40	
	79	31	48	35	
	42	43	43	42	

4.4. Hypothetical HDL cholesterol and triglyceride levels of 18 adult females are provided in the following table.

A. Use these data to compute Pearson's, Spearman's, and Kendall's sample correlation coefficients. In addition to the sample correlation coefficients, compute the 95% CI for ξ, and the p-value testing H_0: $\xi = 0$.

Hypothetical HDL Cholesterol and Triglyceride Levels of 18 Hypothetical Adult Females

Subject	HDL (mg/dL)	Triglycerides (mg/dL)
1	57	34
2	49	118
3	59	83
4	64	101
5	51	143
6	79	63
7	52	164
8	60	141
9	40	245
10	77	54
11	82	79
12	55	207
13	58	112
14	53	191
15	38	290
16	76	39
17	42	202
18	58	118

B. Use the data to construct normal density plots (or other graphical display) of the HDL cholesterol and triglyceride levels.

C. Use the data to compute measures of skewness and kurtosis for the HDL cholesterol and triglyceride levels.

D. Use the data to perform the Shapiro–Wilk test to assess the normality of the HDL cholesterol and triglyceride levels.

E. Based on the results from Problems B–D above, which of the three correlation coefficients computed in A is the most appropriate measure of the association between HDL cholesterol and triglycerides?

4.5. Suppose a researcher investigating racial disparities in breast cancer detection obtains the data in the following table from a hospital database for the years 2003–2013. Assuming that these data are a representative sample, is there any evidence of a difference in the cancer stage at diagnosis for Caucasians compared to African Americans?

Cancer Stage at Diagnosis of Breast Cancer for Caucasian and African American Women.

Ethnicity	Cancer Stage: Localized	Regional	Distant	Total Number of Women
Caucasian	217	102	17	336
African American	44	33	9	86

4.6. A researcher wants to use the data from the following table to compare the level of a newly discovered biomarker in obese adults diagnosed with diabetes mellitus Type II to obese adults free of diabetes.

A. Using the data in the following table, determine the appropriate statistical method to use to compare the biomarker level of obese adults with and without diabetes.

Biomarker Levels (μg/dL) in Obese Adults With and Without Diabetes Mellitus Type II

Biomarker Level (μg/dL)	
Disease Free	Diabetics
120	265
88	267
120	277
120	326
111	300
117	291
112	249
124	313
121	318
113	292
116	293
122	325
123	290
121	322
122	296
101	243
99	303
119	
109	
112	
111	
107	
122	
106	
122	

B. Use the appropriate statistical method to compare the biomarker levels of obese adults with and without diabetes mellitus Type II.

4.7. A researcher wants to examine the concentrations of an enzyme involved with the metabolism of toxins in workers at a petrochemical company.

A. Determine the appropriate statistical method to use to compare the enzyme concentrations in workers in the PVC production unit of the petrochemical company compared to office workers at the same company using the data in the following table.

B. Use the appropriate statistical method to compare the biomarker concentrations of production workers and office workers.

Enzyme Levels (μg/L) in PVC Production Unit Workers and Office Workers

Enzyme Level (μg/L)	
PVC Production Unit Workers	Office Workers
55	118
54	74
57	133
56	136
54	144
59	102
57	147
57	111
58	106
58	74
63	155
64	135
	143
	144
	178
	112
	77

4.8. Suppose an investigator conducts a study to compare a new chemotherapy regimen for the treatment of colorectal cancer to the standard chemotherapy regimen. Upon enrollment into the study, subjects are assembled into matched pairs so that both subjects in the pair have the same TNM classification. One outcome to be compared is carcinoembryonic antigen (CEA) level 1 month after initiation of chemotherapy. CEA is a biomarker of cancer progression (lower is better). Apply the paired *t*-test, Wilcoxon signed ranks test, and sign test to the data in the following table to compare the CEA levels of subjects treated with the two chemotherapy regimens. Of these three methods, which should be used to compare the chemotherapies' CEA levels and what is the justification for this choice?

CEA Levels in Matched Pairs of Colorectal Cancer Receiving a New Chemotherapy Regimen or the Standard Chemotherapy Regimen

	CEA Level (ng/mL)	
Pair	"New" Treatment Patient	"Standard of Care" Patient
1	17	22
2	29	31
3	14	22
4	5	16
5	2	9
6	7	14
7	25	21
8	3	8
9	11	7
10	33	38

4.9. Use the hypothetical data in the following table to compare the results of three methods for screening patients for Alzheimer's disease (AD): the apolipoprotein E (Apo E) allele test, magnetic resonance imaging (MRI) of the brain, and the cognitive function test (CFT).

Apo E, MRI, and CFT Test Results on Hypothetical Patients

Test Result			Frequency
Apo E	MRI	CFT	
+	+	+	56
−	−	−	119
+	+	−	23
+	−	−	11
+	−	+	25
−	+	+	7
−	+	−	5
−	−	+	44

4.10. A researcher wants to examine the correlation between two biomarkers that pilot data suggest are normally distributed with a Pearson correlation of $r = 0.51$. How many observations are needed in the study to estimate Pearson's correlation coefficient with a precision of $\pm$ 0.1 at the 95% confidence level?

4.11. A researcher wants to examine the correlation between tumor stage and serum carcinoembryonic antigen (CEA) level in patients with urachal adenocarcinoma, a rare form of bladder cancer. For pilot data, the Spearman correlation coefficient (SCC) was 0.82 and Kendall's concordance coefficient (KCC) was 0.60. How many observations are needed in the study to estimate the SCC and KCC with a precision of $\pm$ 0.15 at the 95% confidence level?

4.12. A researcher wants to examine the correlation between two biomarkers that pilot data suggest are normally distributed with a Pearson correlation of $r=0.51$. How many observations are needed in the study to achieve 80% power to test $H_0 : \rho \leq 0.2$ vs. $H_0 : \rho > 0.2$ at the 5% significance level?

4.13. A researcher wants to examine the correlation between tumor stage and serum carcinoembryonic antigen (CEA) level in patients with urachal adenocarcinoma, a rare form of bladder cancer. For pilot data, the Spearman correlation coefficient (SCC) was 0.82 and Kendall's concordance coefficient (KCC) was 0.60. How many observations are needed in the study to achieve 80% power to test $H_0 : \rho \leq 0.5$ vs. $H_0 : \rho > 0.5$ at the 5% significance level?

4.14. A researcher obtains a Spearman's correlation of $r_{sh}=0.15$ for the association between serum concentrations of two liver enzymes in 34 healthy babies and a Spearman's correlation of $r_{sn}=0.66$ in 18 babies with Type B Niemann–Pick disease. Does the correlation of the two enzymes differ significantly between healthy babies and babies with Type B Niemann–Pick disease?

4.15. In serum samples of 104 healthy adults, a researcher obtains a Pearson's correlation of $r_{\text{AB}}=0.78$ between biomarkers A and B, a Pearson's correlation of $r_{\text{AC}}=0.53$ between biomarkers A and C, and a Pearson's correlation of $r_{\text{BC}}=0.31$ between biomarkers B and C. Is there a significant difference in the correlation between biomarkers A and B compared to the correlation between A and C?

4.16. A researcher obtains a baseline Spearman's correlation of $r_{xy}=0.66$ for the association between serum concentrations of two liver enzymes, A and B, in 18 babies with Type B Niemann–Pick disease. After treating these 18 babies with a bone marrow transplant (BMT), suppose the Spearman's correlation of the two liver enzymes is $r_{uv}=0.23$. Given the information below, determine if there is a significant difference in the correlations between the two enzymes before and after the BMT:

- Spearman's correlation between Enzyme A at pre-BMT and at post-BMT is $r_{xu}=0.48$.
- Spearman's correlation between Enzyme A at pre-BMT and Enzyme B at post-BMT is $r_{xv}=0.16$.
- Spearman's correlation between Enzyme A at post-BMT and Enzyme B at pre-BMT is $r_{yu}=0.11$.
- Spearman's correlation between Enzyme B at pre-BMT and at post-BMT is $r_{yv}=0.37$.

4.17. An oncologist wants to compare the correlation of expression of the microRNAs miR-181b and miR-340 in patients with chronic lymphocytic leukemia

(CLL) to the expression of these same two microRNAs in chronic myelogenous leukemia (CML) patients. Pilot data yielded a Spearman's correlation coefficient of $r_{sl} = 0.8762$ for CLL patients and $r_{sm} = 0.7217$ for CML patients. Using estimates of the true correlation from the pilot data, how many patients are needed per group to achieve 80% power to detect a difference between the CML and CLL microRNA correlations at the 5% significance level?

4.18. Suppose researchers want to compare the expression of osteonectin in paired ovarian and omental tissue samples from women diagnosed with high-grade ovarian cancer. The hypothetical study results are shown in the following table. Is there a difference in osteonectin expression in ovarian vs. omental tissue samples?

Osteonectin Expression in Ovarian and Omental Tissue Samples from 206 Women Diagnosed with High-Grade Ovarian Cancer.

		Ovarian Sample	
		Expressed	Not Expressed
Omental sample	Expressed	39	32
	Not Expressed	11	124

4.19. Suppose serum blood urea nitrogen (BUN) levels (mg/dL) were ordered routinely for all patients' annual physical examination as part of an assessment of kidney function. The BUN levels of nine randomly selected patients are shown in the following table. Subject number 6 was taking antibiotics known to increase BUN levels when her blood sample was drawn. Is the BUN of subject number 6 an outlier?

The BUN Levels of Nine Randomly Selected Patients

Subject	BUN (mg/dL)
1	11.3
2	10.1
3	13.0
4	12.3
5	10.5
6	14.8
7	12.6
8	12.8
9	13.7

5

VALIDATION OF BIOMARKERS

5.1 OVERVIEW OF METHODS FOR ASSESSING CHARACTERISTICS OF BIOMARKERS

In this chapter, we provide an overview of methods for what is commonly referred to as "validation" of a biomarker. We restrict our consideration of the process of validating a biomarker to establishing that it has both adequate reliability and adequate validity.

According to the *Dictionary of Epidemiology*, *reliability* refers to "the degree to which the results obtained by a measurement procedure can be replicated" (Porta 2008, p. 214). Thus, "reliability" is often used interchangeably with "repeatability" and "reproducibility." On the other hand, the *validity* of a biomarker is defined to be the extent to which it measures what it is intended to measure. Here, we are thinking in terms of *measurement validity*; there are many other types of validity, including analytical validity, clinical validity, study validity, etc. (Porta 2008, p. 251).

In our view, one must establish that the biomarker is reliable before dealing with issues of validity; if once cannot safely assume that the biomarker will provide equivalent results upon repeated determinations using the same biological specimen, it will not be suitable for practical use. Two important aspects of the reliability of any measurement process are *intra-rater* and *inter-rater* reliability (IER). The intra-rater reliability (IAR) (also called *intra-observer agreement*) of a biomarker describes the degree of agreement between two determinations made by the same individual

Analysis of Biomarker Data: A Practical Guide, First Edition. Stephen W. Looney and Joseph L. Hagan.

on the same biological specimen under "identical" conditions. The IER (sometimes called *inter-observer agreement*) of a biomarker describes the degree of agreement between the determinations made by two different individuals on the same biological specimen under "identical" conditions. A reliable biomarker must exhibit adequate levels of both types of reliability.

Interchangeability is a fundamental concept underlying both reliability and validity. For a biomarker to have adequate IAR, it must be the case that, regardless of when the analyst performs the determination, it is safe to assume that an equivalent result will be obtained. For a biomarker to have adequate IER, it must be the case that, regardless of which analyst performs the biomarker determination, it is safe to assume that equivalent results will be obtained. For a biomarker to have adequate validity, it must be the case that the biomarker determination can be substituted in place of the gold standard result (assuming that there is a gold standard) or in place of the standard test result (if there is no gold standard).

Other terms are also used to describe desirable properties for a biomarker. *Accuracy* is often used interchangeably with validity; for example, the validity of a diagnostic test (as measured by sensitivity and specificity when a gold standard is available) is often referred to as *diagnostic accuracy*. *Precision* is another desirable characteristic of any biomarker. According to the *Dictionary of Epidemiology*, precision is the "relative lack of random error" (Porta 2008, p. 190). In statistics, we often think of summary measures of variability such as the standard deviation, inter-quartile range, and coefficient of variation as measures of precision. More precisely, the inverse of any such measure of the variability of a biomarker could be used to measure the precision of the biomarker (Porta p. 191). Similarly, the standard error could be thought of as a measure of the *imprecision* of a sample estimate. We do not consider assessment of precision in our discussion of the process of validating a biomarker. Shoukri (2011, Chapter 4) provides a very thorough coverage of this topic, as do many textbooks that deal with the statistical validation of measurement processes in clinical chemistry (Jones and Payne 1997; Fritsma and McGlasson 2012).

In terms of the organization of this chapter, in Section 5.2 we begin with a discussion of measures of agreement in general, separately for discrete variables (Section 5.2.1) and for continuous variables (Section 5.2.2). Next, in Section 5.3, we discuss the use of these general measures of agreement in assessing the reliability of biomarkers, first for dichotomous biomarkers (Section 5.3.2), and then for continuous biomarkers (Section 5.3.3). In Section 5.4, we discuss the use of measures of agreement in assessing the validity of biomarkers, first in the case where a gold standard is available (Section 5.4.2), separately for dichotomous (Section 5.4.2.1) and continuous biomarkers (Section 5.4.2.2). In Section 5.4.3, we discuss the use of measures of agreement in assessing validity when a gold standard is not available, separately for dichotomous (Section 5.4.3.1) and continuous (Section 5.4.3.2) biomarkers. Finally, in Sections 5.4.4 and 5.4.5, we discuss the assessment of criterion and construct validity for biomarkers. These concepts are usually thought of as being specific to the psychometric evaluation of measurement scales, but they are also applicable to the validation of biomarkers and assessment of them should be considered for inclusion any time the validity of a new biomarker is being evaluated.

5.2 GENERAL DESCRIPTION OF MEASURES OF AGREEMENT

5.2.1 Discrete Variables

5.2.1.1 Cohen's Kappa Consider Table 5.1, which shows agreement between two "judges," each of whom has evaluated n "targets" as being either "positive" or "negative."

For example, each "judge" could be a psychiatrist and each "target" could be a patient who is being diagnosed as either neurotic or psychotic, as in the hypothetical data given in Table 5.2.

The two most commonly used measures of agreement between two dichotomous variables are the *Index of Crude Agreement*, given by

$$p_0 = \frac{a+d}{n}, \tag{5.1}$$

and *Cohen's kappa*, given by

$$\hat{\kappa} = \frac{p_0 - \hat{p}_e}{1 - \hat{p}_e}, \tag{5.2}$$

where p_e is the percentage agreement between the two variables that "can be attributed to chance" (Cohen 1960). If the evaluation by Judge A is truly independent of the evaluation by Judge B (i.e., the only way they could agree is by random chance), the degree of agreement attributable to chance can be estimated using the Law of Probability for Independent Events by

$$\hat{p}_e = p_{1\bullet}p_{\bullet 1} + p_{2\bullet}p_{\bullet 2},$$

where the estimated probabilities that Judge A classifies a target as either "positive" or "negative" are given by $p_{1.} = \frac{f_1}{n}$ and $p_{2.} = 1 - p_{1.}$, respectively. Similarly, $p_{.1} = \frac{g_1}{n}$ and $p_{.2} = 1 - p_{.1}$ are the estimated probabilities that Judge B will classify a target as either "positive" or "negative." After substituting the above result for $\hat{p}_e$ into (5.2) and simplifying, the formula for Cohen's kappa can now be written as

$$\hat{\kappa} = \frac{2\,(ad - bc)}{n^2(f_1 g_2 + f_2 g_1)}, \tag{5.3}$$

using the notation in Table 5.1.

TABLE 5.1 Agreement Between Two Dichotomous Variables

	Judge B		
Judge A	Positive	Negative	Total
Positive	a	b	f_1
Negative	c	d	f_2
Total	g_1	g_2	n

TABLE 5.2 Agreement Between Two Psychiatrists on 85 Patients

	Psychiatrist B		
Psychiatrist A	Neurotic	Psychotic	Total
Neurotic	75	1	76
Psychotic	5	4	9
Total	80	5	85

Kappa = 1 if there is perfect agreement ($b = c = 0$), kappa = −1 if there is perfect disagreement ($a = d = 0$), and kappa = 0 if agreement is no better than chance ($p_0 = \hat{p}_e$). Landis and Koch (1977, p. 165) provide guidelines for interpreting the magnitude of kappa, which are provided in Table 5.3.

Alternatively, Fleiss et al. (2003, p. 604) characterize values greater than 0.75 as representing "excellent agreement beyond chance," values between 0.40 and 0.75 as "fair to good," and values below 0.40 as "poor agreement beyond chance."

The approximate variance of $\hat{\kappa}$ is given by

$$\widehat{\text{Var}}(\hat{\kappa}) = \frac{1}{n(1-\hat{p}_e)^2}\left(\sum_{i=1}^{2} p_{ii}\{1-(p_{i.}+p_{.i})(1-\hat{\kappa})\}^2 + (1-\hat{\kappa})^2 \sum_{i\neq j}^{2} p_{ij}(p_{i.}+p_{.j})^2 - \{\hat{\kappa}-\hat{p}_e(1-\hat{\kappa})\}^2\right) \tag{5.4}$$

where n is the number of targets being rated by the two judges, and $p_{ij} = \frac{n_{ij}}{n}$, $i = 1, 2; j = 1, 2$. Approximate $100(1-\alpha)\%$ Wald-type confidence limits for κ are given by $\hat{\kappa} \pm z_{\alpha/2}\widehat{\text{Var}}(\hat{\kappa})$.

The FREQ procedure in SAS can be used to calculate $\hat{\kappa}$ and find the approximate Wald confidence limits.

TABLE 5.3 Guidelines for Interpreting Coefficient Kappa

Value of Kappa	Interpretation
<0.00	Poor
0.00–0.20	Slight
0.21–0.40	Fair
0.41–0.60	Moderate
0.61–0.80	Substantial
0.81–1.00	Almost perfect

Example 5.1 Coefficient Kappa

For the data in Table 5.2, we obtain $p_0 = \frac{a+d}{n} = \frac{75+4}{85} = 0.9294$ and $\hat{p}_e = p_{1.}p_{.1} + p_{2.}p_{.2} = (0.8941)(0.9412) + (0.1059)(0.0588) = 0.8478$. Applying Equation (5.2), we obtain $\hat{\kappa} = \frac{p_0 - \hat{p}_e}{1 - \hat{p}_e} = \frac{0.9294 - 0.8478}{1 - 0.8478} = 0.54$, which indicates that there is "moderate" agreement between the two judges using the Landis and Koch criteria (Table 5.3). Using (5.4), we obtain $\widehat{\text{Var}}(\hat{\kappa}) = 0.02713$. This yields an approximate 95% confidence interval (CI) for κ of $0.54 \pm 1.96\sqrt{0.010641} = (0.21, 0.86)$. Note how wide this CI is, in spite of the relatively large sample size ($n = 85$). Based on the endpoints of this CI, the true agreement could be anywhere from "fair" to "almost perfect."

The following SAS code can be used to perform the calculations in Example 5.1:

```
options formchar="|----|+|---+=|-/\<>*";

data  kappa;
      input A B count @ @;
      datalines;
1 1 75  1 2 1
2 1 5   2 2 4
;

proc  format;
      value firstfmt
   1='Neurotic'
   2='Psychotic';

proc  format;
    value secondfmt
   1='Neurotic'
   2='Psychotic';

proc  freq order=data; weight count;
      format A firstfmt.;
      format B secondfmt.;
      tables A*B / nopercent nocol norow agree;
      title1 'Coefficient kappa';
      run;
```

Despite its popularity, various authors have noted several deficiencies with coefficient kappa (Feinstein and Cicchetti 1990, p. 545; Byrt et al. 1993, p. 425). These deficiencies include the following: (1) if no targets are classified into one of the two categories ("positive" or "negative") by either judge, kappa = 0. (2) If there are no agreements between the two judges for either of the two categories, kappa < 0. (3)

The value of kappa is affected by any imbalance in the relative frequency of "positive" and "negative" in the sample. (Rather large imbalances of this nature are commonly encountered with biomarker data in practice.) The larger the imbalance, the larger the value of $\hat{p}_e$ and the smaller the value of kappa. (4) The value of kappa is affected by any imbalance in the relative frequencies of "positive" for Judge A and "positive" for Judge B. The larger the imbalance, the smaller the expected agreement, and the larger the value of kappa.

In order to adjust for these deficiencies, Byrt et al. (1993) proposed an alternative measure of agreement, the *prevalence-adjusted and bias-adjusted kappa* (*PABAK*),

$$\text{PABAK} = \frac{(n_{11} + n_{22}) - (n_{12} + n_{21})}{n} = 2p_0 - 1, \qquad (5.5)$$

where p_0 is the index of crude agreement given in Equation (5.1). (Note that PABAK is equivalent to the proportion of "agreements" between the variables minus the proportion of "disagreements.") The approximate variance of PABAK is given by $\widehat{\text{Var}}(PABAK) = \frac{4p_0(1-p_0)}{n}$ and approximate $100(1-\alpha)\%$ confidence limits for the true value of PABAK are given by $\text{PABAK} \pm z_{\alpha/2}\sqrt{\widehat{\text{Var}}(\text{PABAK})}$. The value of PABAK can be interpreted using the Landis and Koch or Fleiss et al. criteria for interpreting kappa (Table 5.3).

Example 5.2 Deficiencies of Coefficient Kappa

As an illustration of some of the deficiencies of κ, consider the hypothetical data on the agreement between two judges given in Table 5.4.

Even though the two judges agree on 80% of the targets, the value of kappa is only –0.08 (95% CI −0.25, 0.08), indicating poor agreement according to the Landis and Koch criteria. This illustrates two of the previously mentioned deficiencies: (1) Since the two judges did not agree on any of the targets that they classified as negative, kappa < 0. (2) The value of kappa is also adversely affected by the difference in the relative frequencies of positive (90%) and negative (10%) targets in the sample. The PABAK coefficient, which adjusts for both of these shortcomings, is equal to $2p_0 - 1 = 2(0.80) - 1 = 0.60$ (Equation (5.5). Using the formula for $\widehat{\text{Var}}$(PABAK) given

TABLE 5.4 Hypothetical Data Showing Agreement Between Two Judges

	Judge B		
Judge A	Positive	Negative	Total
Positive	80	15	95
Negative	5	0	5
Total	85	15	100

above, we find $\widehat{\text{Var}}(\text{PABAK}) = \frac{4p_0(1-p_0)}{n}$ =0.0064, and an approximate 95% CI for the true PABAK value of $0.60 \pm 1.96\sqrt{.0064} = (0.44, 0.76)$. This indicates "fair to good" agreement using the Fleiss et al. criteria. We feel these results provide a much more accurate representation of the degree of agreement between the two judges than the results for kappa. We recommend that the PABAK coefficient be reported in addition to coefficient kappa any time there is an indication that kappa does not adequately measure the degree of agreement between the dichotomous ratings of two "judges."

The following SAS code can be used to perform the calculations for PABAK for the data in Table 5.4. It also produces exact confidence limits for PABAK using the exact CI procedure for a binomial proportion.

```
options formchar="|----|+|---+=|-/\<>*";

data  table5_4;
      input judge_a judge_b count @@;
      cards;
      1 1 80   1 0 15
      0 1 5   0 0 0
      ;

data  crude;
      set table5_4;
      if ((judge_a = 1 and judge_b = 1) or (judge_a = 0 and
      judge_b = 0)) then correct = 1; else correct = 0;

proc  freq data=crude;
   weight count;
   tables correct / binomial(level="1" p = .75);
   exact binomial;
      output out = pabak binomial;
   run;

data  pabak;
      set pabak;
      crude = _bin_;
      pabak = 2*_bin_-1;
      se_pabak = 2*e_bin;
      lcl_pabak_a = 2*l_bin-1;
      ucl_pabak_a = 2*u_bin-1;
      lcl_pabak_e = 2*xl_bin-1;
      ucl_pabak_e = 2*xu_bin-1;
      keep crude pabak se_pabak lcl_pabak_a ucl_pabak_a
      lcl_pabak_e ucl_pabak_e;
```

```
proc print data = pabak;
     var crude pabak se_pabak lcl_pabak_a ucl_pabak_a
     lcl_pabak_e ucl_pabak_e;
     title1 'PABAK';
     run;
```

In addition to using κ and PABAK to measure overall agreement, it is also advisable to assess the agreement separately for those targets that appear to be positive and those that appear to be negative. Such measures can be used to help diagnose the type(s) of disagreement that may be present.

Cicchetti and Feinstein (1990) proposed indices of *average positive agreement* (p_{pos}) and *average negative agreement* (p_{neg}) for this purpose. Using the same notation as in Table 5.1, p_{pos} and p_{neg} are calculated as follows:

$$p_{\text{pos}} = \frac{a}{(f_1 + g_1)/2} \tag{5.6}$$

$$p_{\text{neg}} = \frac{d}{(f_2 + g_2)/2}.$$

Note that the denominators of p_{pos} and p_{neg} are the average number of targets that the two methods classify as positive and negative, respectively. Following Graham and Bull (1998), let

$$\phi_{11} = [2/(2p_{11} + p_{12} + p_{21}] - [4p_{11}/(2p_{11} + p_{12} + p_{21})^2], \tag{5.7}$$

$$\phi_{12} = \phi_{21} = -2p_{11}/(2p_{11} + p_{12} + p_{21})^2,$$

and

$$\phi_{22} = 0.$$

Then the variance of p_{pos} can be estimated using

$$\widehat{\text{Var}}(p_{\text{pos}}) = \frac{1}{n}\left(\sum_{i=1}^{2}\sum_{j=1}^{2}\phi_{ij}^2 p_{ij} - \left(\sum_{i=1}^{2}\sum_{j=1}^{2}\phi_{ij}p_{ij}\right)^2\right).$$

Similarly, let

$$\gamma_{11} = 0, \tag{5.8}$$

$$\gamma_{12} = \gamma_{21} = -2p_{22}/(2p_{22} + p_{12} + p_{21})^2,$$

and

$$\gamma_{22} = [2/(2p_{22} + p_{12} + p_{21})] - [4p_{22}/(2p_{22} + p_{12} + p_{21})^2].$$

Then the variance of p_{neg} can be estimated using

$$\widehat{\text{Var}}(p_{\text{neg}}) = \frac{1}{n}\left(\sum_{i=1}^{2}\sum_{j=1}^{2}\gamma_{ij}^2 p_{ij} - \left(\sum_{i=1}^{2}\sum_{j=1}^{2}\gamma_{ij}p_{ij}\right)^2\right).$$

Approximate $100(1-\alpha)\%$ Wald-type CIs for the true values of p_{pos} and p_{neg} are given by $p_{\text{pos}} \pm z_{\alpha/2}\sqrt{\widehat{\text{Var}}(p_{\text{pos}})}$ and $p_{\text{neg}} \pm z_{\alpha/2}\sqrt{\widehat{\text{Var}}(p_{\text{neg}})}$, respectively.

Simulation results due to Graham and Bull (1998) suggest that these approximate CIs provide adequate coverage for $n > 200$. For smaller n, they recommend that a bootstrap or Bayesian procedure be used to construct the CI. However, they do not provide software for implementing either of these approaches, both of which require rather extensive programming.

Example 5.3 Indices of Positive and Negative Agreement

For the data in Table 5.4, applying the formulas in (5.6) yields $p_{\text{pos}} = \frac{80}{(95+85)/2} = 88.9\%$ and $p_{\text{neg}} = \frac{0}{(5+15)/2} = 0.0\%$. Thus, there is moderate overall agreement between the two judges (as measured by the PABAK coefficient of 0.60), "almost perfect agreement" on targets that appear to be positive, and no agreement on targets that appear to be negative. Using the formulas in (5.7), we obtain an approximate 95% CI for the true value of p_{pos} of $p_{\text{pos}} \pm z_{\alpha/2}\sqrt{\widehat{\text{Var}}(p_{\text{pos}})} = 88.9\% \pm 1.96(2.5\%) = (84.0\%, 93.7\%)$. Of course, this interval may be inaccurate since $n < 200$. For p_{neg}, the formulas in (5.8) yield $\widehat{\text{Var}}(p_{\text{neg}}) = 0$. Thus, we cannot obtain a meaningful CI for the true value of p_{neg}.

The following SAS code can be used to find the estimates of p_{pos} and p_{neg} and the associated Wald CIs for the data in Table 5.4. This code is also provided on the companion website.

```
/*
p_pos, p_neg and their 95% CIs can be calculated by inputting the
data corresponding to the four cell counts (a b c d) for any
2x2 table.
*/

title1 'Calculation of SE and CI for p_pos & p_neg';

data ci;
input a b c d;
```

```
datalines;
80 15 5 0
;

data ci;
  set ci;
n = a+b+c+d;
p11 = a/n;
p12 = b/n;
p21 = c/n;
p22 = d/n;

/*p_pos calculation*/

o1 = 2/(2*p11+p12+p21)-4*p11/((2*p11+p12+p21)**2);
o2 = -2*p11/((2*p11+p12+p21)**2);
o3 = o2;
o4 = 0;
var_ppos  =  (1/n)*((o1**2)*(p11)+(o2**2)*(p12)+(o3**2)*(p21)+
(o4**2)*(p22)) - ((o1)*(p11)+(o2)*(p12)+(o3)*(p21)+
(o4)*(p22))**2;
se_ppos = sqrt(var_ppos);
ppos = a/(((a+ b)+(a+c))/2);
u_ci_ppos = ppos+(1.96)*(se_ppos);
l_ci_ppos = ppos-(1.96)*(se_ppos);
/*p_neg calculation*/

y1 = 0;
y2 = (-2*p22)/(2*p22+p12+p21)**2;
y3 = y2;
y4 = 2/(2*p22+p12+p21)-((4*p22)/(2*p22+p12+p21)**2);

var_pneg = (1/n)*((y1**2)*(p11)+ (y2**2)*(p12)+ (y3**2)*(p21)+
(y4**2)*(p22) ) - ((y1)*(p11)+ (y2)*(p12)+ (y3)*(p21)+
(y4)*(p22))**2;
se_pneg = sqrt(var_pneg);
pneg=d/(((c+ d)+(b+ d))/2);
u_ci_pneg = pneg+(1.96)*(se_pneg);
l_ci_pneg = pneg-(1.96)*(se_pneg);

run;
proc print data=ci;
var ppos se_ppos l_ci_ppos u_ci_ppos pneg se_pneg l_ci_pneg
u_ci_pneg ;
run;
```

5.2.1.2 Extensions of Coefficient Kappa

Two Categories, More than Two Judges The method of Fleiss (1971) can be used to calculate an overall measure of agreement among $k > 2$ "judges" making dichotomous determinations. For example, consider the hypothetical data in Table 5.5, which shows the results of 20 psychiatric patients who were diagnosed as depressed (coded as "1") or not depressed (coded as "0") by four different psychiatrists.

Let n denote the number of targets, and k denote the number of judges. Let y_{ij} denote the determination (either "positive" or "negative") based on the jth judge for the ith target, where $y_{ij} = 1$ for "positive" and $y_{ij} = 0$ for "negative," and let

$$y_i = \sum_{j=1}^{k} y_{ij}$$

denote the number of positive ratings on the ith target. Fleiss (1971) generalized Cohen's kappa to a new measure, $\hat{\kappa}_f$ as follows:

$$\hat{\kappa}_f = \frac{p_0 - \hat{p}_e}{1 - \hat{p}_e},$$

TABLE 5.5 Agreement Among 4 Psychiatrists in the Diagnosis of 20 Patients

	Psychiatrist				
Patient	1	2	3	4	Total
1	0	0	0	0	0
2	0	0	1	0	1
3	1	1	1	1	4
4	1	1	1	1	4
5	1	1	0	1	3
6	0	0	0	0	0
7	1	0	0	0	1
8	0	0	0	0	0
9	1	1	1	1	4
10	1	0	1	1	3
11	1	1	1	1	4
12	1	1	0	1	3
13	1	1	0	0	2
14	1	0	1	0	2
15	1	0	0	0	1
16	0	0	1	0	1
17	1	1	1	1	4
18	1	0	0	0	1
19	1	1	1	1	4
20	1	1	1	1	4
Total	15	10	11	10	46

Source: Adapted from Table 4.4 of Shoukri (2004, p. 50). Reproduced with permission of CRC Press in the format Republish in a Book via Copyright Clearance Center.

where

$$p_0 = 1 - \frac{2}{n} \sum_{i=1}^{n} \frac{y_i(k - y_i)}{k(k-1)}, \tag{5.9}$$

$$\hat{p}_e = 1 - 2\hat{\pi}(1 - \hat{\pi}),$$

and

$$\hat{\pi} = \frac{\sum_{i=1}^{n} y_i}{nk}.$$

Example 5.4 Generalized Coefficient Kappa (Two Categories, Four Judges)

For the hypothetical data in Table 5.5, the formulas in (5.9) yield $p_0 = 0.733$, $\hat{\pi} = 0.575$, $\hat{p}_e = 0.511$, and $\hat{\kappa}_f = 0.454$, indicating only "moderate" agreement among the four psychiatrists. Of course, Cohen's kappa (or the PABAK coefficient) could be used to measure the agreement between any two of the psychiatrists.

The value of $\hat{\kappa}_f$ can be calculated for the data in Table 5.5 using R, as indicated below. The R code given below is also provided in the companion website.

```
# Read in Table 5.5 data
Psych_1 <- c(0, 0, 1, 1, 1, 0, 1, 0, 1, 1, 1, 1, 1, 1, 1, 0, 1,
1, 1, 1)
Psych_2 <- c(0, 0, 1, 1, 1, 0, 0, 0, 1, 0, 1, 1, 1, 0, 0, 0, 1,
0, 1, 1)
Psych_3 <- c(0, 1, 1, 1, 0, 0, 0, 0, 1, 1, 1, 0, 0, 1, 0, 1, 1,
0, 1, 1)
Psych_4 <- c(0, 0, 1, 1, 1, 0, 0, 0, 1, 1, 1, 1, 0, 0, 0, 0, 1,
0, 1, 1)
Table5.5 <- cbind(Psych_1, Psych_2, Psych_3, Psych_4)

Check data
Table5.5
install.packages("irr", dependencies=TRUE)

library(irr)
# Table 5.5 data analysis
# Fleiss' Kappa
kappam.fleiss(Table5.5, exact = FALSE, detail = FALSE)
```

Fleiss and Cuzick (1979) generalized $\hat{\kappa}_f$ to the situation where there is a variable number of evaluations (e.g., targets are possibly evaluated by differing numbers of judges.). Letting k_i denote the number of judges for target i, this generalized version of $\hat{\kappa}_f$ is given by the following:

$$\hat{\kappa}_f = 1 - \left\{ \left[\sum_{i=1}^{n} \frac{y_i(k_i - y_i)}{k_i} \right] / n(\bar{k} - 1)\hat{\pi}(1 - \hat{\pi}) \right\}, \tag{5.10}$$

where $\bar{k} = \sum_{i=1}^{n} k_i/n$ is the average number of ratings per target and $\hat{\pi} = \sum_{i=1}^{n} y_i/n\bar{k}$ is the overall proportion of targets scored as "1."

It is sometimes useful to express coefficient kappa or one of its generalizations in terms of an appropriate intra-class correlation coefficient (ICC) calculated on the 0/1 agreement data. For example, Fleiss and Cuzick (1979) showed that the generalized version of $\hat{\kappa}_f$ given in (5.10) is asymptotically equivalent to the estimated ICC obtained if one uses a particular random effects model to describe the variation in the observed values y_{ij}. As shown by Fleiss and Cuzick (1979), if n is sufficiently large, there is very little difference between $\hat{\kappa}_f$ in (5.10) and the ICC approximation, so it makes little difference which one is used in terms of the estimated degree of agreement. An advantage of using the ICC-based version of $\hat{\kappa}_f$ is that a formula for an approximate variance (and hence an approximate CI) is available (Mak, 1988). As best we can determine, there is no closed-form expression for the variance (either exact or approximate) of $\hat{\kappa}_f$. (A formula is available under the assumption that the true value of κ_f is zero. While such a variance estimate would be useful if the primary goal of the analysis is to test H_0: $\kappa_f = 0$, it is of no use if one wishes to find a CI for κ_f in the general estimation setting when there is no particular interest in testing a specific hypothesis concerning κ_f. Typically, when evaluating a new biomarker, there is no underlying hypothesis of interest.)

The ICC-based approximation to $\hat{\kappa}_f$ is given by

$$\hat{\rho}_{\mathrm{I}} = \frac{\mathrm{MST} - \mathrm{MSE}}{\mathrm{MST} + (k_o - 1)\mathrm{MSE}}, \tag{5.11}$$

where MSE denotes the mean square for error, MST denotes the mean square for targets, and k_0 denotes the appropriate summary measure of the number of judges who evaluated the targets. Note that this corresponds to ICC(1,1) in Shrout and Fleiss (1979). When calculated from continuous data, this version of the ICC would be appropriate for a method comparison study (see Section 5.4.3.2), in which each of n targets is evaluated by a different set of k judges, who are randomly selected from a larger population of judges.

The formulas for calculating the quantities in (5.11) using the 0/1 data are as follows:

$$\mathrm{MST} = \left[\sum_{i=1}^{n} \frac{y_i^2}{k_i} - \frac{\left(\sum_{i=1}^{n} y_i \right)^2}{K} \right] / (n - 1), \tag{5.12}$$

$$\text{MSE} = \left(\sum_{j=1}^{n} y_i - \sum_{i=1}^{n} \frac{y_i^2}{k_i} \right) / (K - n),$$

$$k_0 = \left(K - \frac{\sum_{j=1}^{n} k_i^2}{K} \right) / (n - 1),$$

where $K = \sum_{i=1}^{n} k_i$ is the total number of ratings of the n targets. (Note that if each target is evaluated by the same number of judges, k, then $k_0 = k$).

Using the notation in Shoukri (2004, p. 49), the estimated variance of $\hat{\rho}_{\text{I}}$ is given by the following:

$$\text{Var}(\hat{\rho}_{\text{I}}) = (V_{11}C_1^2 - 2C_1C_2V_{12} + V_{22}C_2^2)/n, \tag{5.13}$$

where

$$C_1 = 1/(\bar{k} - 1)\hat{\pi}(1 - \hat{\pi}),$$

$$C_2 = \frac{C_1\{1 + (\bar{k} - 1)[\hat{\rho}_{\text{I}} + 2\hat{\pi}(1 - \hat{\rho}_{\text{I}})]\}}{\bar{k}},$$

$$V_{11} = \sum_{i=1}^{n} \left(\frac{y_i^4}{n_i^2} - f_i^2 \right) / n,$$

$$V_{12} = \sum_{i=1}^{n} \left(\frac{y_i^3}{n_i} - n_i f_i \hat{\pi} \right) / n,$$

$$V_{22} = \sum_{i=1}^{n} \left(y_i^2 - n_i^2 \hat{\pi}^2 \right) / n,$$

and $f_i = \hat{\pi}(1 - \hat{\pi})[1 + (k_i - 1)\hat{\rho}_{\text{I}}] + n_i \hat{\pi}^2$.

As before, $\bar{k}$ is the average number of ratings per target and $\hat{\pi}$ is the overall proportion of targets scored as "1."

Example 5.5 The ICC-Based Approximation to Generalized Kappa

Applying the formulas in (5.11)–(5.13) to the hypothetical data in Table 5.5, we obtain $\hat{\rho}_{\text{I}} = 0.471$, with an approximate variance of 0.01514. This yields a Wald-type approximate 95% CI of $\hat{\rho}_{\text{I}} \pm z_{\alpha/2}\sqrt{\text{Var}\left(\hat{\rho}_{\text{I}}\right)} = 0.471 \pm 1.96\left(\sqrt{0.01514}\right) = (0.230, 0.712)$. Note that there is very little practical difference between the ICC-based estimate of 0.471 and the value of $\hat{\kappa}_f = 0.454$ obtained using (5.10).

The value of $\hat{\rho}_I$ can be calculated for the data in Table 5.5 using either the SPSS syntax or R code given below, or the SAS code given on the companion website. Note, however, that the CIs that are available using SPSS or R code *are not correct* for these data since they are based on the assumption that the data are normally distributed. Since the data in Table 5.5 are 0/1, this cannot be the case.

```
SPSS

RELIABILITY
 /VARIABLES=Psych_1 Psych_2 Psych_3 Psych_4
 /SCALE('ALL VARIABLES') ALL
 /MODEL=ALPHA
 /ICC=MODEL(ONEWAY).

R code

# Read in Table 5.5 data
Psych_1 <- c(0, 0, 1, 1, 1, 0, 1, 0, 1, 1, 1, 1, 1, 1, 1, 0, 1,
1, 1, 1)
Psych_2 <- c(0, 0, 1, 1, 1, 0, 0, 0, 1, 0, 1, 1, 1, 0, 0, 0, 1,
0, 1, 1)
Psych_3 <- c(0, 1, 1, 1, 0, 0, 0, 0, 1, 1, 1, 0, 0, 1, 0, 1, 1,
0, 1, 1)
Psych_4 <- c(0, 0, 1, 1, 1, 0, 0, 0, 1, 1, 1, 1, 0, 0, 0, 0, 1,
0, 1, 1)

Table5.5 <- cbind(Psych_1, Psych_2, Psych_3, Psych_4)

Table5.5

install.packages("irr", dependencies=TRUE)
library(irr)

# Table 5.5 data analysis

# ICC
icc(Table5.5, model = ("oneway"),
type = c("agreement"),
unit = c("single"))
```

Two judges, more than two nominal categories In some instances, each "judge" is asked to classify a "target" as belonging to one of c nominal categories, where $c \geq 3$. For example, consider the hypothetical data in Table 5.6 on the diagnoses of 100 patients by two psychiatrists (Fleiss et al. 2003, p. 599).

TABLE 5.6 Hypothetical Data Showing Diagnoses of 100 Patients by 2 Psychiatrists

	Psychiatrist B			
Psychiatrist A	Psychotic	Neurotic	Organic	Total
Psychotic	75	1	4	80
Neurotic	5	4	1	10
Organic	0	0	10	10
Total	80	5	15	100

Source: Adapted from Table 18.1 of Fleiss et al. (2003, p. 599). Used with permission from John Wiley & Sons.

In this more general setting, it is useful to represent the cross-classification data between the two judges in the general form given in Table 5.7, in which the numbers falling into the different cells have now been replaced by the estimated probabilities, obtained by dividing the cell counts n_{ij} by the total sample size, n. Using this notation, the index of crude agreement (i.e., the overall proportion of observed agreement) is given by $p_0 = \sum_{i=1}^{c} p_{ii}$ and the estimated proportion of agreement that can be attributed to chance is given by $\hat{p}_e = \sum_{i=1}^{c} p_{i.}p_{.i}$. Equation (5.2) can now be used to measure agreement between the two judges across all categories: $\hat{\kappa} = \frac{p_0 - \hat{p}_e}{1 - \hat{p}_e}$. The approximate variance of $\hat{\kappa}$ is given by a generalization of Equation (5.4):

$$\widehat{\text{Var}}(\hat{\kappa}) = \frac{1}{n(1-\hat{p}_e)^2}\left(\sum_{i=1}^{c} p_{ii}\{1-(p_{i.}+p_{.i})(1-\hat{\kappa})\}^2 + (1-\hat{\kappa})^2 \sum_{i \neq j}^{c} p_{ij}(p_{i.}+p_{.j})^2 - \{\hat{\kappa} - \hat{p}_e(1-\hat{\kappa})\}^2\right), \quad (5.14)$$

where n is the number of targets evaluated by the two judges, and $p_{ij} = \frac{n_{ij}}{n}$, $i = 1, 2, \ldots, c$; $j = 1, 2$. As in the case of two categories, approximate $100(1-\alpha)\%$ Wald confidence limits for κ are given by $\hat{\kappa} \pm z_{\alpha/2}\sqrt{\widehat{\text{Var}}(\hat{\kappa})}$.

TABLE 5.7 Agreement Between Two Judges for More than Two Categories

	Judge B				
Judge A	1	2	...	c	Total
1	p_{11}	p_{12}	...	p_{1c}	$p_{1.}$
2	p_{21}	p_{22}	...	p_{2c}	$p_{2.}$
.	.	.		.	.
.	.	.		.	.
.	.	.		.	.
c	p_{c1}	p_{c2}	...	p_{cc}	$p_{c.}$
Total	$p_{\cdot 1}$	$p_{\cdot 2}$	...	$p_{\cdot c}$	1

Example 5.6 Generalized Coefficient Kappa (Three Nominal Categories, Two Judges)

For the data given in Table 5.6, $p_0 = \sum_{i=1}^{c} p_{ii} = 0.89$, $\hat{p}_e = 0.66$, and $\hat{\kappa} = \frac{p_0 - \hat{p}_e}{1 - \hat{p}_e} = 0.68$. Applying Equation (5.14), we obtain $\widehat{\text{Var}}(\hat{\kappa}) = 0.007569$, which yields an approximate 95% CI(κ) of $0.68 \pm 1.96\sqrt{0.007569} = (0.51\text{–}0.85)$, indicating "moderate-to-substantial" agreement between the two psychiatrists, according to the Landis and Koch criteria.

The value of $\hat{\kappa}$ can be calculated for the data in Table 5.6 using R, as indicated below. This R code is also provided on the companion website.

```
# Generate Table 5.6 data
PsychiatristA  <-  c(rep("Psychotic",  80), rep("Neurotic",  10),
rep("Organic", 10))
PsychiatristB  <-  c(rep("Psychotic",  75), rep("Neurotic",  1),
rep("Organic",  4), rep("Psychotic",  5), rep("Neurotic",  4),
rep("Organic",  11))

# Check data
table(PsychiatristA, PsychiatristB)

Table5.6 <- cbind(PsychiatristA, PsychiatristB)

# Table 5.6 data analysis
kappam.fleiss(Table5.6, exact = FALSE, detail = FALSE)
```

More than Two Judges, More than Two Nominal Categories In this scenario, each of n "targets" is classified by some number of "judges" as belonging to one of c nominal categories, where $c \geq 3$. For example, consider the hypothetical data in Table 5.8, in which 20 psychiatric patients were assigned to one and only one of the following diagnoses: (1) depression, (2) personality disorder, (3) schizophrenia, (4) neurosis, (5) other. Six psychiatrists were potentially available to evaluate each patient; however, not all patients were evaluated by all six.

Fleiss (1971) proposed a generalized version of coefficient kappa that is applicable in this situation. Let k_{ij} denote the number of judges who assign subject i to category j ($i = 1, 2, \ldots, n$; $j = 1, 2, \ldots, c$). Fleiss proposed the following measure of overall agreement that is equivalent to the index of crude agreement when $k = 2$, $c = 2$, and all targets are evaluated by all judges:

$$p_0 = \frac{\sum_{i=1}^{n}\sum_{j=1}^{c} k_{ij}^2 - nk}{nk(k-1)}. \tag{5.15}$$

TABLE 5.8 Agreement Among 6 Psychiatrists in the Diagnosis of 20 Patients

	Diagnosis				
Patient	Depression	Personality Disorder	Schizophrenia	Neurosis	Other
1	0	0	0	6	0
2	0	3	0	0	0
3	0	1	4	0	0
4	0	0	0	0	6
5	0	3	0	0	0
6	2	0	4	0	0
7	0	0	4	0	0
8	2	0	3	0	0
9	2	0	0	4	0
10	0	0	0	0	6
11	1	0	0	5	0
12	1	1	0	0	0
13	0	3	3	0	0
14	1	0	0	5	0
15	0	2	0	3	0
16	0	0	5	0	0
17	3	0	0	1	0
18	5	1	0	0	0
19	0	2	0	4	0
20	1	0	2	0	0
Total	18	16	25	28	12

Source: Adapted with permission from Table 1 of Fleiss (1971). Copyright © (1971) by the American Psychological Association.

The estimated proportion of agreement that can be attributed to chance is given by

$$\hat{p}_e = \sum_{j=1}^{c} p_j^2,$$

where

$$p_j = \frac{\sum_{i=1}^{n} k_{ij}}{nk}.$$

Equation (5.2) can now be used to measure agreement between the two judges across all categories: $\hat{\kappa}_{mc} = \frac{p_0 - \hat{p}_e}{1 - \hat{p}_e}$. (The subscript mc denotes "multiple categories.")

Example 5.7 Generalized Coefficient Kappa (Five Nominal Categories, Six Judges)

For the hypothetical data given in Table 5.8, the formula in Equation (5.15) yields $p_0 = \frac{\sum_{i=1}^{n} \sum_{j=1}^{c} k_{ij}^2 - nk}{nk(k-1)} = \frac{383 - (20)(6)}{(20)(6)(5)} = 0.438$. Furthermore, $\hat{p}_1 = 0.150$, $\hat{p}_2 = 0.133$,

$\hat{p}_3 = 0.208$, $\hat{p}_4 = 0.100$, and $\hat{p}_e = \sum_{j=1}^{c} p_j^2 = 0.148$. Thus, $\hat{\kappa}_{mc} = \frac{p_0 - \hat{p}_e}{1 - \hat{p}_e} = \frac{0.438 - 0.148}{1 - 0.148}$ $= 0.341$.

5.2.1.3 Weighted Kappa It is sometimes desired to measure agreement between two judges on a collection of n targets, each of which is assigned an ordinal score by each judge. If we label these ordinal scores by 1, 2, ... , c, then the observed proportions of agreement and disagreement for the c ordinal categories can be put in the format of Table 5.7. As an example, consider the data in Table 5.9 on the agreement between two neurologists who independently classified 149 possible multiple sclerosis (MS) patients into one of the following ordinal categories: (1) certain MS, (2) probable MS, (3) possible MS, and (4) doubtful, unlikely, or definitely not MS (Westlund and Kurland 1953).

Independent of the data on agreement and disagreement between the two judges, *agreement weights*, denoted by w_{ij}, $i = 1, 2, \ldots, c; j = 1, 2, \ldots, c$, are also assigned to each of the c^2 cells in Table 5.7, where it is understood that the rows and columns have been ordered. These weights are assigned so that $0 \leq w_{ij} < 1$ for $i \neq j$ (i.e., the judges are treated symmetrically) and $w_{ii} = 1$ (i.e., exact agreement is given maximal weight). The estimated weighted agreement between the two judges is given by

$$p_{0w} = \sum_{j=1}^{c} \sum_{i=1}^{c} w_{ij} p_{ij},$$

and the estimated weighted proportion of agreement that can be attributed to chance is given by

$$p_{ew} = \sum_{j=1}^{c} \sum_{i=1}^{c} w_{ij} p_{i.} p_{.j}.$$

Then, using Equation (5.2), weighted kappa is given by

$$\hat{\kappa}_w = \frac{p_{0w} - \hat{p}_{ew}}{1 - \hat{p}_{ew}}, \tag{5.16}$$

TABLE 5.9 Agreement Between 2 Neurologists on 149 Possible MS Patients

	Neurologist B				
Neurologist A	Certain	Probable	Possible	Unlikely	Total
Certain	38	5	0	1	44
Probable	33	11	3	0	47
Possible	10	14	5	6	35
Unlikely	3	7	3	10	23
Total	84	37	11	17	149

Source: Adapted from Table 1 of Landis and Koch (1977, p. 161). Used with permission from John Wiley & Sons.

with approximate variance

$$\widehat{\text{Var}}(\hat{\kappa}_{\text{w}}) = \frac{1}{n(1-\hat{p}_{\text{ew}})^2}\left(\sum_{i=1}^{c}\sum_{j=1}^{c} p_{ij}[w_{ij} - (\overline{w}_{i.} + \overline{w}_{.j})(1-\hat{\kappa}_{\text{w}})]^2 - [\hat{\kappa}_{\text{w}} - \hat{p}_{\text{ew}}(1-\hat{\kappa}_{\text{w}})]^2\right),$$

and $100(1 - \alpha)\%$ Wald-type approximate confidence limits for κ_{w} given by $\hat{\kappa}_{\text{w}} \pm z_{\alpha/2}\sqrt{\widehat{\text{Var}}(\hat{\kappa}_{\text{w}})}$. Note that when $w_{ij} = 0$ for $i \neq j$ (i.e., all disagreements are given an equal weight of zero), weighted kappa is equivalent to unweighted kappa.

The weights in weighted kappa are intended to give more weight to disagreements near the main diagonal than those further away from the diagonal. Various weights have been proposed (Fleiss et al. 2003, p. 609), but the most commonly used weights are given by

$$w_{ij} = 1 - \frac{(i-j)^2}{(c-1)^2}. \tag{5.17}$$

For example, since there are four ordered categories in Table 5.9, a disagreement occurring in the (1,2), (2,1), (2,3), (3,2), (3,4), or (4,3) positions would be given a weight of 8/9. A disagreement occurring in the (1,3), (3,1), (2,4), or (4,2) positions would be given a weight of 5/9, and a disagreement occurring in the (1,4) or (4,1) positions would be given a weight of 0.

Example 5.8 Weighted Kappa

For the data in Table 5.9, applying the formulas in (5.16) yields $\hat{\kappa}_{\text{w}} = 0.38$, $\widehat{\text{Var}}(\hat{\kappa}_{\text{w}}) = 0.002673$, and an approximate 95% CI(κ_{w}) of (0.28, 0.48). If the ordinal nature of the categories is ignored, we obtain $\hat{\kappa} = 0.21$, $\widehat{\text{Var}}(\hat{\kappa}) = 0.002550$, and an approximate 95% CI(κ_{w}) of (0.11, 0.31). Thus, taking the ordinal nature of the classifications into account results in a somewhat larger estimate of the agreement between the neurologists.

The following SAS code can be used to perform the calculations for weighted kappa (and unweighted kappa) for the data in Table 5.9:

```
options formchar="|----|+|---+=|-/\<>*";

proc  format;
      value MSfmt
   1='Certain'
   2='Probable'
   3='Possible'
   4='Unlikely';
```

```
data   weighted_kappa;
       input A B count @@;
       format A B MSfmt.;
       datalines;
       1 1 38 1 2 5 1 3 0 1 4 1
       2 1 33 2 2 11 2 3 3 2 4 0
       3 1 10 3 2 14 3 3 5 3 4 6
       4 1 3  4 2 7 4 3 3 4 4 10
       ;

proc   freq data=weighted_kappa;
       tables A*B / nopercent nocol norow agree;
       weight count;
       title1 'Weighted kappa';
       run;
```

Weighted kappa based on the weights given in (5.17) can be shown to be equivalent to other possible measures of agreement between two ordinal variables. Fleiss and Cohen (1973) showed that $\hat{\kappa}_{\mathrm{w}}$ can be interpreted as an ICC based on a random effects ANOVA model in which the values $1, 2, \ldots, c$ are treated as *bona fide* data, under the assumption that the n targets and the two judges are both random samples from larger populations of targets and judges, respectively. This corresponds to the ICC(2,1) in Shrout and Fleiss (1979). (See Section 5.2.2.2 for a description of the ICC.) In addition, Shoukri (2004, pp. 41–42) has shown that $\hat{\kappa}_{\mathrm{w}}$ using the weights in (5.17) is equivalent to Lin's coefficient of concordance (LCC) between two ordinal variables whose possible values are $1, 2, \ldots, c$. (See Section 5.2.2.2 for a description of the LCC.) Because of these equivalencies and since the weights given in (5.17) are the most commonly used, we will not consider other possible choices for the weights in weighted kappa. Note, however, that if the ordinal categories are assigned values other than $1, 2, \ldots, c$, the equivalence between $\hat{\kappa}_{\mathrm{w}}$ and the ICC no longer holds.

5.2.2 Continuous Variables

5.2.2.1 Pearson's Correlation Coefficient Agreement between two continuous variables X and Y is most commonly measured using Pearson's correlation coefficient (PCC), typically denoted by r (see Section 3.8). However, it has been known since at least 1973 that this is not an appropriate use for the PCC (Westgard and Hunt, 1973). As is commonly known, the PCC measures the *strength of linear association* between two variables, not agreement. It is important to distinguish between *agreement* and *correlation*. There is perfect *agreement* between two variables X and Y if and only if all points in a scatterplot of Y versus X fall exactly on the line $Y = X$; however, there is perfect *correlation* between Y and X if all points in the scatterplot fall exactly on *any* straight line. See Westgard and Hunt (1973) and Altman and Bland (1983) for discussions of other shortcomings of the PCC as a measurement of agreement.

TABLE 5.10 Hypothetical Data on Agreement Between Judges A and B

Target	Judge A(X)	Judge B(Y)
1	206	31
2	28	4
3	112	17
4	98	14
5	104	16
6	47	7
7	73	11
8	43	4
9	93	14
10	57	7
11	87	10

To illustrate how misleading the PCC can be as a measure of agreement, consider the hypothetical data presented in Table 5.10. As a first step in assessing agreement between X and Y, we recommend that one always construct the scatterplot between Y and X and then superimpose the line $Y = X$ on the scatterplot to get an idea of how much the agreement between X and Y deviates from 1.0. The recommended scatterplot for the data in Table 5.10 is provided in Figure 5.1.

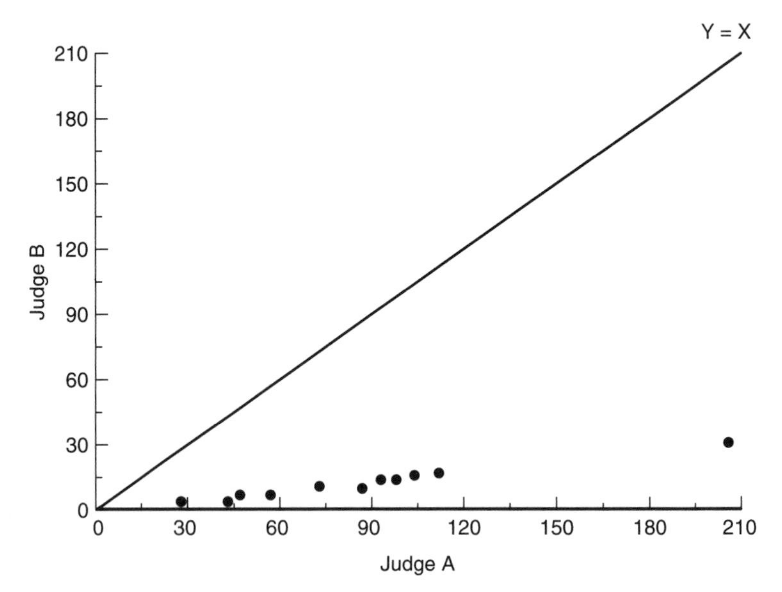

FIGURE 5.1 Scatterplot of hypothetical data on agreement between Judges A and B with the line of perfect agreement ($Y = X$) superimposed. Reprinted from Looney and Hagan (2008), with permission from Elsevier.

For the hypothetical data in Table 5.10, the PCC between X and Y is almost perfect, $r = 0.989$. However, there is an obvious deviation from perfect agreement, with each value for X being consistently less than the corresponding value for Y. In the sections that follow, we will describe various alternatives to the PCC for measuring agreement between continuous variables and illustrate them using the data in Table 5.10.

5.2.2.2 Alternatives to Pearson's Correlation Coefficient

Intra-class Correlation Coefficient The most commonly recommended alternative to the PCC for measuring agreement between continuous measurements is the ICC, denoted by r_I (Shrout and Fleiss 1979). Using an example presented by Shrout and Fleiss, suppose that one wishes to measure the agreement among k "judges," each of whom has evaluated n "targets" on some continuous scale. For example, each "judge" could be a psychiatrist and each "target" could be a patient who is being evaluated on a measurement scale (e.g., severity of depression) by each psychiatrist. Table 5.11 contains some hypothetical data illustrating this scenario.

The ICC is a measure of the size of the *within* variability (i.e., variability attributed to the heterogeneity among the judges' evaluations of the targets) relative to the *between* variability (i.e., variability attributed to the heterogeneity among the targets being analyzed by the judges).

The ICC ranges between 0 and 1, inclusive, with $r_I = 0$ indicating no agreement at all (large within-target variability and zero between-target variability), and $r_I = 1$ indicating perfect agreement (zero within-target variability and large between-target variability). Fleiss et al. (2003, p. 604) provided guidelines for interpreting the magnitude of the value of r_I as a measure of agreement (Table 5.12).

Suppose that n targets are each evaluated by k judges, with each judge assigning a value of some continuous variable to each target. There are several versions of the ICC, each of which can provide a valid measure of agreement depending on which set of underlying assumptions is most appropriate (Shrout and Fleiss 1979). The version of the ICC that is used most commonly to measure reliability of a continuous

TABLE 5.11 Agreement Among Four Judges on Six Targets

	Judge				
Target	1	2	3	4	Mean
1	9	2	5	8	6.0
2	6	1	3	2	3.0
3	8	4	6	8	6.5
4	7	1	2	6	4.0
5	10	5	6	9	7.5
6	6	2	4	7	4.8
Mean	7.7	2.5	4.3	6.7	5.3

Source: Adapted with permission from Table 2 of Shrout and Fleiss (1979). Copyright © (1979) by the American Psychological Association.

biomarker (see Section 5.3.3) is based on the assumption that the n targets constitute a random sample of all possible targets and that the k judges constitute a random sample of all possible judges. (This is denoted by ICC (2,1) in Shrout and Fleiss.) The most commonly used method for calculating the appropriate ICC under these assumptions is to further assume that the observed values of the evaluations of the targets by the judges follow a two-way random effects model with interaction:

$$Y_{ij} = \mu + \alpha_i + \beta_j + (\alpha\beta)_{ij} + \varepsilon_{ij}; \quad 1 \le i \le n; \quad 1 \le j \le k; \tag{5.18}$$

where

Y_{ij} = evaluation value for target i by judge j,
μ = population mean response,
α_i = offset in mean response for target i,
β_j = offset in mean response for judge j,
$(\alpha\beta)_{ij}$ = degree to which the ith judge departs from their usual rating when confronted by the jth target,
ε_{ij} = evaluation measurement error.

The assumptions that underlie this model are as follows: for $1 \le i \le n$, $1 \le j \le k$, α_i, β_j, $(\alpha\beta)_{ij}$, and ε_{ij} are all independent; $\alpha_i \sim N(0, \sigma_T^2)$, $\beta_j \sim N(0, \sigma_J^2)$, $(\alpha\beta)_{ij} \sim N(0, \sigma_I^2)$, and $\varepsilon_{ij} \sim N(0, \sigma_\varepsilon^2)$, where $N(\theta, \delta^2)$denotes the normal distribution with mean θ and variance δ^2. All of these assumptions taken together imply that $Y_{ij} \sim N(\mu, \sigma^2)$, where $\sigma^2 = \sigma_T^2 + \sigma_J^2 + \sigma_I^2 + \sigma_\varepsilon^2$. The population value of the ICC is defined to be $\rho_I = \max[0, \sigma_T^2/\sigma^2]$ and the sample value r_I is obtained by replacing the variance components σ_T^2 and σ^2 by their sample estimates obtained from the least-squares fit of the two-way random effects model in (5.18). After some simplification,

$$r_I = \frac{\text{MST} - \text{MSE}}{\text{MST} + (k-1)\text{MSE} + k(\text{MSJ} - \text{MSE})/n}, \tag{5.19}$$

where MSE denotes the mean square for error, MST denotes the mean square between targets, MSJ denotes the mean square for judges, k denotes the number of judges who evaluate each target, and n denotes the number of targets. The formulas for calculating these mean squares are as follows:

$$\text{MST} = k \sum_{i=1}^{n} (\bar{y}_{i.} - \bar{\bar{y}})^2/(n-1), \tag{5.20}$$

$$\text{MSJ} = n \sum_{j=1}^{k} (\bar{y}_{.j} - \bar{\bar{y}})^2/(k-1),$$

$$\text{MSE} = \left(\sum_{i=1}^{n} \sum_{j=1}^{k} (y_{ij} - \bar{\bar{y}})^2 - (n-1)\text{MST} - (k-1)\text{MSJ} \right) / (nk - n - k + 1)$$

where

$$\bar{y}_{i.} = \sum_{j=1}^{k} y_{ij}/m, \ \ \bar{y}_{.j} = \sum_{i=1}^{n} y_{ij}/n, \ \ \bar{\bar{y}} = \sum_{i=1}^{n} \bar{y}_{i.}/n.$$

Let

$$\upsilon = \frac{(k-1)(n-1)\{kr_{\text{I}}F_{\text{J}} + n[1 + (k-1)r_{\text{I}}] - kr_{\text{I}}\}^2}{(n-1)k^2 r_{\text{I}}^2 F_{\text{J}}^2 + \{n[1 + (k-1)r_{\text{I}}] - kr_{\text{I}}\}^2},$$

where $F_{\text{J}} = \text{MSJ/MSE}$. Define $F^* = F_{\alpha/2,\, n-1,\, \upsilon}$ and $F_* = F_{\alpha/2,\, \upsilon,\, n-1}$, where $F_{\gamma,\, df1,\, df2}$ is the general notation for the upper-γ percentage point of the F distribution with df_1 and df_2 degrees of freedom. Then, following Shrout and Fleiss (1979), an approximate 95% CI for ρ_{I} is given by (LCL, UCL), where:

$$\text{LCL} = \frac{n(\text{MST} - F^*\text{MSE})}{F^*[k\text{MSJ} + (kn - k - n)\text{MSE}] + n\text{MST}}, \tag{5.21}$$

and

$$\text{UCL} = \frac{n(F_*\text{MST} - \text{MSE})}{k\text{MSJ} + (kn - k - n)\text{MSE}] + nF_*\text{MST}}.$$

Example 5.9 Intra-Class Correlation Coefficient, *ICC*(2,1)

For the data in Table 5.11, Equations (5.19) and (5.20) yield $r_{\text{I}} = 0.290$, indicating "poor" agreement according to the Fleiss criteria. Using (5.21), an approximate 95% CI (ρ_{I}) is given by (0.019, 0.761). Note the adverse effect that the small sample size ($n = 6$ targets) has on the width of the CI.

There is an alternative version of the ICC that would be appropriate for a method comparison study (see Section 5.4.3.2), in which each of n targets is evaluated by the same k judges, who are the only judges of interest. (This is denoted by ICC(3,1) in Shrout and Fleiss (1979).) The estimated ICC can be derived using a slightly different version of the two-way ANOVA model given in (5.18), in which judges are no longer treated as a random effect. This alternative mixed effects model is given by

$$Y_{ij} = \mu + \alpha_i + \beta_j + (\alpha\beta)_{ij} + \varepsilon_{ij}; \ \ 1 \le i \le n; \ \ 1 \le j \le k; \tag{5.22}$$

where

Y_{ij} = evaluation value for target i by judge j,
μ = population mean response,
α_i = offset in mean response for target i,

β_j = offset in mean response for judge j,

$(\alpha\beta)_{ij}$ = degree to which the jth judge departs from their usual rating when confronted by the ith target,

ε_{ij} = evaluation measurement error.

The assumptions that underlie this model are as follows: for $1 \le i \le n$, $1 \le j \le k$, α_i and ε_{ij} are independent; $\alpha_i \sim N(0, \sigma_T^2)$, $(\alpha\beta)_{ij} \sim N(0, \sigma_{\mathrm{I}}^2)$, and $\varepsilon_{ij} \sim N(0, \sigma_\varepsilon^2)$. Note that "judges" is no longer a random effect; rather, it is a fixed effect subject to the constraint $\sum_{j=1}^{k} \beta_j = 0$. Only the interaction components for different targets are independent; for the same target, say the ith, the interaction components are assumed to satisfy $\sum_{j=1}^{k} (\alpha\beta)_{ij} = 0$. A consequence of this constraint is that the covariance between any two interaction components for the same target, $(\alpha\beta)_{ij}$ and $(\alpha\beta)_{ij'}$, say, is equal to $-\sigma_{\mathrm{I}}^2/(k-1)$. All of these assumptions taken together imply that $Y_{ij} \sim N(\mu, \sigma^2)$, where $\sigma^2 = \sigma_T^2 + \sigma_{\mathrm{I}}^2 + \sigma_\varepsilon^2$. As before, the population value of this alternative ICC is defined to be $\rho_{\mathrm{I}}^* = \max[0, \sigma_T^2/\sigma^2]$ and the sample value r_{I}^* is obtained by replacing the variance components σ_T^2 and σ^2 by their sample estimates obtained from the least-squares fit of the two-way mixed effects model in (5.22). The alternative version of the sample ICC is given by

$$r_{\mathrm{I}}^* = \frac{\mathrm{MST} - \mathrm{MSE}}{\mathrm{MST} + (k-1)\mathrm{MSE}}, \tag{5.23}$$

where MST and MSE are calculated as in Equation (5.20).

To find an approximate $\mathrm{CI}(\rho_{\mathrm{I}}^*)$, let $F_{\mathrm{T}} = \mathrm{MST/MSE}$, $F_{\mathrm{L}} = F_T/F_{\alpha/2, n-1, (n-1)(k-1)}$, and $F_{\mathrm{U}} = F_T F_{\alpha/2, (n-1)(k-1), (n-1)}$. Then, again following Shrout and Fleiss (1979), an approximate 95% CI for ρ_{I}^* is given by (LCL*, UCL*), where

$$\mathrm{LCL}^* = \frac{F_{\mathrm{L}} - 1}{F_{\mathrm{L}} + (k-1)} \text{ and } \mathrm{UCL}^* = \frac{F_{\mathrm{U}} - 1}{F_{\mathrm{U}} + (k-1)}. \tag{5.24}$$

This version of the ICC takes into account the fact that the judges are fixed, and not a random sample from some hypothetical population of judges.

There is a third type of ICC described by Shrout and Fleiss (1979). It is based on a scenario in which each of n targets is evaluated by a different set of k judges, who are randomly selected from a larger population of judges. The underlying random effects ANOVA model differs from the models in (5.18) and (5.22), namely,

$$Y_{ij} = \mu + \beta_j + w_{ij}; \quad 1 \le i \le n; \quad 1 \le j \le k;$$

where

Y_{ij} = evaluation value for target i by judge j,

μ = population mean response,

β_j = offset in mean response for judge j,

w_{ij} = residual component.

TABLE 5.12 Guidelines for Interpreting the Intra-class Correlation Coefficient (ICC)

Value of ICC	Interpretation
<0.40	Poor
0.40–0.75	Fair to good
0.75	Excellent

The "residual component," as described by Shrout and Fleiss, is equal to the sum of the judge effect, the judge × target interaction, and the error term. The assumptions that underlie this model are as follows: for $1 \le i \le n$, $1 \le j \le k$, β_j and ε_{ij} are independent; $\beta_j \sim N(0, \sigma_{\mathrm{J}}^2)$, $\varepsilon_{ij} \sim N(0, \sigma_{\varepsilon}^2)$.

Because the scenario underlying this model (each of n targets is evaluated by a different set of k judges) is rarely, if ever, used in biomarker validation studies, the ICC resulting from it (denoted ICC(1,1) by Shrout and Fleiss) is generally not useful when analyzing biomarker data. However, the point estimate of ICC(1,1) is computationally equivalent to the ICC that Fleiss and Cuzick (1979) showed is asymptotically equivalent to the generalized version of $\hat{\kappa}_f$ described in Section 5.2.1.2. (See Example 5.5.) However, the CI for the true ICC(1,1) provided in Shrout and Fleiss (1979) is not appropriate for the ICC described by Fleiss and Cuzick.

Example 5.10 Intra-Class Correlation Coefficient, ICC(3,1)

For the data in Table 5.11, Equation (5.23) yields $r_{\mathrm{I}}^* = 0.715$, indicating "fair to good" agreement according to the Fleiss et al. criteria (Table 5.12). Using Equation (5.24), an approximate 95% CI (ρ_I) is given by (0.342, 0.946). This is quite a departure from the results obtained if the judges are assumed to be a random sample and r_{I} is used to measure agreement instead of r_{I}^* (see Example 5.9).

The SAS code that can be used to calculate the estimates of the ICC for the data in Examples 5.9 and 5.10 is provided on the companion website. It can also be downloaded from http://support.sas.com/documentation/onlinedoc/stat/ex_code/121/intracc.html.

The following SPSS syntax can be used to calculate the ICCs and the corresponding CIs for Examples 5.9 and 5.10:

***Example 5.9* This syntax produces ICC(2,1).**

```
RELIABILITY
 /VARIABLES=judge1 judge2 judge3 judge4
 /SCALE('ALL VARIABLES') ALL
 /MODEL=ALPHA
 /ICC=MODEL(RANDOM) TYPE(ABSOLUTE) CIN=95 TESTVAL=0.
```

*** Example 5.10* This syntax produces ICC(3,1).**

```
RELIABILITY
 /VARIABLES=judge1 judge2 judge3 judge4
 /SCALE('ALL VARIABLES') ALL
 /MODEL=ALPHA
 /ICC=MODEL(MIXED) TYPE(CONSISTENCY) CIN=95 TESTVAL=0.
```

The following R code will also produce the ICCs and the corresponding CIs for Examples 5.9 and 5.10:

```
# Read in Table 5.11 data
Judge_1 <- c(9, 6, 8, 7, 10, 6)
Judge_2 <- c(2, 1, 4, 1, 5, 2)
Judge_3 <- c(5, 3, 6, 2, 6, 4)
Judge_4 <- c(8, 2, 8, 6, 9, 7)
Table5.11 <- cbind(Judge_1, Judge_2, Judge_3, Judge_4)

Table5.11
install.packages("irr", dependencies=TRUE)
library(irr)

# Example 5.9 data analysis

# ICC(2,1)

icc(Table 5.11, model = c("twoway"),
type = c("agreement"),
unit = c( "single"), r0 = 0, conf.level = 0.95)

# Example 5.10 data analysis

# ICC(3,1)

icc(Table5.11, model = c("twoway"),
type = c("consistency"),
unit = c( "single"), r0 = 0, conf.level = 0.95)
```

The SPSS syntax and R code given above are also provided on the companion website.

Lin's Coefficient of Concordance Lin (1989, 2000) proposed an alternative to the ICC that is also useful for measuring agreement between two continuous variables: LCC. The sample value of the LCC, denoted by r_c, is given by

$$r_c = \frac{2\,s_{12}}{s_1^2 + s_2^2 + (\bar{x}_1 - \bar{x}_2)^2} \tag{5.25}$$

where

s_{12} = covariance of X_1 and X_2,
$\bar{x}_1$ = mean of X_1,
$\bar{x}_2$ = mean of X_2,
s_1^2 = variance of X_1,
s_2^2 = variance of X_2.

It can be shown that if there is perfect agreement between X_1 and X_2, $r_c = 1$; if there is perfect disagreement, $r_c = -1$; and, for all other situations, $-1 < r_c < 1$. The value of the LCC can be interpreted using the Fleiss et al. criteria given in Table 5.12 for the ICC.

The approximate variance of Lin's coefficient is given by

$$\widehat{\text{Var}}(r_c) = \frac{1}{n-2}\left[\left(\frac{1-r^2}{r^2}r_c^2(1-r_c^2)\right) + \left(2r_c^3(1-r_c)\frac{(\bar{x}_1-\bar{x}_2)^2}{s_1 s_2 r}\right) - r_c^4\frac{(\bar{x}_1-\bar{x}_2)^4}{2s_1^2 s_2^2 r^2}\right], \tag{5.26}$$

where r is the Pearson correlation coefficient (PCC) for X_1 and X_2, and n is the number of targets for which paired observations for X_1 and X_2 are obtained. When $n \geq 30$, an approximate $100(1 - \alpha)\%$ Wald-type CI for the population value of LCC, denoted by ρ_c, can be obtained using $r_c \pm z_{\alpha/2}\sqrt{\widehat{\text{Var}}(r_c)}$. When $n < 30$, an approximate CI based on the bootstrap approach is recommended (Cheng and Gansky 2006).

Example 5.11 Lin's Coefficient of Concordance

To illustrate a situation in which there is strong correlation, but poor agreement, again consider the hypothetical data in Table 5.10. For these data, $n = 11$, $\bar{x} = 12.27$, $\bar{y} = 86.18$, $s_x = 7.70$, $s_y = 48.31$, $s_{xy} = 367.85$, $r = 0.989$. Therefore, from Equations (5.25) and (5.26),

$$r_c = \frac{2s_{12}}{s_x^2 + s_y^2 + (\bar{x}-\bar{y})^2} = \frac{2(367.85)}{(7.70)^2 + (48.31)^2 + (12.27 - 86.18)^2} = 0.088$$

and $\hat{se}(r_c) = 0.037$. An approximate 95% CI for ρ_c based on 1000 bootstrap samples is given by (0.024, 0.126). (Note that this CI will be slightly different each time the SAS code is run, since it is based on randomly generated bootstrap samples.) For the data in Table 5.10, the 95% Wald interval is given by (0.015, 0.160), which would not be appropriate since $n < 20$.

As pointed out previously, the PCC between X and Y for these data is almost perfect, $r = 0.989$, 95% CI (0.957, 0.997); however, LCC is only 0.088. For the ICCs (Section 5.2.2.2), $r_I = 0.095$, 95% CI (–0.087, 0.446) and $r_I^* = 0.307$, 95%

CI (–0.326, 0.751). The PCC indicates near-perfect *linear association*, but the LCC and both ICCs indicate extremely poor *agreement* between the two measurements, a much more accurate depiction of what is indicated in Figure 5.1. In Section 5.4.3.2 below, we present a method that can be used to ascertain the nature and extent of the disagreement between any two measurements on the same scale, such as that indicated by Figure 5.1.

The SAS code (Cheng and Gansky 2006) that can be used to calculate the sample estimate of the LCC and find the bootstrap CI using the data in Table 5.10 is provided on the companion website. The SPSS syntax and the R code provided with Examples 5.9 and 5.10 (and available on the companion website) can also be used to calculate the ICCs for these data.

Spearman's Correlation *Spearman's rank correlation coefficient (SCC)*, denoted by r_S, measures the "agreement in ranks" between two sets of measurements, after the measurements have been ordered ("ranked") from smallest to largest. (See Section 4.5.1.1.) This method is particularly useful, and to be preferred over PCC, when examining the agreement between two continuous variables that do not follow a bivariate normal distribution (i.e., either X or Y or both are non-normally distributed). However, there often is very little difference between the values of PCC and SCC even when the data are non-normal and there is a nonlinear relationship between X and Y. Typically, the CI for the SCC will be wider than the corresponding CI for the PCC when the two sample correlations are equal.

Example 5.12 Spearman's Correlation Coefficient

For the data in Table 5.10, the value of SCC is very close to that of PCC: $r_S = 0.984$, 95% CI (0.954, 1.000). These results are not surprising since the plot in Figure 5.1 indicates a very strong linear relationship between the ratings of Judge A and the ratings of Judge B. Note that the CI for the SCC is slightly wider than that for the PCC.

St. Laurent's Coefficient As an alternative to PCC and LCC, St. Laurent (1998) proposed a new coefficient for quantifying the agreement between an approximate measurement X and the gold standard G. As St. Laurent pointed out, method comparison studies in which a gold standard is present are common in the literature, and he cites several examples, including the study by Prigent et al. (1991), in which the percentage of heart muscle mass affected by an induced myocardial infarction as estimated by planar imaging (denoted by X), was compared against that measured by pathology (the gold standard, denoted by G) for $n = 12$ dogs. Prigent et al. (1991) did not provide their raw data; however, Table 5.13 contains a close approximation to their data obtained by visually estimating the values of X and G from the scatterplot given in Figure 3 of their article.

To derive his measure of agreement, St. Laurent considers the model

$$X_i = G_i + \varepsilon_i, \tag{5.27}$$

TABLE 5.13 Approximate Data Estimated Graphically from Prigent et al. (1991)

Dog	Pathology (G)	Planar Imaging (X)
1	7.8	14.4
2	9.3	17.9
3	12.4	22.4
4	12.6	30.3
5	17.9	46.1
6	19.7	20.0
7	21.4	35.7
8	23.9	38.9
9	25.9	39.4
10	29.2	46.1
11	30.0	42.2
12	31.4	41.7

where X_i is the approximate measurement and G_i is the corresponding gold-standard measurement on the ith target, $i = 1, \ldots, n$. It is assumed that G is a random variable with mean μ and variance σ_G^2, and ε_i is the measurement error associated with X_i, which is assumed to have mean 0 and variance σ^2. This is essentially a one-way random effects model, except that the random effect G_i is observed. Thus, G_i accounts for the unit-to-unit variability in the population of gold-standard measurements. According to the model given in (5.27), the approximate measurement X_i would be in perfect agreement with the corresponding gold standard value G_i for each unit were it not for an additive measurement error.

From (5.27), $\text{Cov}(X_i, G_i) = \text{Var}(G_i) = \sigma_G^2$ and $\text{Var}(X_i) = \sigma_G^2 + \sigma^2$, from which it follows that

$$\rho_G^2 = \sigma_G^2/(\sigma_G^2 + \sigma^2) \tag{5.28}$$

is the square of the correlation between X and G. St. Laurent proposed ρ_G, the correlation between X and G as a new measure of the agreement between the approximate measurement X and the gold standard G. To obtain the sample estimate r_G, St. Laurent recommended that the variance components in (5.28) be replaced by their sample estimates. Following St. Laurent's development, let $D_i = X_i - G_i$ denote the ith difference between the approximate measurement and the gold standard, and let $S_{DD} = \sum_{i=1}^{n} D_i^2, S_{GG}^2 = \sum_{i=1}^{n} (G_i - \bar{G})^2$. Then $S_{GG}/(n-1)$ is an unbiased estimator of σ_G^2 and S_{DD}/n is an unbiased estimator of σ^2 since $E(D_i) = 0$ and $\text{Var}(D_i) = \text{Var}(\varepsilon_i) = \sigma^2$. Thus, rewriting ρ_G^2 as $\rho_G^2 = 1/[1 + (\sigma^2/\sigma_G^2)]$, St. Laurent proposed

$$1/\{1 + [(n-1)S_{DD}]/(nS_{GG})\},$$

or the "asymptotically equivalent" (and simpler) estimator

$$r_G^2 = 1/[1 + (S_{DD}/S_{GG})], \quad (5.29)$$

as his new measure of agreement with a gold standard. He also showed that

$$r_G^2 = 1/[1 + 2b_1(1/r_c - 1)], \quad (5.30)$$

where b_1 is the estimated slope of the regression of the approximate measurement X on the gold standard measurement G, and r_c is the value of LCC (Section 5.2.2.2) for the agreement between X and G.

As indicated by St. Laurent, if ε_i and G_i are both assumed to be normally distributed, then r_G^2 is the maximum likelihood estimator of ρ_G^2. Under these assumptions, $(1 - 1/n)[(1/r_G^2) - 1)]$ is distributed as $[(1/\rho) - 1]F_{n,n-1}$, where $F_{n,n-1}$ has an F distribution with n and n–1 degrees of freedom. Thus, a $100(1 - \alpha)\%$ CI for ρ_G^2 is given by (LCL, UCL), where

$$\text{LCL} = \frac{F_L}{F_L + [(1/r_G^2) - 1](n-1)/n}, \quad (5.31)$$

$$\text{UCL} = \frac{F_U}{F_U + [(1/r_G^2) - 1](n-1)/n},$$

and F_U and F_L are the upper and lower α/2-percentage points of an F distribution with n and n–1 *df*, respectively. (Note that an approximate bootstrap CI for ρ_G^2 could be obtained by applying (5.30) to the endpoints of an approximate bootstrap CI for the true value of LCC.) St. Laurent's coefficient and the approximate CI in (5.31) can be calculated using the freely available WINPEPI software, which can be downloaded from http://www.brixtonhealth.com/pepi4windows.html. WINPEPI is also capable of performing many of the other analyses described in this chapter, as well as sample size calculations for them.

Example 5.13 St. Laurent's Coefficient

For the data in Table 5.13, Equations (5.29) and (5.31) yield $r_G^2 = 0.481$, 95% CI (0.300–0.728), indicating only fair agreement between planar imaging and the pathology gold standard. This is not surprising, since an examination of the data in Table 5.13 indicates that the percentage of heart muscle mass is always overestimated using planar imaging and this is confirmed in the scatterplot of these data given in Figure 5.2. For comparison purposes, LCC indicates even less agreement than St. Laurent's coefficient: $r_c = 0.405$ (95% bootstrap CI, 0.133–0.619). (Note that we do not recommend that the LCC be used for these data since a gold standard is available.) The PCC between X and Y is quite strong ($r = 0.809$; 95% CI, 0.439–0.944); however, as discussed previously, PCC cannot be recommended as a measure of agreement.

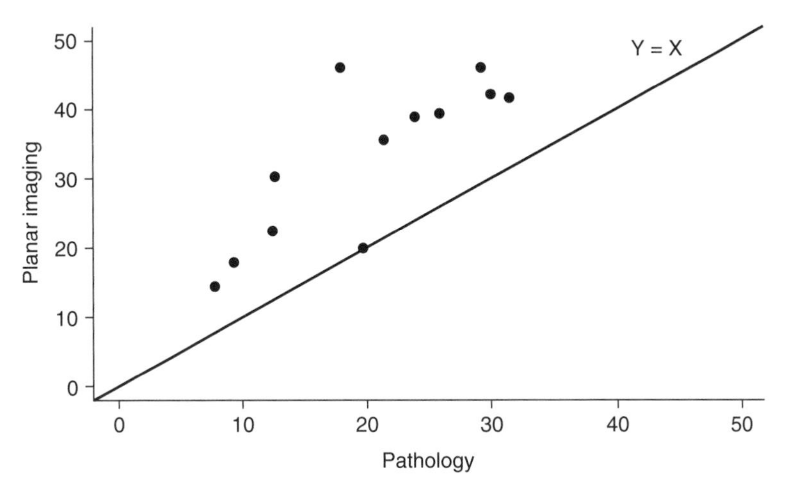

FIGURE 5.2 Scatterplot of data on agreement between estimated percentage of heart muscle mass affected by an induced myocardial infarction as determined by planar imaging versus that measured by pathology (the gold standard) with the line of perfect agreement superimposed.

5.3 ASSESSING RELIABILITY OF A BIOMARKER

5.3.1 General Considerations

The general methods for measuring agreement between two variables described in Sections 5.1 and 5.2 can be used to assess the IAR and IER of a biomarker. Both types of reliability require that one be able to measure the agreement between two different determinations of the biomarker for the same biological specimen. To assess intra-rater reliability, the same analyst would determine the value of the biomarker (either a continuous "reading" such as concentration or a dichotomous "reading" such as present/absent) using the same specimen of material under "identical" conditions. This determination must be blinded, of course, so that the analyst is unaware on the second occasion that he or she is examining the same experimental material that he or she examined before. To assess inter-rater reliability, two different analysts would make the determination using the same specimen of material under "identical" conditions. This determination should also be blinded so that Analyst A is unaware of the result of Analyst B and vice versa.

5.3.2 Assessing Reliability of a Dichotomous Biomarker

To assess both the IAR and IER of a dichotomous biomarker, one uses a 2×2 table to show the agreement (and disagreement) between the two determinations. To assess IAR, one constructs the 2×2 table given in Table 5.14. To assess IER, one constructs a similar 2×2 table to show the agreement (and disagreement) between the two determinations made by different analysts on the same biological specimens. To determine the level of inter-rater or intra-rater reliability, the measures of agreement

TABLE 5.14 2 × 2 Table Showing Agreement Between Two Determinations by the Same Analyst of the Same Biological Specimens

	Determination 2		
Determination 1	Positive	Negative	Total
Positive	a	b	f_1
Negative	c	d	f_2
Total	g_1	g_2	n

for dichotomous variables described in Section 5.2.1 are applied. Because of its widespread use and general acceptability, we recommend that coefficient kappa (along with a 95% CI, if desired) be calculated as the "first-line" measure of agreement (and hence, reliability). If, based on scientific grounds, kappa appears to provide a distorted picture of the degree of agreement (due to the shortcomings described in Section 5.2.1.1), then the PABAK coefficient should also be used to measure reliability and the results for both coefficients should be reported. For example, in their examination of interobserver agreement, Preusser et al. (2008) found that "some observers showed no variation in an assessment run (i.e., always voted solely "yes" or "no"). In such cases, no kappa values were computed." As discussed in Section 5.2.1.1, this is one of the shortcomings of kappa as a measure of agreement: if no specimens are classified into one of the two categories ("positive" or "negative") by either rater, kappa = 0. In this situation, kappa is meaningless as a measure of agreement, and the value of PABAK (and its CI, if desired) should be reported.

In addition to reporting PABAK whenever kappa appears to be inadequate as a measure of agreement, we also recommend that one assess the agreement separately for those specimens that appear to be positive and those that appear to be negative. (Note that the availability of a gold standard is irrelevant to assessing reliability.) Using measures of positive agreement and negative agreement in assessing reliability is analogous to using sensitivity and specificity in assessing validity in the presence of a gold standard. Such measures can be used to help diagnose the type(s) of disagreement that may be present in the reliability assessments.

For example, Tockman et al. (1988) evaluated the use of murine monoclonal antibodies to a glycolipid antigen of human lung cancer as a biomarker for detecting early lung cancer. As part of their assessment of the agreement between raters in the scoring of stained specimens, they compared the results obtained on 123 slides read by both a pathologist and a cytotechnologist. Their results are given in Table 5.15.

As part of their assessment of the IER, Tockman et al. (1988) stated that "Interobserver variability of scored specimens was assessed for 123 independently doubly read slides.... The McNemar's χ^2 probability was 1.000 that no difference exists between the independent scoring interpretations of pathologist and cytotechnologist." The obvious misinterpretation of the p-value of McNemar's test (see Section 4.4.3.1) notwithstanding, what Tockman et al. actually did was to test for what Shoukri calls "interrater bias" (Shoukri 2004, pp. 49–51); in other words, they performed an hypothesis test to compare the percentage classified as positive by the pathologist with the percentage classified as positive by the cytotechnologist. While such a test

TABLE 5.15 2 × 2 Table Showing Agreement Between a Pathologist and a Cytotechnologist When Scoring the Same Stained Specimen

	Cytotechnologist		
Pathologist	Positive	Negative	Total
Positive	31	1	32
Negative	0	91	91
Total	31	92	123

Source: Adapted from Table 4 of Tockman et al. (1988). Reprinted with permission.

is often informative, one should also measure the degree of agreement between the raters (Kraemer 1980).

Example 5.14 Use of Kappa with Biomarker Data

For the data in Table 5.15, we obtain $\hat{\kappa} = 0.979$ using equation (5.3) and $\widehat{\text{Var}}(\hat{\kappa}) = 0.0004494$ using (5.4). This yields an approximate 95% CI for κ of (0.94, 1.00). These results indicate excellent IER for the biomarker proposed by Tockman et al. (1988). In this situation, there is very little reason to doubt the usefulness of kappa as a measure of agreement, so it is unlikely that PABAK and the indices of positive and negative agreement will provide any additional insight into the degree of inter-rater agreement. In fact, applying the formulas in (5.5) and (5.6) to the data in Table 5.15, we see that the sample value of PABAK (0.984) is almost identical to that of kappa, as are the indices of positive agreement and negative agreement: $p_{\text{pos}} = 0.984$ and $p_{\text{neg}} = 0.995$. Thus, there is nothing to indicate anything other than excellent IER for the biomarker proposed by Tockman et al.

5.3.2.1 Dichotomous Biomarker, More Than Two Raters When it is desired to assess agreement among more than two raters when assessing IER, Cochran's Q test (see Section 4.4.3.2) can be used to compare all of the raters simultaneously in terms of the proportion of specimens that each one classified as "positive" to assess what Shoukri calls "inter-rater bias." If Cochran's Q test rejects the null hypothesis of no inter-rater bias, then McNemar's test with a Bonferroni adjustment can be used to compare each pair of raters, or, it can be sufficient to simply conclude that there is significant disagreement among the raters. (Note that this approach could also be used when assessing intra-rater reliability when an individual rater has been asked to classify each specimen on more than two occasions. Then, one would be testing for significant "intra-rater bias.")

Example 5.15 Use of Cochran's Q with Biomarker Data

Reid et al. (2012) examined the validity and reliability of urine cytology as a biomarker for grading urothelial carcinoma. In this study, urine samples from 41 subjects with known urothelial carcinoma were used to grade the urothelial tumors as "low grade" or "high grade." Each urine sample was independently graded by three pathologists.

TABLE 5.16 Agreement Among Three Pathologists in Terms of Classification Results Based on Urine Cytology

Pattern[a]	Frequency
1 1 1	23
1 0 1	4
0 1 1	5
0 1 0	4
0 0 1	3
0 0 0	2

[a]The first value in each pattern indicates the classification result for Pathologist 1, the second value for Pathologist 2, and the third value indicates the result for Pathologist 3. The pattern 1 0 1, for example, indicates that Pathologists 1 and 3 both classified the patient as having a high-grade tumor, whereas Pathologist 2 classified the patient as having a low-grade tumor.
Source: Data courtesy of Dr. Michelle Reid.

One of the goals of the study was to examine IER among the pathologists. Consider the data in Table 5.16 , which shows the results of the grading by the three pathologists: "0" indicates that the pathologist scored the tumor as "low grade," whereas "1" indicates that the tumor was scored as "high grade." Note that, for 23 of the 41 patients with urothelial cancer, all three raters agreed that the tumor was high grade; for two patients, all three raters agreed that the tumor was low grade. For the remaining 16 patients, there was disagreement among the three pathologists.

Using Equation (4.52), the value of the test statistic for Cochran's Q for these data is $Q_0 = 6.13$ and, with $df = 2$, the approximate chi-squared p-value is 0.047. The exact p-value is 0.059, but the mid p adjustment yields a result that is very similar to the chi-squared approximation (mid-p value $= 0.048$). Thus, there appears to be significant inter-rater bias. With regard to determining the source of this bias, pairwise comparisons based on McNemar's test with a Bonferroni adjustment yield only one significant pairwise difference: Pathologist 1 differed significantly from Pathologist 3 ($\chi_0^2 = 8.00$, $df = 1$, $p = 0.0047$; exact p-value $= 0.0078$; mid-p value $= 0.0039$).

While test results such as these are informative, one should also measure the degree of agreement among the raters (Kraemer 1980). As discussed in Section 5.2.1.2, the method of Fleiss (1971) can be used to calculate an overall measure of agreement among $k > 2$ raters who are performing dichotomous classifications.

Example 5.16 Generalized Coefficient kappa Applied to Biomarker Data

Using the formulas in Equation (5.9), the data in Table 5.16 yield $p_0 = 0.740$, $\hat{\pi} = 0.764$, $\hat{p}_e = 0.639$, and $\hat{\kappa}_f = 0.278$. To obtain an approximate CI using the ICC approximation to $\hat{\kappa}_f$,we apply the formulas in (5.11)–(5.13) to the data in Table 5.16 and obtain $\hat{\rho}_I = 0.287$ and an estimated $\text{Var}\left(\hat{\rho}_I\right)$ of 0.0130. This yields an approximate 95% CI of $\hat{\rho}_{\mathrm{I}} \pm z_{\alpha/2}\sqrt{\mathrm{Var}\left(\hat{\rho}_{\mathrm{I}}\right)} = 0.287 \pm 1.96\,(0.114) = (0.064, 0.510)$. Note that there is very little meaningful difference between the ICC-based estimate of $\hat{\rho}_{\mathrm{I}} = 0.287$ and the value $\hat{\kappa}_f = 0.278$ obtained using (5.9). These results indicate that there is poor agreement among the three pathologists based on the Fleiss criteria (Table 5.12). In terms of the pairwise kappa coefficients, there is unacceptably low inter-rater agreement between Pathologists 1 and 2 ($\hat{\kappa} = 0.229$) and between Pathologists 2 and 3 ($\hat{\kappa} = 0.111$). There is moderate inter-rater agreement between Pathologists 1 and 3 ($\hat{\kappa} = 0.497$) according to the Landis–Koch criteria (Table 5.3).

5.3.3 Assessing Reliability of a Continuous Biomarker

To assess either IAR or IER, a biomarker determination is repeated for each of n specimens. For intra-rater reliability, the same analyst evaluates the same specimen on two separate occasions under "identical" conditions. For inter-rater reliability, two different analysts evaluate the same specimen, each under "identical" conditions.

Example 5.17 Inter-rater Reliability for Biomarker Data

Consider the data in Table 5.17 that were taken from a study of a bile acid-induced apoptosis assay for colon cancer risk (Carol Bernstein, personal communication, October 17, 2000). The goal was to assess IER. The method most commonly used to measure IER for the data in Table 5.17 is PCC, as was done by Bernstein et al. (2000), who obtained $r = 0.884$ (95% CI 0.679–0.961). However, as discussed in Section 5.2.2.1, the PCC is not an appropriate measure of agreement. Valid alternative measures of agreement for the data in Table 5.17 include the ICC and LCC (see Section 5.2.2.2).

TABLE 5.17 Inter-rater Reliability Data

Specimen	Analyst A	Analyst B
1	11	27
2	9	15
3	54	72
4	55	63
5	50	65
6	44	49
7	58	51
8	5	8
9	21	30
10	58	43
11	41	40
12	59	62
13	39	52
14	34	49
15	23	21

Source: Carol Bernstein, personal communication, October 17, 2000.

Since there are 15 specimens and 2 analysts, $n = 15$ and $k = 2$, using our notation from Section 5.2.2.2. As is usually done in reliability studies, we assume that the 2 analysts are a random sample from the hypothetical population of all possible analysts; therefore, the correct version of the ICC to use is ICC(2, 1) and the formulas are given in Equations (5.19) and (5.20). The following results are obtained: MST = 698.919, MSJ = 246.533, MSE = 43.176, and

$$r_{\mathrm{I}} = \frac{698.919 - 43.176}{698.919 + (2-1)(43.176) + 2(246.533 - 43.176)/15} = 0.852.$$

Using Equation (5.21), a 95% CI for the true ICC is given by (0.553, 0.951).

The intermediate results required to calculate the LCC for the data given in Table 5.17 are as follows:

$$\bar{x}_1 = 37.40,\ \bar{x}_2 = 43.13, s_1 = 19.1975,\ s_2 = 19.3275,\ s_{12} = 327.8714.$$

Applying (5.25), we obtain:

$$r_c = \frac{2s_{12}}{s_1^2 + s_2^2 + (\bar{x}_1 - \bar{x}_2)^2} = \frac{2(327.999)}{368.544 + 373.5523 + (37.4 - 43.13)^2} = 0.844,$$

an almost identical result to the ICC of 0.852. Since $n = 15$, we use a 95% bootstrap CI for the true LCC based on 1000 samples; this is given by (0.628, 0.914). The values of the ICC and the LCC are only slightly smaller than the PCC and both measures indicate "excellent" IER according to the Fleiss et al. criteria (Table 5.12). However, note the extreme width of the CIs for both the ICC and the LCC (owing to the small value of n). The lower limits of these CIs indicate only "fair to good" IER, according to the Fleiss criteria.

5.3.4 Assessing Inter-Subject, Intra-Subject, and Analytical Measurement Variability

The presentation in this section very closely follows the description by Taioli et al. (1994) of their proposed scheme for evaluating the reliability of a biomarker. Taioli et al. state that, in addition to IAR and IER, there are three major components of biomarker variability that must be considered when evaluating reliability. These are: (1) *Inter-subject* variability, which could be attributable to race, gender, diet, etc.; (2) *Intra-subject* variability, which could be attributable to random biologic variation, change in diet, change in exposure, time of observation, etc.; and (3) *Analytical* or *laboratory* variability, which could be attributable to variation between analytical batches, variation within analytical batches, and/or random variation within the measurement process itself. Even if a biomarker has acceptable validity, an excess of intra-individual and/or laboratory variability could render it unusable for practical purposes (Taioli et al. 1994, p. 308).

The experimental setup required to evaluate each of the three sources of variability mentioned above is as follows: biological specimens from each of n subjects are obtained on m occasions (e.g., *weeks*), and the biomarker determination is repeated for each of r replicate samples (e.g., *aliquots*) from each specimen on each occasion. Under the framework proposed by Taioli et al., replicate samples *must* be used in order to perform a proper evaluation of all three aspects of biomarker reliability.

The data from the repeated biomarker determinations are used to estimate the three components of biomarker variability identified by Taoli et al. Inter-subject variability is assessed using the data from multiple subjects, intra-subject variability is assessed using the data from multiple occasions, and analytical variability is assessed using the data from the replicate samples. Once an estimate of analytical variability (or "error variance") has been obtained using the analysis proposed by Taoli et al., it can be used in method comparison studies (see Section 5.4.3.2). An estimate of the total variance of the biomarker determination, which is useful in calculating the appropriate sample size required for future studies involving the biomarker, can be obtained by combining the estimates of inter-subject variability, intra-subject variability, and analytical variability resulting from their proposed analysis.

The statistical model underlying the methods proposed by Taioli et al. (1994) is very similar to the random-effects model that underlies the derivation of the ICC when measuring agreement between continuous variables (see Section 5.2.2.2). The main difference is that the replicate observations must now be accounted for:

$$Y_{ijk} = \mu + \alpha_i + \beta_j + (\alpha\beta)_{ij} + \varepsilon_{ijk}; \quad 1 \leq i \leq n; \quad 1 \leq j \leq m; \quad 1 \leq k \leq r \qquad (5.32)$$

where

Y_{ijk} = biomarker value for subject i on occasion j and replicate k,
μ = population mean response,
α_i = offset in mean response for subject i,
β_j = offset in mean response for occasion j,
$(\alpha\beta)_{ij}$ = offset in mean response for the interaction between subject i and occasion j,
ε_{ijk} = biomarker measurement error.

(A significant interaction term indicates that the differences among subjects vary from one occasion to the next.)

The assumptions that underlie the model in Equation (5.32) are as follows: for $1 \leq i \leq n, 1 \leq j \leq m, 1 \leq k \leq r, \alpha_i, \beta_i, (\alpha\beta)_{ij}$, and ε_{ijk} are all independent; $\alpha_i \sim N(0, \sigma_\alpha^2)$, $\beta_i \sim N(0, \sigma_\beta^2)$, $(\alpha\beta)_{ij} \sim N(0, \sigma_{\alpha\beta}^2)$, and $\varepsilon_{ijk} \sim N(0, \sigma_\varepsilon^2)$. All of these assumptions taken together imply that $Y_{ijk} \sim N(\mu, \sigma^2)$, where $\sigma^2 = \sigma_\alpha^2 + \sigma_\beta^2 + \sigma_{\alpha\beta}^2 + \sigma_\varepsilon^2$.

As in Section 5.2.2, the appropriate statistical method for analyzing data that follow this model is two-way random-effects analysis of variance (ANOVA). This analysis yields tests of significance for each main effect (subjects and occasions) and a test of the significance of the interaction between subjects and occasions. It also provides estimates of each variance component (inter-subject variability, intra-subject variability, and analytical variability).

TABLE 5.18 Random-Effects ANOVA for DNA-Protein Cross-link Data

Variance Component	Variance Estimate	F (df)	p-value
Week	0.0545	13.68 (2, 7)	<0.010
Between subject	0.0176	3.45 (4, 7)	0.073
Week * subjects	0.0110	2.33 (7, 40)	0.045
Error	0.0317	–	–

Source: Adapted from Table 2 of Taioli et al. (1994, p. 307). Public Domain.

Example 5.18 Assessment of Sources of Variability for Biomarker Data

Taioli et al. illustrate their approach in an example that involves the assessment of the reliability of four biomarkers for exposure to carcinogenic metals. The biomarkers they examine are: (1) DNA-protein cross-link (DNA-PC), (2) DNA-amino acid cross-link (DNA-AA), (3) metallothionein gene expression (MT), and (4) autoantibodies to oxidized DNA bases (DNAox). We restrict our discussion to the results from only one of their studies here (DNA-PC). In that study, weekly blood samples were drawn three times ($m = 3$) from each of five healthy, unexposed subjects ($n = 5$) and each blood sample was divided into either three or four aliquots ($r = 3$ or 4) for analysis. The blood samples were analyzed during the week in which they were drawn. The results of fitting the random-effects ANOVA model in (5.32) are given in Table 5.18. The error variance for the DNA-PC determination is estimated to be 0.0317 and the estimated total variance is $(0.0545 + 0.0176 + 0.0110 + 0.0317) = 0.1148$.

Based on the results in Table 5.18, there is a significant "week" effect (i.e., intra-subject variability); however, the "subject" effect (i.e., inter-subject variability) does not quite reach statistical significance. There is also a significant interaction between "week" and "subjects"; this suggests that the "week" effect varies across subjects. As indicated by Taioli et al., by analyzing the blood samples in the week in which they were drawn, the investigators may have introduced a possible batch effect that is confounded with the "week" effect. Therefore, the significant intra-subject variability could be due to the batch effect and not to true week-to-week variation. To eliminate this batch effect in the future, the investigators modified their assay so that the DNA-PC determination could be performed for all samples at one time, rather than during the week in which they were drawn.

5.4 ASSESSING VALIDITY

5.4.1 General Considerations

Just as general methods for measuring agreement between two variables can be used to assess the IAR and IER of a biomarker, the same methods can be used to assess the validity of a biomarker. In this section, we will distinguish between *conformity* and *consistency* as they relate to assessing validity. Conformity is used to describe the agreement between the biomarker and the gold standard for the outcome of interest.

Note that this term applies in situations when the biomarker and the gold standard determinations are both dichotomous, as well as situations in which the biomarker and the gold standard determinations are both continuous. We will treat each of the situations separately in this section.

If a gold standard is not available for the exposure or outcome that the biomarker is intended to measure, the term *consistency* is used to describe the agreement between the biomarker and some other method. Again, the determinations using the biomarker and the "other method" can both be dichotomous, or they can both be continuous. (It can also happen that both the biomarker and the other method are ordinal.) The "other method" could be the standard method which a new biomarker is intended to replace, or a competing biomarker.

5.4.2 Assessing Validity When a Gold Standard Is Available

5.4.2.1 Dichotomous Biomarkers

Estimating Sensitivity and Specificity Just as in the assessment of reliability of a dichotomous biomarker described in Section 5.3.2, the assessment of the validity of a dichotomous biomarker requires the use of a 2×2 table. If a gold standard is available for the exposure or outcome that the dichotomous biomarker determination is intended to represent (the "event"), then, as stated previously, the term "conformity" is used to describe the agreement between the biomarker determination and the occurrence of the event. The 2×2 table that summarizes the cross-classification between the biomarker and the gold standard is called the "truth table."

Example 5.19 Assessment of Conformity for Biomarker Data

Consider the study by Qiao et al. (1997), who examined the agreement between the biomarker proposed by Tockman et al. (1988) and the gold standard method for diagnosing lung cancer. The truth table for their data is given in Table 5.19.

Three measures of conformity can be obtained from this table: (1) *sensitivity* = 42/57 = 73.7%, the percentage of those who experienced the event that the biomarker correctly identifies as "positive"; (2) *specificity* = 53/76 = 69.7%, the percentage of those who did not experience the event that the biomarker correctly identifies as

TABLE 5.19 Truth Table for Tumor-Associated Antigen as a Biomarker for Lung Cancer

	Gold Standard		
Tumor-Associated Antigen	Positive	Negative	Total
Positive	42	23	65
Negative	15	53	68
Total	57	76	133

Source: Adapted from Table 3 of Qiao et al. (1997), with permission from AACR.

"negative"; and (3) *overall accuracy* = (42 + 53)/133 = 71.4% , the percentage of all subjects that the biomarker correctly identifies. Generally speaking, the classifier is considered to have adequate validity if each of sensitivity, specificity, and overall accuracy are at least 75%. In this example, each of these measures just misses the desirable cutoff.

Qiao et al. compared these results for the new biomarker with those for the "standard methods" (chest x-ray and sputum cytology) for diagnosing lung cancer and concluded that their proposed biomarker was more sensitive but had lower specificity than both of the standard methods (Qiao et al. 1997, p. 893). However, the authors did not perform any statistical tests to support their conclusions regarding the relative sensitivities and specificities of the three methods for diagnosing lung cancer that they compared. We discuss this topic in Section 5.4.2.1.

Predictive value, a criterion that is almost always used to evaluate the performance of diagnostic tests in clinical medicine, is often overlooked when evaluating the utility of a biomarker as a diagnostic tool. Predictive value is an alternative way of looking at the validity of a diagnostic test based on a biomarker when a gold standard is available: of those specimens for which the result of the biomarker determination was positive, what percentage were confirmed to indicate disease using the gold standard? This is known as *positive predictive value* (PPV). Similarly, of those specimens for which the result of the biomarker determination was negative, what percentage were confirmed to not have the disease using the gold standard? This is known as *negative predictive value* (NPV).

Using the entries in the truth table given in Table 5.19, PPV = 42/65 = 64.6%, the percentage of those the biomarker identified as "positive" who actually had lung cancer, and NPV = 53/68 = 77.9%, the percentage of those the biomarker identified as "negative" who actually did not have lung cancer. Many clinicians would consider PPV and NPV to be more useful as measures of the clinical utility of a diagnostic test than sensitivity and specificity. Note that Qiao et al. did not evaluate their biomarker in terms of predictive value.

In addition to reporting the point estimates of the measures of conformity that we have discussed, it is considered good statistical practice to also present CIs for the true values. However, in many published evaluations of new biomarkers, CIs were not presented (as in Qiao et al.). Since sensitivity, specificity, and overall accuracy are all proportions, standard methods for finding a CI for a proportion can be applied. However, finding CIs for PPV and NPV is more complicated since these estimates are not proportions in the truest sense. The usual approach for finding a CI for a proportion is to apply methods based on the binomial distribution, as described in Section 3.6.1. For these methods to be valid, the denominator of the estimated proportion (i.e., the sample size) must be a known constant. However, the denominator of PPV (and of NPV) is not a constant, but a random variable, since it is equal to the number of specimens classified as positive by the biomarker in the particular sample that one is analyzing. Therefore, special methods must be used in order to account for the random nature of the denominators of PPV and NPV.

Estimating Positive and Negative Predictive Value Mercaldo et al. (2007) compared various methods for finding CIs for PPV and NPV and recommended a method based on the *logit* transformation, which in general is defined by logit(p) = log[$p/(1-p)$], where $0 < p < 1$, and "log" denotes the natural logarithm. This method is valid provided that the estimated sensitivity and specificity are both strictly between 0 and 1. If either the sensitivity or specificity of the test are equal to 0 or 1, they recommend that their "adjusted logit" method be used. Both methods are described below.

Let Se and Sp denote the estimated sensitivity and specificity, respectively, of the diagnostic test, and let p denote the estimated prevalence of the disease in the population under study. Then it can be shown that

$$\text{PPV} = \frac{p \bullet \text{Se}}{p \bullet \text{Se} + (1-p) \bullet (1-\text{Sp})} \tag{5.33}$$

and

$$\text{NPV} = \frac{(1-p) \bullet \text{Sp}}{p \bullet (1-\text{Se}) + (1-p) \bullet \text{Sp}}.$$

After some algebra, it can be seen that:

$$\text{logit(PPV)} = \log\left[\frac{p \bullet \text{Se}}{(1-p) \bullet (1-\text{Sp})}\right] \tag{5.34}$$

and

$$\text{logit(NPV)} = \log\left[\frac{(1-p) \bullet \text{Sp}}{p \bullet (1-\text{Se})}\right].$$

Applying the delta method (Casella and Berger, 2002, pp. 240–245), Mercaldo et al. derive the following approximate variances:

$$\text{Var[logit(PPV)]} \approx \frac{1}{n_1}\left[\frac{1-\text{Se}}{\text{Se}}\right] + \frac{1}{n_0}\left[\frac{\text{Sp}}{1-\text{Sp}}\right] \tag{5.35}$$

and

$$\text{Var[logit(NPV)]} \approx \frac{1}{n_1}\left[\frac{\text{Se}}{1-\text{Se}}\right] + \frac{1}{n_0}\left[\frac{1-\text{Sp}}{\text{Sp}}\right],$$

where n_1 is the number of study subjects with the disease and n_0 is the number of study subjects without the disease. Using these results, one can derive the following Wald-type CIs for the true values of logit (PPV) and logit (NPV):

$$\log\text{it(PPV)} \pm z_{\alpha/2}\sqrt{\text{Var[logit(PPV)]}} \tag{5.36}$$

TABLE 5.20 Summary of Conformity Results for Tumor-Associated Antigen as a Biomarker for Lung Cancer

Measure of Conformity	Point Estimate (%)	95% Confidence Interval
Overall accuracy	71.4	(63.8%, 79.1%)
Sensitivity	73.7	(62.3%, 85.1%)
Specificity	69.7	(59.4%, 80.1%)
Positive predictive value	64.6	(55.7%, 72.7%)
Negative predictive value	77.9	(69.1%, 84.8%)

and

$$\log \text{it}(\text{NPV}) \pm z_{\alpha/2}\sqrt{\text{Var}[\text{logit}(\text{NPV})]}.$$

The final step is to "back transform" the endpoints of the intervals in (5.36) to obtain approximate CIs for PPV and NPV. Thus, the CI for PPV is given by the following:

$$\left[\frac{e^{\log \text{it}(\text{PPV})-z_{\alpha/2}\sqrt{\text{Var}[\text{logit}(\text{PPV})]}}}{1+e^{\log \text{it}(\text{PPV})-z_{\alpha/2}\sqrt{\text{Var}[\text{logit}(\text{PPV})]}}}, \frac{e^{\log \text{it}(\text{PPV})+z_{\alpha/2}\sqrt{\text{Var}[\text{logit}(\text{PPV})]}}}{1+e^{\log \text{it}(\text{PPV})+z_{\alpha/2}\sqrt{\text{Var}[\text{logit}(\text{PPV})]}}}\right]. \quad (5.37)$$

The corresponding approximate CI for NPV is obtained by simply replacing PPV in Equation (5.37) by NPV.

Table 5.20 contains point estimates and CIs for the various measures of conformity we have discussed in this section using the data for the new biomarker for lung cancer proposed by Qiao et al. (see Table 5.19). The CIs for overall accuracy, sensitivity, and specificity in Table 5.20 were calculated using the Wald method for finding CIs for proportions (Section 3.6.1); the CIs for PPV and NPV were calculated using the logit method proposed by Mercaldo et al. that we have just described.

The following SAS code can be used to find Wald-type and exact CIs for sensitivity, specificity, and overall accuracy, and to perform tests of the null hypothesis that the true value of each of these measures is at least 75%. It can also be used to calculate PPV and NPV. Note that CIs based on the binomial are *not* appropriate for the PPV and NPV, as we have discussed previously. The SAS code given below is also available on the companion website. SAS code for calculating CIs for PPV and NPV using the logit method proposed by Mercaldo et al. (2007) is also provided there.

```
options formchar="|----|+|---+=|-/\<>*";

data  lung_CA;
      input biomarker gold_standard count @@;
      cards;
      1 1 42  1 0 23
      0 1 15  0 0 53
      ;
```

```
title 'Sensitivity';
proc  freq data=lung_CA;
      where gold_standard=1;
   weight Count;
   tables biomarker / binomial(level="1" p = .75);
   exact binomial;
   run;

title 'Specificity';
proc  freq data=lung_CA;
   where gold_standard=0;
   weight Count;
   tables biomarker / binomial(level="0" p = .75);
   exact binomial;
   run;

data  accuracy;
      set lung_CA;
      if ((biomarker = 1 and gold_standard = 1) or (biomarker = 0
      and gold_standard = 0)) then correct = 1; else correct = 0;

title1 'Accuracy';
proc  freq data=accuracy;
   weight Count;
   tables correct / binomial(level="1" p = .75);
   exact binomial;
   run;

data  lung_CA;
      set lung_CA;
      id=1;
      row+1;

proc  sort data = lung_CA;
      by row;
      run;

data  cells;
      array size(4) a b c d;
      retain a b c d;
      set lung_CA;
      by id;
      if first.id = 1 then do i = 1 to 4;
      size(i) = .;
      end;
```

```
        size(row) = count;
        if last.id = 1 then output;

        keep id a b c d;
        run;

data    cells;
        set cells;
        ppv = a / (a+b);
        npv = d / (c+d);

        title1 'Positive and Negative Predictive Value';
proc    print data = cells;
        run;
```

As we mentioned earlier in this section, the CIs given in (5.37) are valid provided that neither *Se* nor *Sp* are equal to 1.0. If either the sensitivity or the specificity are equal to 1.0, then the *adjusted logit* method can be applied, which involves replacing *Se* and *Sp* in (5.33) by more robust estimates of sensitivity and specificity that account for the degenerate behavior of estimated proportions when a binomial sample consists entirely of successes (or failures). In particular, *Se* is replaced by $\tilde{Se}$ and *Sp* is replaced by $\tilde{Sp}$, where

$$\tilde{Se} = \frac{n_1 Se + (k^2/2)}{\tilde{n}_1}, \tag{5.38}$$

$$\tilde{Sp} = \frac{n_0 Sp + (k^2/2)}{\tilde{n}_0},$$

where

$$\tilde{n}_1 = n_1 + k^2,$$

$$\tilde{n}_0 = n_0 + k^2,$$

and

$$k = z_{\alpha/2}.$$

Here, $z_{\alpha/2}$ denotes the upper $\alpha/2$-percentage point of the standard normal distribution. The adjusted estimates of PPV and NPV are then used in Equations (5.34)–(5.37) to obtain the adjusted logit confidence limits for the true PPV and NPV. SAS code that can be used to calculate the adjusted estimates of PPV and NPV, as well as the adjusted logit confidence limits, is provided on the companion website.

TABLE 5.21 Truth Table for Sputum Cytology in Diagnosing Lung Cancer

	Gold Standard		
Sputum Cytology	Positive	Negative	Total
Positive	12	0	12
Negative	45	76	121
Total	57	76	133

Source: Adapted from Table 3 of Qiao et al. (1997), with permission from AACR.

Following Mercaldo et al. (2007), we recommend that the logit method be used unless either PPV or NPV are equal to 100%, in which case the adjusted logit method should be used.

Example 5.20 Positive and Negative Predictive Value for Biomarker Data

Table 5.21 contains the truth table for the use of sputum cytology in diagnosing lung cancer for the study by Qiao et al. (1997). Based on the results in Table 5.21, PPV = 100%. Since the estimated specificity $Sp = 100\%$, the estimated Var[logit(PPV] in Equation (5.35) is infinite, and the confidence limits in (5.37) do not exist. Applying the adjusted logit method of Mercaldo et al., we obtain PPV = 87.7% with 95% confidence limits of (61.2%, 97.0%). Note that the estimate of NPV for these data is essentially unaffected if we use the adjusted logit method: 62.8% (59.6%, 65.9%) using the logit approach versus 62.8% (59.3%, 66.1%) using the adjusted logit.

Another factor that must be considered when estimating predictive value is that the estimates of NPV and PPV are heavily dependent on the estimated prevalence of the disease in the population being studied. This is particularly important when a case-control study is used (Section 2.2.3), since the data from a case-control study cannot be used to estimate prevalence. To estimate PPV and NPV using data from a case-control study, an external estimate of the prevalence, p, must be used in Equation (5.33). Even if the data come from a cross-sectional or prospective study design, it is still preferable to use a (possibly external) estimate of the prevalence that accurately describes the population being studied (Gordis 2004, pp. 83–86).

Example 5.21 Effect of Estimated Prevalence on Positive and Negative Predictive Value

To get a sense of how dependent the estimates of PPV and NPV are on the estimated prevalence, consider the truth table for the new biomarker for lung cancer given in Table 5.19. Based on these data, the estimated prevalence of lung cancer is $p = 57/133 = 42.9\%$ and the point estimates and CIs for PPV and NPV in Table 5.20 incorporate this estimate. Since the population studied by Qiao et al. consisted of tin miners who were exposed to high levels of tobacco smoke, radon, and arsenic, an estimated prevalence this high is probably reasonable. However, suppose that the results in Table 5.19 were obtained from a population-based sample, in which the prevalence of lung cancer is only 1%. This does not affect the results for sensitivity, specificity, and overall accuracy given in Table 5.20; however, quite different results are obtained for PPV and NPV: PPV = 2.4% (1.7%–3.5%); NPV = 99.6% (99.4%–99.8%). We strongly recommend that one use the most accurate estimate of prevalence that is available when finding point estimates and confidence limits for PPV and NPV. The sample-based estimate of prevalence should be used only if no other estimate is available and under no circumstances should the sample-based estimate be used if the data were obtained from a case-control study. If no external estimate of prevalence is available, then PPV and NPV should not be reported for a case-control study.

5.4.2.2 Comparing Several Dichotomous Biomarkers If a gold standard is available and there are two or more competing dichotomous biomarkers, it is usually of interest to compare these biomarkers in terms of sensitivity, specificity, and overall accuracy. One might also be interested in comparing a new biomarker with one or more "standard" diagnostic tests in terms of these measures of conformity. For example, Qiao et al. (1997) used the "paired χ^2 test" to compare the sensitivity, specificity, and accuracy of their new biomarker based on immunocytochemistry with two "routine clinical detection methods" for lung cancer (sputum cytology and chest x-ray). When analyzing paired data of this type, the appropriate method for comparing two biomarkers in terms of classification accuracy is McNemar's test (McNemar 1947). There is no statistical method that is commonly known as the "paired χ^2 test." Although a χ^2 approximation is available for McNemar's test, it is preferable to use the exact version of the test (Siegel and Castellan 1988, pp. 78–79; Suissa and Shuster 1991). When comparing three or more diagnostic tests in terms of conformity (as in Qiao et al.), the preferred method is the Cochran Q test (Cochran 1950). McNemar's test and the Cochran Q test are more generally known as tests for comparing "dependent proportions" (Agresti 2007, pp. 245–246, 252) and they are covered in detail in Section 4.4.3. In this section, we focus on the use of these tests in validating a dichotomous biomarker when a gold standard is available.

Comparing Two Dichotomous Biomarkers As described in Section 4.4.3.1, in order to perform McNemar's test, one must arrange the cross-classified data in the "canonical form" for dependent proportions. Qiao et al. (1997) did not provide the data in this form in their article. However, the hypothetical 2 × 2 table given in Table 5.22 for the comparison of their biomarker with chest x-ray in terms of sensitivity yields approximately the same test statistic for the chi-square approximation to McNemar's test ($\chi^2 = 11.6$) as that presented in their article ($\chi^2 = 12.0$). (Note, that it is unclear if Qiao et al. (1997) used McNemar's test since they referred to their method as the "paired χ^2 test.")

It is important to note the special structure of Table 5.22. The rows and columns are each labeled "correct" and "incorrect." Each cell entry in the 2 × 2 table represents the number of specimens that the newly proposed biomarker *and* the more traditional

TABLE 5.22 Hypothetical 2 × 2 Table for Comparing the Sensitivities of a New Biomarker for Lung Cancer Versus Chest X-ray

	Biomarker		
Chest X-Ray	Correct	Incorrect	Total
Correct	19	5	24
Incorrect	23	10	33
Total	42	15	57

method of chest x-ray both correctly classified into that category. Out of the 57 confirmed cases of lung cancer in Qiao et al. (1997), 42 were correctly classified by the new biomarker, whereas only 24 were correctly classified by chest x-ray. The biomarker and x-ray agreed on a correct positive diagnosis for only 19 of these 57 confirmed cases, and they agreed on an incorrect negative diagnosis for 10 of the 57. However, as discussed in Section 4.4.3.1, these *concordant* cases of the disease are irrelevant as far as the statistical analysis is concerned, since the test statistic for McNemar's test is calculated using only the *discordant* cases of lung cancer; that is, those for which the biomarker and chest x-ray disagreed: 23 cases out of the 57 which the biomarker correctly identified as lung cancer, but the chest x-ray did not, and the 5 cases out of the 57 which the chest x-ray correctly identified as lung cancer, but the biomarker did not.

Example 5.22 McNemar's Test Applied to Biomarker Data

Using the notation in Section 4.4.3.1, for the data in Table 5.22, we have $n_{21} = 23$, $n_{12} = 5$, and $n^* = 28$. The reference distribution (conditional on the value of n^*) is therefore binomial with $n^* = 28$ and $\pi = 0.5$. The exact two-tailed p-value is $2 \cdot \Pr(n_{21} \geq 23 \mid n^* = 28, \pi = 0.5) = 0.00091$, with mid-$p$ value of 0.00055. Thus, there is very strong evidence of a difference in diagnostic accuracy between the new biomarker and chest x-ray. For the approximate test based on chi-square, $\chi_0^2 = 11.6$, $df = 1$, 2-tailed p-value = 0.00067, a result that is very similar to the mid-p value.

Comparing More Than Two Dichotomous Biomarkers When there are more than two dichotomous biomarkers or diagnostic tests to be compared, Cochran's Q test (see Section 4.4.3.2) could be used to compare all of the diagnostic tests simultaneously in terms of sensitivity, specificity, and/or overall accuracy. If Cochran's Q test rejects the null hypothesis that the diagnostic tests are equivalent in terms of any of these measures of conformity, then McNemar's test with a Bonferroni adjustment could be used to compare each pair of diagnostic tests. If a new biomarker is being compared with a "standard" biomarker, or another commonly used test, then the pairwise comparisons of greatest interest would more than likely be the comparisons of the new biomarker with each of the tests already in use.

TABLE 5.23 Hypothetical Data for Comparison of Three Diagnostic Tests for Lung Cancer in Terms of Sensitivity

Pattern[a]	Frequency
1 1 1	12
1 1 0	7
1 0 0	5
0 1 0	23
0 0 0	10

[a]The first value in each pattern indicates the accuracy result for x-ray, the second value for the new biomarker, and the third value indicates the result for the test based on sputum cytology. The pattern 1 1 0, for example, indicates that x-ray and the biomarker were both correct in classifying the patient as having lung cancer, whereas sputum cytology was incorrect.

Example 5.23 Cochran's Q Test Applied to Biomarker Data

In the study by Qiao et al. (1997), one could use Cochran's Q test to compare the three diagnostic tests (the new biomarker, the test based on sputum cytology, and chest x-ray) simultaneously in terms of sensitivity. Qiao et al. did not present sufficient data in their article for us to be able perform Cochran's test. However, for illustration purposes, we constructed a hypothetical data set that yields McNemar test results similar to the "paired χ^2" test results presented by Qiao et al. for the pairwise comparisons of the new biomarker with each of sputum cytology and x-ray in terms of sensitivity. This hypothetical data set is given in Table 5.23. A "1" indicates that the diagnostic test correctly classified the patient as having lung cancer, whereas a "0" indicates that the diagnostic test incorrectly classified the patient as not having lung cancer. Note that, for 12 of the 57 patients with lung cancer, all 3 diagnostic tests were correct; for 10 of the patients, all 3 diagnostic tests were incorrect.

Using Equation (4.52), the value of the test statistic for Cochran's Q test for the data in Table 5.23 is $Q_0 = 39.09$ with $df = 2$, and the approximate chi-squared p-value is < 0.001. Thus, there appears to be a significant difference among the three diagnostic tests in terms of sensitivity. In terms of pairwise comparisons among the three diagnostic tests using the approximate version of McNemar's test, one finds that there are strongly significant differences between all possible pairs: biomarker versus x-ray ($\chi^2 = 11.57$, $df = 1$, $p < 0.001$); biomarker versus sputum cytology ($\chi^2 = 30.00$, $df = 1$, $p < 0.001$); and x-ray versus sputum cytology ($\chi^2 = 12.00$, $df = 1$, $p < 0.001$). (Note that the "paired χ^2" test statistics presented in Qaio et al. were 12.0 for biomarker vs. x-ray and 40.2 for biomarker vs. sputum cytology.) These results are not surprising in view of the rather large differences in sensitivity among the three diagnostic tests: biomarker (73.7%), x-ray (42.1%), and sputum cytology (21.1%).

5.4.2.3 Continuous Biomarkers The assessment of the validity of a continuous biomarker in the presence of a gold standard is equivalent to the calibration of the biomarker (Bland and Altman 1986). Numerous detailed accounts of methods for calibrating a biomarker are already available (e.g., Strike 1991; Jones and Payne 1997; Fritsma and McGlasson 2012). In this section, we focus on the application of two methods that can be used to assess the validity of a continuous biomarker: ROC curve analysis and St. Laurent's coefficient of agreement.

ROC Curve Analysis In some instances, a biomarker yields only an indication that a specimen is positive or negative, as in the study by Qiao et al. (see Table 5.19). However, it is more common for the biomarker determination to be on an ordinal or continuous scale. For example, Weiss et al. (2003–2004) evaluated several potential biomarkers for lung cancer that are measured on a continuous scale, including epidermal growth factor receptor (EGFR) and fatty acid synthase (FASE). The problem is that determining the sensitivity and specificity of a diagnostic test based on a continuous or ordinal biomarker requires a cutpoint so that the biomarker can be used to classify the subject as either positive or negative. The sensitivity and specificity of a diagnostic test based on a continuous or ordinal biomarker are therefore tied to the cutpoint that is selected. A natural question to ask is "how does one determine the "optimal" cutpoint? Weiss et al. (2003–2004) selected the optimal cutpoints for the biomarkers they considered based on "levels of each biomarker that provide the best balance of sensitivity [and] specificity…."; that is, they used receiver operating characteristic (ROC) curve analysis to select their cutpoints.

A single cutpoint must be selected for all future applications of the continuous or ordinal biomarker as a diagnostic tool; however, many possible cutpoints (sometimes called *thresholds*) could be used. An ROC curve overcomes this limitation by considering all possible cutpoints (or at least a scientifically meaningful selection of cutpoints) for the biomarker.

An ROC curve is a plot of the sensitivity of the biomarker on the y-axis *versus* (1-specificity) on the x-axis. Each point on the plotted curve corresponds to a different cutpoint used to determine if the specimen should be classified as positive or negative using the biomarker after it has been dichotomized at that particular cutpoint.

Example 5.24 ROC Curve Analysis for Biomarker Data

Consider the study by Jayakumar et al. (2013), who examined the use of semaphorin (SEMA) concentration (pg per mg urinary creatinine) at 2 hours after cardiopulmonary bypass as a diagnostic test for acute kidney injury (AKI). The sample consisted of 26 children who experienced AKI and 34 children who did not. Table 5.24 contains the classification results when various cutpoints were used for SEMA concentration. The choice of a cutpoint to classify the SEMA test result as positive or negative is relatively arbitrary. Suppose that a SEMA reading of 246.7 or more, for example, is defined to be a positive test result. Then the sensitivity and specificity would be 0.92 and 0.44, respectively (Table 5.24). Alternatively, if a SEMA reading of 576.7 or more is defined to be a positive test result, then the sensitivity and specificity would be 0.69 and 0.97. Obviously, both sensitivity and specificity are highly dependent on the selected cutpoint.

TABLE 5.24 Semaphorin Test Characteristics at Different Cutoff Values

Cutoff Value for Semaphorin, pg/mg Urinary Creatinine	Sensitivity	Specificity
33.8	1.00	0.00
58.3	1.00	0.03
123.3	0.96	0.06
246.7	0.92	0.44
357.5	0.89	0.77
492.1	0.81	0.94
576.7	0.69	0.97
1125.7	0.62	1.00
9534.8	0.04	1.00

The ROC curve based on the sensitivity and specificity results for SEMA contained in Table 5.24 is given in Figure 5.3. Any plot of an ROC curve has two components: the empirical ROC curve that is obtained by joining the plotted points that represent (sensitivity, 1-specificity) for each cutpoint, together with the "chance diagonal," which is the 45 degree line drawn through the coordinates (0,0) and (1,1). If the biomarker determination diagnoses patients as positive or negative for the disease purely by chance, the ROC curve will coincide exactly with this diagonal line. Generally speaking, the most desirable cutpoint to use in the practical application of a biomarker is the value that achieves the best balance between sensitivity and specificity. This corresponds to the cutpoint that minimizes the Euclidean (straight-line) distance between the upper left-hand corner of the axes of the plot of the ROC

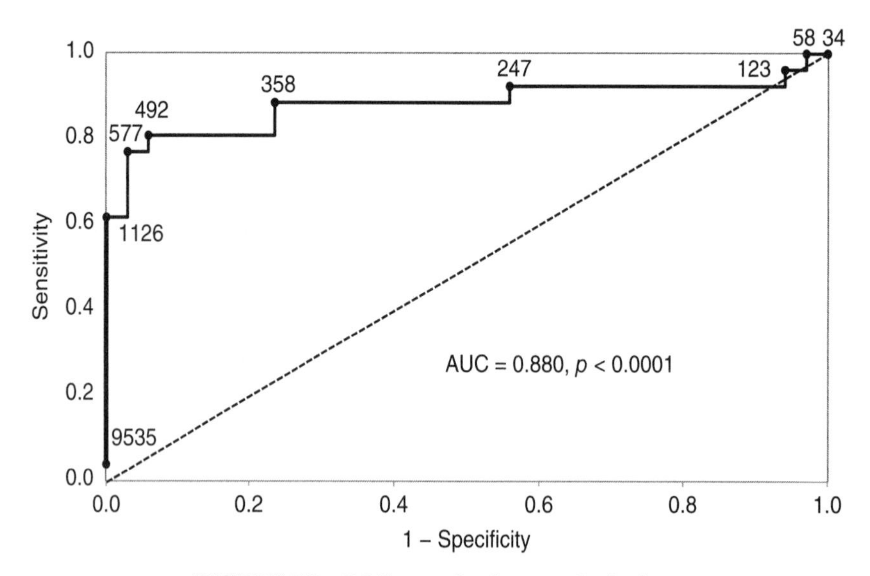

FIGURE 5.3 ROC curve for the semaphorin data.

TABLE 5.25 Guidelines for Interpreting the Area Under the ROC Curve (AUC)

Value of AUC	Interpretation
≤0.50	No discrimination
0.51–0.69	Unacceptably low
0.70–0.79	Acceptable
0.80–0.89	Excellent
0.90–1.00	Outstanding

curve (corresponding to 100% sensitivity and 100% specificity) and the ROC curve itself. We have sometimes found it useful to use a drafting compass to draw an arc through the points on the ROC curve that appear to be closest to the upper left-hand corner. It should then be obvious what value to use for the optimal cutoff.

For the ROC curve in Figure 5.3, the optimal cutpoint for SEMA is 492.1, yielding a sensitivity of 0.81 and a specificity of 0.94.

An exception to the general guideline for determining the optimal cutpoint would occur in situations in which it is desirable for the sensitivity (or specificity) to be no smaller than a certain value (e.g., a sensitivity of 90%). Then, one would choose the cutpoint that achieves this level of sensitivity and the largest possible level of specificity. For the ROC curve in Figure 5.3, the cutpoint for SEMA that maximizes specificity while yielding no less than 90% sensitivity is 246.7 pg/mg urinary creatinine, with a sensitivity of 0.92 and a specificity of 0.44 (Table 5.24).

The area under the ROC curve (AUC) is an effective way to summarize the overall diagnostic accuracy of the test based on the biomarker determination (Hanley and McNeil 1982). The AUC can be any value between 0 and 1, where a value of 0 indicates a perfectly inaccurate test and a value of 1 reflects a perfectly accurate test. If the area under the ROC curve is exactly 1, then it consists of two line segments joining the coordinates (0,0), (0,1), and (1,1). Clearly, this represents an ideal situation where both the sensitivity and the specificity of the diagnostic test based on the biomarker are 100%. Likewise, if the area under the ROC curve is exactly 0, then it represents the situation where the test based on the biomarker incorrectly classifies all patients with the disease/condition as negative and all patients without the disease/condition as positive. (In this case, the predicted categories could simply be reversed, thus achieving 100% accuracy.) In general, a value of 0.5 for the AUC is considered to be the meaningful lower bound, representing a diagnostic test with discriminating ability that is no better than chance. (In this case, the ROC curve would correspond to the "chance diagonal" in Figure 5.3.) Hosmer and Lemeshow (2000, p. 162) provide general guidelines for interpreting the AUC, as given in Table 5.25.

Since a value of 0.5 for the AUC is considered to be the lower bound for meaningful discriminating ability, it is natural to perform a hypothesis test to determine if the true area under the ROC curve is greater than 0.5. Specifically, the null and alternate hypotheses are H_0: AUC = 0.5 vs. H_a: AUC > 0.5. In this section, we describe how to obtain the estimated area, denoted by $\widehat{\text{AUC}}$, and its approximate standard error (ASE), as well as how to perform statistical inference for the true AUC using these estimates.

Several methods have been proposed for estimating the AUC, including the trapezoidal rule (Hanley and McNeil 1982). One can also fit a binormal distribution to the ROC curve and estimate the AUC using the area under the fitted curve (Zhou et al. 2011, pp. 118–133). All of these methods are rather intensive computationally and require the use of a computer. For general ROC curve analysis, we highly recommend the collection of SAS programs developed by Gönen (2007). The SAS code can be downloaded from http://support.sas.com/publishing/authors/gonen.html or http://www.mskcc.org/research/epidemiology-biostatistics/biostatistics/downloads.

R code for performing these analyses can be downloaded from the latter website.

Perhaps the easiest way to obtain the estimated AUC based on the trapezoidal rule is to note its similarity to the Mann–Whitney–Wilcoxon (M-W-W) test statistic (Hanley and McNeil 1982). The M-W-W test (Section 4.2.3.3) is a distribution-free test used to compare two samples of continuous or ordinal data that is based on counting the number of pairs for which the value of the biomarker for an "abnormal" individual exceeds the biomarker value for a "normal" individual, assuming that higher levels of the biomarker are associated with greater likelihood of being "abnormal."

Let x_A denote a biomarker reading obtained from an abnormal individual and x_N a reading obtained from a normal individual. Let

$$S(x_A, x_N) = \left\{ \begin{array}{lll} 1 & \text{if} & x_A > x_N \\ \frac{1}{2} & \text{if} & x_A = x_N \\ 0 & \text{if} & x_A < x_N \end{array} \right\}.$$

For a sample consisting of n_A abnormal individuals and n_N normal individuals, the area under the ROC curve, as approximated by the trapezoid rule, can be estimated using

$$\widehat{\text{AUC}} = \frac{1}{n_\text{A} n_\text{N}} \sum_1^{n_A} \sum_1^{n_B} S(x_A, x_B). \tag{5.39}$$

The sum $\sum_1^{n_A} \sum_1^{n_B} S(x_A, x_B)$ appearing in (5.39) is directly related to the M-W-W test statistic (Lehmann 1975, pp. 21–22).

Calculation of the ASE for $\widehat{\text{AUC}}$ is not straightforward. Hanley and McNeil describe a method that is fairly easy computationally, but is known to produce biased estimates under certain conditions. DeLong et al. (1988) proposed an alternative method that is implemented in PROC LOGISTIC in SAS and is also available in the collection of SAS programs developed by Gönen (2007) mentioned previously. The complex calculations required for this method are beyond the scope of this text; however, we do provide SAS code that can be used to calculate ASE($\widehat{\text{AUC}}$).

TABLE 5.26 Semaphorin Concentration for Children With and Without Acute Kidney Injury (AKI)

Group	Semaphorin Concentration (per pg/mg Urinary Creatinine)					
With AKI	1758.40	2178.46	1280.00	628.33	1390.00	2555.71
	492.11	1208.33	3885.00	1125.71	361.61	3772.22
	855.81	123.33	2015.00	1286.67	9534.78	58.33
	2050.00	357.50	850.00	576.67	5192.11	5411.90
	1520.00	246.67				
Without AKI	285.00	251.43	290.00	210.63	139.04	380.63
	415.50	300.00	346.88	137.50	109.77	266.25
	281.75	147.87	402.27	575.96	172.50	382.86
	252.86	170.00	169.38	910.00	299.55	33.75
	158.57	182.50	230.00	181.67	300.00	315.00
	226.25	226.67	425.71	458.89		

Source: Data courtesy of Dr. Ganesan Ramesh.

Once the ASE is obtained, an approximate Wald-type CI for the true AUC can be found by using:

$$\widehat{\text{AUC}} \pm z_{\alpha/2}\text{ASE}(\widehat{\text{AUC}}), \tag{5.40}$$

where $z_{\alpha/2}$ denotes the upper $\alpha/2$-percentage point of the standard normal distribution. The Wald method can also be used to perform a formal hypothesis test of $H_0 : \text{AUC} = 0.5$ versus $H_1 : \text{AUC} > 0.5$. The Wald-type test statistic is given by

$$z_{0\text{w}} = \frac{(\widehat{\text{AUC}} - 0.5)}{\text{ASE}(\widehat{\text{AUC}})} \tag{5.41}$$

and the upper-tailed p-value is calculated using the standard normal distribution.

Example 5.25 Estimating Area Under the ROC Curve for Biomarker Data

Consider Table 5.26, in which the SEMA concentration (per pg/mg urinary creatinine) at 2 hours after cardiopulmonary bypass is given for each child in the study by Jayakumar et al. (2013). For these data, the area under the ROC curve is estimated to be $\widehat{\text{AUC}} = 0.880$ using Equation (5.39). This means that if one uses SEMA to diagnose AKI, then one has an 88% chance of correctly distinguishing a child with the disease from a child without the disease. For these data, the method of Delong et al., as implemented in PROC LOGISTIC in SAS, yields $\text{ASE}(\widehat{\text{AUC}}) = 0.0551$,and an approximate 95% Wald CI for the true AUC of (0.772, 0.988). This indicates that SEMA provides excellent discriminating ability between those children with AKI and those without, according to the Hosmer–Lemeshow criteria. For the data in

Table 5.26, the formula in Equation (5.41) yields a test statistic of $z_{0w} = 6.90$ (p-value < 0.0001), very strong evidence that the true AUC exceeds the minimally acceptable level of 0.5.

The following SAS code can be used to perform the calculations for AUC for the data in Table 5.26. It is also available on the companion website.

```
data sema_y;
input sema_pg_creat2h @@;
datalines;
1758.40 2178.46 1280.00 628.33 1390.00 2555.71
492.11 1208.33 3885.00  1125.71 361.61 3772.22
855.81 123.33 2015.00   1286.67 9534.78 58.33
2050.00 357.50 850.00   576.67 5192.11 5411.90
1520.00 246.67
;

data sema_n;
input sema_pg_creat2h @@;
datalines;
285.00 251.43 290.00 210.63 139.04 380.63
415.50 300.00 346.88 137.50 109.77 266.25
281.75 147.87 402.27 575.96 172.50 382.86
252.86 170.00 169.38 910.00 299.55  33.75
158.57 182.50 230.00 181.67 300.00  315.00
226.25 226.67 425.71 458.89
;

data sema_y;
       set sema_y;
       aki_y = 1;

data sema_n;
       set sema_n;
       aki_y = 0;

data sema;
       set sema_y sema_n;

proc  logistic data = sema outest = coeff covout nos descending;
      model aki_y (event='1') = sema_pg_creat2h;
      roc 'SEMA at 2 hr' sema_pg_creat2h;
      title1 'Wald Interval for True AUC';
      title2 'DeLong et al. (1988) Method'
      run;
```

It is important to note that estimating the AUC has *nothing* to do with the particular cutpoint that is chosen. Rather, $\widehat{\text{AUC}}$ is simply a measure of the quality of a diagnosis based on the continuous or ordinal biomarker, without reference to which cutpoint is used.

By definition, AUC is restricted to the interval (0, 1), and there is nothing to guarantee that the endpoints of the interval given in Equation (5.40) will satisfy this restriction, especially if $\widehat{\text{AUC}}$ is close to 1.0. For this reason, several authors (Zhou et al. 2011, p. 130; Pepe, 2003, p. 107) have recommended that a logit transformation be applied to $\widehat{\text{AUC}}$ before deriving the Wald-type CI. (The logit transformation was used in Section 5.4.2.1 to derive approximate CIs for PPV and NPV.) For the estimated area under the ROC curve, the logit transformation is given by

$$\text{logit}(\widehat{\text{AUC}}) = \log\left[\frac{\widehat{\text{AUC}}}{1-\widehat{\text{AUC}}}\right], \tag{5.42}$$

which is defined provided $0 < \widehat{\text{AUC}} < 1$. Then an approximate $100(1-\alpha)\%$ Wald-type CI for logit(AUC) is given by

$$\text{logit}(\widehat{\text{AUC}}) \pm z_{\alpha/2}\text{ASE}(\text{logit}(\widehat{\text{AUC}})), \tag{5.43}$$

where $\text{ASE}(\text{logit}(\widehat{\text{AUC}}))$ denotes the approximate standard error of $\text{logit}(\widehat{\text{AUC}})$ and is given by

$$\text{ASE}(\text{logit}(\widehat{\text{AUC}})) = \frac{\text{ASE}(\widehat{\text{AUC}})}{\widehat{\text{AUC}}(1-\widehat{\text{AUC}})}. \tag{5.44}$$

Letting LL and UL denote the lower and upper confidence limits for logit(AUC) given in Equation (5.43), an approximate $100(1-\alpha)\%$ logit-based CI for AUC is given by

$$\left(\frac{e^{\text{LL}}}{1+e^{\text{LL}}}, \frac{e^{\text{UL}}}{1+e^{\text{UL}}}\right). \tag{5.45}$$

If the method based on the logit transformation is used to find a CI for the true AUC, then the corresponding test statistic is given by

$$z_{\text{ol}} = \frac{\text{logit}(\widehat{\text{AUC}})}{\text{ASE}(\text{logit}(\widehat{\text{AUC}}))}. \tag{5.46}$$

(Note that the null value is zero since $\text{logit}(0.5) = 0.0$.)

Example 5.26 Estimating Area Under the ROC Curve Using the Logit Approach

Applying the formulas in Equations (5.42)–(5.45) to the results obtained in Example 5.25, we obtain:

$$\text{logit}(\widehat{\text{AUC}}) = \log\left(\frac{\widehat{\text{AUC}}}{1 - \widehat{\text{AUC}}}\right) = \log\left(\frac{0.880}{1 - 0.880}\right) = 1.993,$$

$$\text{ASE}[\text{logit}(\widehat{\text{AUC}})] = \frac{\text{ASE}(\widehat{\text{AUC}})}{\widehat{\text{AUC}}(1 - \widehat{\text{AUC}})} = \frac{0.0551}{0.8801(1 - 0.8801)} = 0.522,$$

$$\text{logit}(\widehat{\text{AUC}}) \pm z_{\alpha/2}\text{ASE}(\text{logit}(\widehat{\text{AUC}})) = (0.970,\ 3.017),$$

and

$$\left(\frac{e^{\text{LL}}}{1 + e^{\text{LL}}}, \frac{e^{\text{UL}}}{1 + e^{\text{UL}}}\right) = \left(\frac{e^{0.970}}{1 + e^{0.970}}, \frac{e^{3.017}}{1 + e^{3.017}}\right) = (0.725,\ 0.953).$$

Thus, an approximate 95% logit-based CI for the true AUC is (0.725, 0.953). Note the difference between this interval and the 95% Wald interval presented in Example 5.25: (0.772, 0.988). For these data, the difference between these intervals is not great, but with smaller n or a value of $\widehat{\text{AUC}}$ closer to 1, the difference between the two intervals could be clinically meaningful (Pepe, 2003, p. 107). Using (5.46), the test statistic based on the logit transformation is $z_{\text{ol}} = 3.82$ (compare with the Wald test statistic of $z_{\text{ow}} = 6.90$). The Wald test and the logit-based test both provide very strong evidence that the true AUC is greater than 0.5.

Analysis based on ROC curves is often used to decide which cutpoint to use when developing a diagnostic test based on a continuous biomarker; however, this technique is often misunderstood or misapplied in the biomarker literature. For example, López et al. (2003) stated in their abstract that "On the basis of receiver operating characteristic plot analysis, the normal test threshold was set at 63 U/L" for serum tissue polypeptide antigen, which they were proposing as a biomarker for monitoring bladder tumor recurrence. However, later in their article, they stated that "The cutpoint [63 U/L] was obtained from a control group of 54 healthy subjects, using the value of the 95th percentile of this population." Choosing a cutpoint based on the 95th (or other) percentile in a healthy population (as in López et al. (2003)) is a method commonly used to determine the normal range of a continuous biomarker; however, it has nothing to do with ROC curve analysis. In fact, an examination of the ROC curve presented in Figure 1 of López et al. (2003) indicates that 63 U/L is *not* the value that provides the best balance between sensitivity and specificity (which is what ROC curve analysis would yield). Instead, their Figure 1 indicates that one should choose the cutpoint that provides 55% sensitivity and 60% specificity. (See Figure 5.4.) Because the cutpoints are not labeled on their ROC curve, there is no way to know what serum tissue polypeptide antigen concentration corresponds to this

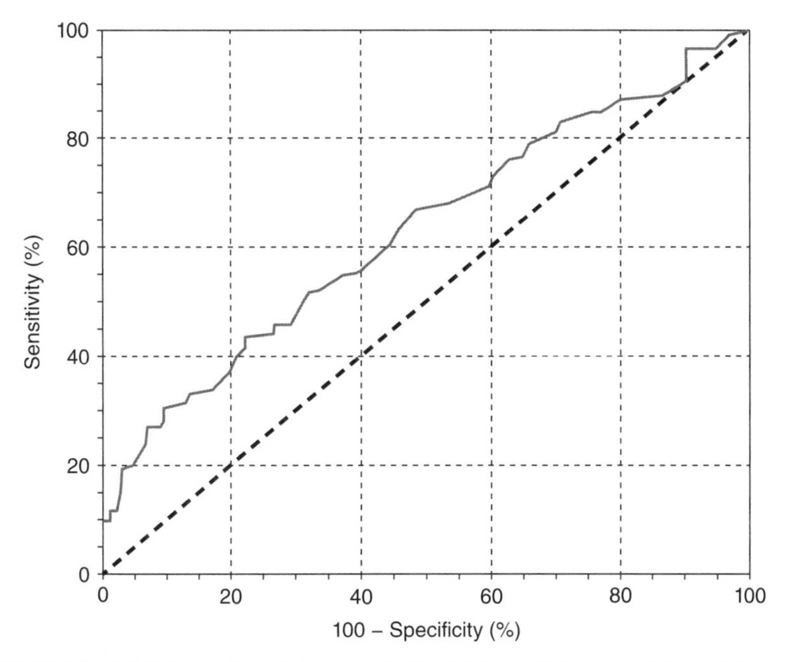

FIGURE 5.4 ROC Curve from López et al. (2003, Figure 1). Reprinted from López et al. (2003), with permission from Elsevier.

cutpoint. Using the cutpoint of 63 U/L recommended by López et al. (2003) yields 45% sensitivity and 73% specificity. Choosing a cutpoint using percentiles from a healthy population is generally not advisable (Knapp and Miller 1992, pp. 31–33); the preferred method is to relate the cutpoint determination to the outcome (typically a disease or disorder) that the biomarker is intended to diagnose, as is done in ROC curve analysis.

St. Laurent's Coefficient For some continuous biomarkers, it is not desirable (or even practical) to dichotomize the result. Rather than validating the biomarker by examining the agreement of the dichotomized version with a dichotomous gold standard, one wishes to examine the agreement between the continuous biomarker determination and a continuous gold standard. The eventual aim, of course, would be to use the continuous biomarker in place of the continuous gold standard, which is typically considered to be too expensive or too invasive to use on a routine basis. Another reason not to dichotomize a continuous biomarker unless absolutely necessary is that information is lost any time a lower level of data is used (e.g., going from an interval-level measurement to a binary-level one). On the other hand, dichotomous biomarkers generally have greater clinical utility since they are easier for clinicians to use when diagnosing a disease or condition.

As an example of the use of a continuous biomarker, Lagorio et al. (1998) evaluated urinary concentration of *trans, trans* muconic acid (*t,t*-MA) as a biomarker to be used in the monitoring of low levels of exposure to benzene. They used urinary concentration of benzene, as quantified by dynamic head-space capillary GC/FID, as the gold standard.

In a more general setting, St. Laurent (1998) describes what he calls "gold-standard comparison problems, in which an approximate method of measurement (such as a biomarker) is compared to a gold standard in order to assess the degree to which the approximate measure agrees with the gold standard." As he states, "this problem differs from calibration ... problems in that it is assumed that the methods being compared yield measurements on the same scale so that no calibration is desired." When validating a continuous biomarker, it is often of interest to conduct such a "gold-standard comparison problem" in order to examine the degree of agreement between the proposed biomarker and a measurement that is acknowledged to be the gold standard (or treated as such for purposes of validating the biomarker, in those cases where no true gold standard exists).

Example 5.27 Use of St. Laurent's Coefficient with Biomarker Data

In a study of Dutch school children (mean age = 11 years), Van Roosbroeck et al. (2008) examined the usefulness of outdoor soot concentration (as measured by diffusion tubes attached to the child's residence) as a surrogate for personal soot exposure (as measured by a badge worn by the child between the chest and head). Consistent with Van Roosbroeck et al., we will treat the outdoor soot concentration as the biomarker (X) and the personal soot exposure as the gold standard (G). The authors did not provide their raw data; however, Table 5.27 contains a close approximation to their data, obtained by visually estimating the values of X and G from the scatterplot given in their article (Figure 5.5). (Note that the original study by Van Roosbroeck et al. (2008) was based on $n = 45$ Dutch school children; however, only 43 unique data points could be identified visually from the scatterplot provided in their article.)

To calculate St. Laurent's coefficient for the data in Table 5.27, we apply Equations (5.29) and (5.31) (see Section 5.2.2.2) and obtain $r_G^2 = 0.297$, 95% CI (0.190–0.443), indicating poor agreement between outdoor soot concentration and the "personal soot" gold standard. For comparison purposes, we calculated LCC and the 95% CI using Equations (5.25) and (5.26) (Section 5.2.2.2). The results indicate slightly greater agreement than St. Laurent's coefficient: $r_c = 0.314$, 95% Wald CI (0.144–0.483). (Note that we do not recommend that the LCC be used for these data since a gold standard is available.) The PCC between X and G indicates stronger association ($r = 0.527$; 95% CI, 0.269–0.714); however, as discussed in Section 5.2.2.1, PCC cannot be recommended as a measure of agreement. Nevertheless, Van Roosbroeck et al. (2008) used the PCC to measure agreement between outdoor soot concentration and the "personal soot" gold standard.

5.4.3 Assessing Validity When a Gold Standard Is Not Available

If a gold standard is not available for the exposure or outcome that the biomarker determination is intended to detect, then the agreement between the biomarker and

TABLE 5.27 Approximate Data Estimated Visually from Van Roosbroeck et al. (2008)

Child	1	2	3	4	5	6	7	8
Personal (*X*)	10.0	10.0	10.0	10.0	10.0	10.0	10.0	10.0
Outdoor (*G*)	20.0	23.5	37.0	38.0	49.0	51.0	65.5	67.0
Child	9	10	11	12	13	14	15	16
Personal (*X*)	10.0	10.0	10.0	10.0	12.0	14.0	14.0	15.0
Outdoor (*G*)	70.0	71.0	76.0	79.0	44.0	46.0	56.0	77.0
Child	17	18	19	20	21	22	23	24
Personal (*X*)	16.0	16.0	16.0	18.0	18.0	18.0	18.0	20.5
Outdoor (*G*)	55.5	70.5	104.5	71.5	74.0	82.5	85.5	26.5
Child	25	26	27	28	29	30	31	32
Personal (*X*)	20.5	20.5	21.5	23.0	27.5	29.0	31.5	31.5
Outdoor (*G*)	31.0	34.0	48.0	55.5	60.0	85.0	65.0	67.5
Child	33	34	35	36	37	38	39	40
Personal (*X*)	31.5	33.0	49.5	62.0	62.0	90.0	102.0	104.5
Outdoor (*G*)	118.0	114.5	54.0	82.0	96.0	121.0	62.5	172.0
Child	41	42	43					
Personal (*X*)	112.0	112.0	116.0					
Outdoor (*G*)	154.0	72.5	59.0					

some other method used to determine the exposure or outcome is referred to as *consistency*. This other method could be the "standard" method or a competing biomarker. For example, suppose that no gold standard had been available in Qiao et al. (1997). Then the investigators could have compared their biomarker based on immunocytochemistry with the two "standard" methods of detecting pre-clinical, localized lung cancer that they considered (chest x-ray and sputum cytology). The consistency among these three diagnostic tests can be assessed using the general methods for assessing agreement that we described in Section 5.2.

5.4.3.1 Dichotomous Biomarkers The first step in assessing consistency between two dichotomous biomarkers or between a dichotomous biomarker and some other dichotomous classifier is to test for significant disagreement; this is analogous to what Shoukri refers to as testing for "interrater bias" when assessing IER (Shoukri 2004, pp. 49–51). In other words, one performs a hypothesis test to compare the percentage classified as positive by the biomarker with the percentage classified as positive by the other classifier. (Note that this is equivalent to comparing the percentage classified as negative by the biomarker with the percentage classified as negative by the other classifier.) As recommended by Kraemer (1980), one should also measure the degree of agreement, in addition to testing for significant disagreement.

When analyzing paired biomarker data of this type, McNemar's test can be used to test for significant disagreement. As described in Section 4.4.3.1, in order to perform McNemar's test, one must arrange the cross-classified data in the "canonical form" for dependent proportions.

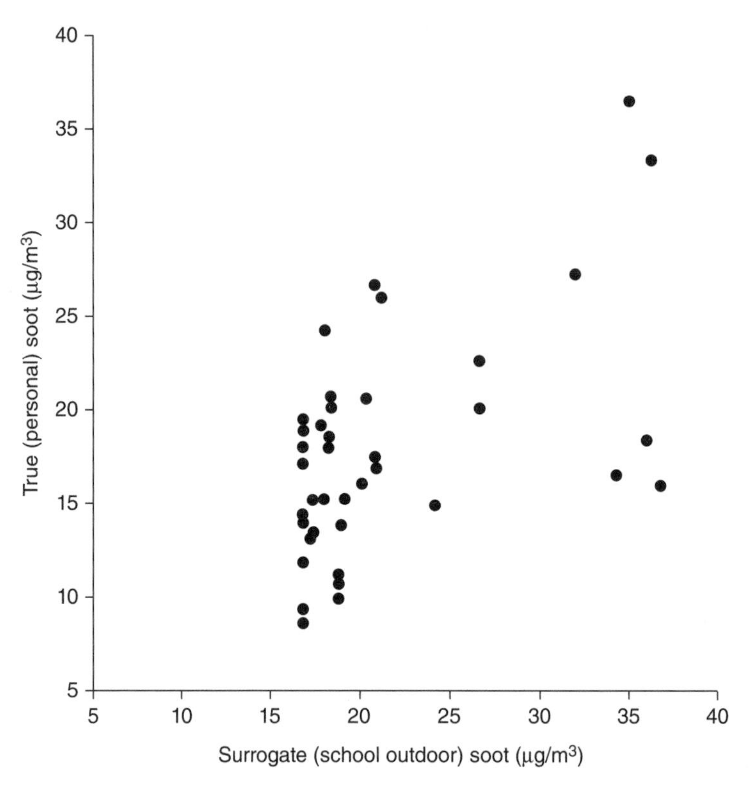

FIGURE 5.5 Scatterplot of average outdoor school soot versus personal soot exposure in the study by Van Roosbroeck et al. (2008, Figure 1). Reprinted with permission from Lippincott Williams and Wilkins/Wolters Kluwer Health: [Epidemiology] Van Roosbroeck et al. (2008), copyright (2008).

Example 5.28 Use of McNemar's Test to Assess Disagreement Between Biomarkers

A hypothetical 2×2 table for the comparison of the new biomarker proposed by Qiao et al. (1997) with chest x-ray is given in Table 5.28. This table was derived using the

TABLE 5.28 Hypothetical 2×2 Table for Comparison of a New Biomarker for Lung Cancer Versus Chest X-Ray

	Chest X-Ray		
Biomarker	Positive	Negative	Total
Positive	24	41	65
Negative	7	61	68
Total	31	102	133

assumption that their new biomarker agreed with the chest x-ray results for the 24 cases diagnosed as positive using chest x-ray.

To perform McNemar's test using the data in Table 5.28, note that $n_{12} = 41$, $n_{21} = 7$, and $n^* = 48$. (Here, we are using the same notation as in Section 4.4.3.1.) The reference distribution (conditional on the value of n^*) is a binomial with $n^* = 48$ and $\pi = 0.5$. The two-tailed exact p-value, given by $2 \cdot \Pr(n_{12} \geq 41 \mid n^* = 48, \pi = 0.5)$ is <0.0001. Thus, there is very strong evidence of significant disagreement between the new biomarker and chest x-ray. (Note that this analysis is *not* equivalent to the analysis in Example 5.22, in which the new biomarker was compared with chest x-ray in terms of sensitivity. In the analysis we are doing here, we are assuming that no gold standard was available, so that we can illustrate how consistency can be assessed by examining the agreement between two classifiers, neither of which is the gold standard.)

As in our discussion of the assessment of IAR and IER for dichotomous variables (Section 5.3.2.), we recommend that coefficient kappa (along with a 95% CI, if desired) be calculated as the "first-line" measure of the consistency between two dichotomous classifiers, neither of which is the gold standard. If, based on scientific grounds, kappa appears to provide a distorted picture of the degree of agreement (due to the shortcomings described in Section 5.2.1.1), then the PABAK coefficient should also be used, as well as p_{pos} and p_{neg}.

Example 5.29 Use of Coefficient kappa to Measure Consistency Between Biomarkers

Applying Equations (5.3) and (5.4) to the data in Table 5.28, the value of Cohen's kappa is only 0.269, with a 95% CI of (0.121–0.417), even though the two methods agree on $(24 + 61)/133 = 64\%$ of the patients. These results indicate poor agreement according to the Fleiss et al. criteria for interpreting kappa (see Table 5.3). The data in Table 5.28 possess two of the characteristics that can lead to a distortion in the performance of kappa as a measure of agreement (Section 5.2.1.1): (1) the value of kappa is affected by any discrepancy in the relative frequency of "disease" and "no disease" in the sample, and (2) the value of kappa is affected by any discrepancy in the relative frequency of "disease" for diagnostic test A and the relative frequency of "disease" for diagnostic test B. For these data, the estimated relative frequency of lung cancer averaged over the two diagnostic tests (the new biomarker and chest x-ray) is 36.1% (and hence the estimated average relative frequency of "no lung cancer" is 63.9%). The estimated relative frequency of lung cancer according to chest x-ray is only 23.3%, whereas it is 48.9% for the new biomarker. Thus, there is reason to believe that kappa is not providing an adequate measure of the agreement between the two biomarkers. However, after applying Equation (5.5) to the data in Table 5.28, we find that the PABAK coefficient provides little improvement over kappa: $PABAK = 2p_0 - 1 = 2(0.639) - 1 = 0.278$, 95% CI (0.114–0.442), results which also indicate poor agreement between the diagnostic tests. Applying the formulas in (5.6)–(5.8), we find that the indices of positive and negative agreement are

$p_{pos} = 2(24)/(31+65) = 0.500$, 95% CI (0.378–0.623) and $p_{neg} = 2(61)/(102+68) = 0.718$, 95% CI (0.641–0.794), respectively. Thus, the disagreement between the two diagnostic tests can be attributed primarily to those subjects that are thought to be positive. This conclusion is reinforced if we make use of the gold standard (as was done in Qiao et al.): the sensitivity of chest x-ray was only 42.1%, whereas it was 73.7% for the new biomarker, a difference that was found to be strongly statistically significant ($p < 0.001$) (see Example 5.23).

When there are more than two dichotomous diagnostic tests to be compared, Cochran's Q test (Section 4.4.3.2) can be used to test for significant disagreement among all of the diagnostic tests simultaneously. If Cochran's Q test fails to reject the null hypothesis that the proportions of specimens classified as "positive" by all of the diagnostic tests are equal, then the generalized version of coefficient kappa (Section 5.2.1.2) can be used to measure the overall agreement among the diagnostic tests. If Cochran's Q test rejects the null hypothesis that the proportions classified as "positive" are all equal, then McNemar's test with a Bonferroni adjustment could be used to compare each pair of diagnostic tests. If a new biomarker is being compared with a "standard" biomarker, or other commonly used tests, then attention would more than likely be focused on the comparison of the new biomarker with the test(s) already in use. We recommend that a Bonferroni adjustment (Section 3.7.2) be used to control the family-wise error rate if the new biomarker is compared with two or more competing diagnostic tests.

Example 5.30 Use of Cochran's Q to Assess Disagreement Among Three Biomarkers

For example, in the study by Qiao et al. (1997), one could use Cochran's Q test to test for significant disagreement among all three of the diagnostic tests for lung cancer (the new biomarker based on immunocytochemistry, the test based on sputum cytology, and the test based on chest x-ray) simultaneously. Qiao et al. (1997) did not present sufficient data in their article for us to be able perform Cochran's test. For illustration purposes, we created a hypothetical data set for the comparison of their new biomarker with sputum cytology and chest x-ray based on the assumption that their biomarker agreed with the sputum cytology and x-ray results on the 12 cases of lung cancer correctly identified by sputum cytology and on the 53 controls correctly identified by the new biomarker. This hypothetical data set is given in Table 5.29. Using Equation (4.52), the value of the test statistic for Cochran's Q test for these data is $Q_0 = 122.43$ and, with $df = 2$, the approximate chi-squared p-value is <0.0001. Thus, there is extremely strong evidence of significant disagreement among the three diagnostic tests. While the results of Cochran's Q test are informative, one should also measure the degree of agreement (or disagreement, in this case) among the three tests (Kraemer 1980).

For the hypothetical data in Table 5.29, applying the formulas in Equation (5.9) yields $\hat{\pi} = 0.2707, \hat{p}_e = 0.6052$, $p_0 = 0.7343$, and $\hat{\kappa}_f = 0.33$, indicating only "fair"

TABLE 5.29 Hypothetical Agreement Among Three Diagnostic Tests for Lung Cancer

Pattern of Agreement[a]	Frequency
Controls	
0 0 0	53
0 0 1	16
1 0 0	7
1 1 1	0
Cases	
0 0 0	15
0 0 1	18
1 0 1	12
1 1 1	12

[a]The first value in each pattern indicates the result for sputum cytology, the second value indicates the result for chest x-ray, and the third value indicates the result of the new biomarker based on immunocytochemistry. The pattern 1 0 1, for example, indicates that sputum cytology classified the specimen as positive, the chest x-ray classified the specimen as negative, and the new biomarker classified the specimen as positive.

agreement among the three diagnostic tests (the new biomarker, sputum cytology, and chest x-ray) using the Landis and Koch criteria (Table 5.3). Of course, Cohen's kappa (or the PABAK coefficient) could also be used to describe the agreement between the new biomarker and either sputum cytology or chest x-ray, as was done for the comparison of the biomarker versus chest x-ray using the data in Table 5.28.

5.4.3.2 Continuous Biomarkers Measuring the consistency between two continuous biomarkers, neither of which is the gold standard, is an example of what is commonly referred to as a "method comparison study" (Altman and Bland 1983; Strike 1996; Westgard and Hunt 1973). For example, Bartczak et al. (1994) compared a high-pressure liquid chromatography (HPLC)-based assay with a gas chromatography (GC) based assay for urinary muconic acid, both of which had been used previously as biomarkers for exposure to benzene. Their data, after omitting an outlier due to an unresolved chromatogram peak, are given in Table 5.30.

Bartczak et al. (1994) used the PCC in their assessment of the agreement between the two methods ($r = 0.969$; 95% CI, 0.890–0.992). However, at least as far back as 1973, it was recognized that r is not appropriate for assessing agreement in a method comparison study. In fact, Westgard and Hunt go so far as to state that "the correlation coefficient . . . is of no practical use in the statistical analysis of comparison data" (1973, p. 53).

Despite the general agreement among statisticians that r is not an acceptable measure of agreement in method comparison studies, its use in this context is still quite prevalent. Hagan and Looney (2004) found that r was used in 28% (53/189) of the method comparison studies published in the clinical research literature in 2001. The prevalence of the use of r in method comparison studies involving biomarkers was not examined separately in their study, but it is unlikely that it differed substantially from

TABLE 5.30 Comparison of Determinations of Muconic Acid (ng/mL) in Human Urine by HPLC-Diode Array and GC-MS Analysis

Specimen Number	HPLC (X_1)	GC-MS (X_2)	$X_1 - X_2$	$(X_1 + X_2)/2$
1	139	151	−12.00	145.00
2	120	93	27.00	106.50
3	143	145	−2.00	144.00
4	496	443	53.00	469.50
5	149	153	−4.00	151.00
6	52	58	−6.00	55.00
7	184	239	−55.00	211.50
8	190	256	−66.00	223.00
9	32	69	−37.00	50.50
10	312	321	−9.00	316.50
11	19	8	11.00	13.50
12	321	364	−43.00	342.50

Source: Adapted from Table 2 of Bartczak et al. (1994), reprinted by permission of Taylor & Francis Ltd.

that found in the clinical research literature as a whole. Acceptable alternatives to Pearson's r that are recommended for assessing agreement between continuous biomarkers include the ICC coefficient, Lin's coefficient of concordance, the Bland-Altman method, and Deming regression (see Sections 5.2.2.2 and 5.4.3.2). It is interesting to note, however, that these methods are rarely used even today in method comparison studies published in the clinical research literature: Hagan and Looney (2004) found that Deming regression was used in none of the 189 method comparison studies published in 2001 and Lin's coefficient was used in only one. The Bland–Altman method was used in only 25 of the published studies (13.2%). The most commonly used method was the ICC, appearing in 118 (62.4%) of the published studies.

While the ICC has been advocated as an alternative to the PCC for measuring agreement between two quantitative variables in method comparison studies (Lee, Koh, and Ong, 1989), its general use for this purpose is not recommended. The primary reason for this is that the version of the ICC recommended by Lee, Koh, and Ong is derived under the assumption that the two biomarkers being considered are a random sample from the population of all biomarkers (Bland and Altman, 1990). This assumption is usually not valid in the typical method comparison study that is used to evaluate a biomarker. Note, however, that the alternative version of the ICC presented in Section 5.2.2.2 (denoted by r_I^*) can be used if this assumption is not valid.

Regardless of the version of the ICC that is used, some of the same disadvantages associated with using the PCC to measure agreement between continuous biomarkers also apply when using the ICC. For example, the ICC, like the PCC, is dependent on the heterogeneity of the sample measurements. Furthermore, the ICC is not dependent on the scale of measurement that is used or on the size of measurement error that might be clinically allowable (Bland and Altman 1990; Atkinson 1995). LCC is also affected by the heterogeneity of the sample (Atkinson and Neville (1997); see Lin and Chinchilli (1997) for a rejoinder). For discussion of other difficulties associated

TABLE 5.31 Comparison of Various Measures of the Agreement Between Determinations of Muconic Acid (ng/mL) in Human Urine by HPLC-Diode Array and GC-MS Analysis

Measure of Agreement	Point Estimate	95% CI
Pearson correlation coefficient, r	0.969	(0.890, 0.992)
Intra-class correlation coefficient, r_I^*	0.968	(0.895, 0.991)
Lin's coefficient of concordance, r_c	0.965	(0.879, 0.985)

with using the ICC in method comparison studies, see Bartko (1994), Lin (1989), and Looney (2001).

Example 5.31 Use of the Intra-class Correlation to Measure Consistency Between Biomarkers

Returning to the method comparison data given in Table 5.30, n = 12, $\bar{x}_1 = 179.75$, $\bar{x}_2 = 191.67$, $s_1 = 137.87$, $s_2 = 134.06$, $s_{12} = 17906.5455$, $r = 0.969$. Applying Equations (5.25) and (5.26), we obtain the following value for Lin's coefficient of concordance:

$$r_c = \frac{2s_{12}}{s_1^2 + s_2^2 + (\bar{x}_1 - \bar{x}_2)^2} = \frac{2(17906.5455)}{(137.87)^2 + (134.06)^2 + (179.75 - 191.67)^2} = 0.965$$

and $\hat{se}(r_c) = 0.022$. An approximate 95% CI for ρ_c based on 1000 bootstrap samples is given by (0.879, 0.985).

For the version of the ICC that does not depend on the assumption that the two biomarkers being considered are a random sample from the population of all biomarkers (ICC(3,1)), Equations (5.23) and (5.24) yield $r_I^* = 0.968$ (95% CI, 0.895–0.991). Recalling our earlier results for the PCC, $r = 0.969$ (95% CI, 0.890–0.992). Thus, the values for the PCC, ICC, and LCC are almost identical and all of them indicate a strong degree of consistency between the two biomarkers for benzene exposure (Table 5.31). However, as we will see in the next section, another assessment method will give us reason to doubt the consistency between these two biomarkers.

In the next three sections, we present alternative methods for assessing agreement that have none of the disadvantages we have described for the PCC, the ICC, and the LCC, and therefore are capable of detecting deficiencies in agreement between two continuous variables in a method comparison study that would not be evident if one of the more traditional measures of agreement were used.

The Bland–Altman Method An alternative approach that can be used to assess consistency between two continuous biomarkers X_1 and X_2 that are both in the same units is the Bland–Altman Method (Altman and Bland 1983; Bland and Altman 1986). The steps involved in this approach are as follows:

(1) Construct the scatterplot of X_2 versus X_1 and superimpose the line $X_2 = X_1$.
(2) Plot the difference between X_1 and X_2 for each subject (denoted by d) versus the mean of X_1 and X_2 for each subject (denoted by m).
(3) Perform a visual check of the assumption that the within-subject repeatability is not correlated with the size of the measurement, that is, that the bias (as measured by d) does not increase (or decrease) systematically as m increases.
(4) Perform a formal hypothesis test to confirm the visual check in Step (3) above by testing H_0: $\rho = 0$, where ρ is the true correlation between d and m. (See Section 3.8.)
(5) If the correlation between d and m is not significant, proceed to Step (6) below. If the correlation is significant, then one should attempt to find a suitable transformation of X_1 or X_2 (or both) so that there is no apparent association between d and m when they are calculated using the transformed data. This is accomplished by repeating Steps (2)–(4) above for the transformed data. The logarithmic transformation has been found to be most useful transformation for this purpose, but other transformations should also be considered. (See Section 4.2.3.1 for general advice on finding a transformation.) If no transformation can be found, Altman and Bland (1983) recommend describing the differences between the two methods being compared by regressing ($X_1 - X_2$) on $(X_1 + X_2)/2$.
(6) Calculate the "limits of agreement": $\bar{d} - 2s_d$ *to* $\bar{d} + 2s_d$, where $\bar{d}$ is the mean difference between X_1 and X_2 ands_d is the standard deviation of the differences (or the corresponding quantities if either X_1 or X_2 were transformed).
(7) Approximately 95% of the differences d should fall within the limits of agreement (assuming a normal distribution). If the differences within these limits are not considered to be clinically relevant, then the two methods X_1 and X_2 can be used interchangeably. However, it is important to emphasize that this method is applicable *only* if both X_1 and X_2 are measured in the same units.

Example 5.32 Use of the Bland–Altman Method to Examine Consistency Between Biomarkers

Consider again the data in Table 5.30 that examined the agreement between two biomarkers of exposure to benzene. Figure 5.6 shows the scatterplot of X_2 versus X_1 with the line $X_2 = X_1$ superimposed. This plot indicates fairly good agreement between X_1 and X_2 except that 9 of the 12 data points are below the line of perfect agreement. The Bland–Altman plot of the difference (HPLC – GC) versus the mean of HPLC and GC is given in Figure 5.7. A visual inspection of this plot suggests that the within-subject repeatability is not associated with the size of the measurement; in other words, d = (HPLC – GC) does not appear to increase (or decrease) systematically as m = (HPLC + GC)/2 increases. There is no evidence of a departure from the normality assumption using the Shapiro–Wilk test (Section 4.2.2.3) for either d ($W_0 = 0.97, p = 0.890$) or m ($W_0 = 0.94, p = 0.455$). The sample correlation between d and m is $r = 0.113$ and the p-value for the test of H_0: $\rho = 0$ is

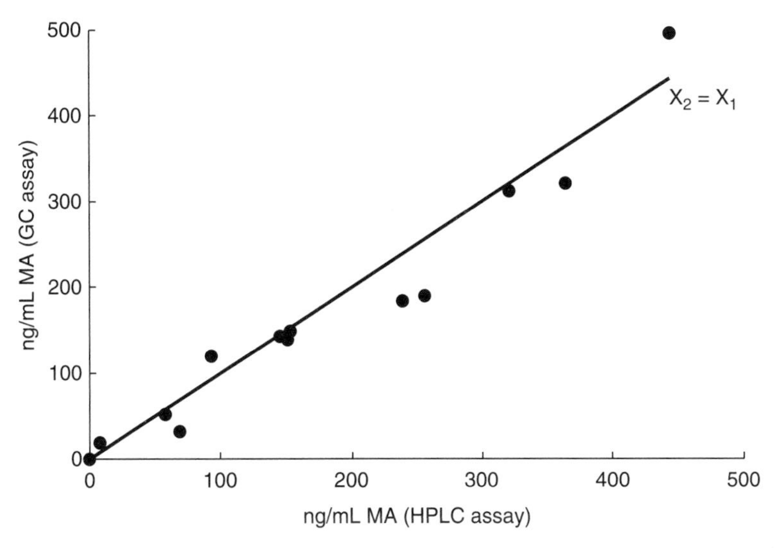

FIGURE 5.6 Scatterplot for assessing agreement between two biomarkers of exposure to benzene: X_1 = high-pressure liquid chromatography (HPLC)-based assay and X_2 = gas chromatography (GC)-based assay for urinary muconic acid. Reprinted from Looney and Hagan (2008), with permission from Elsevier.

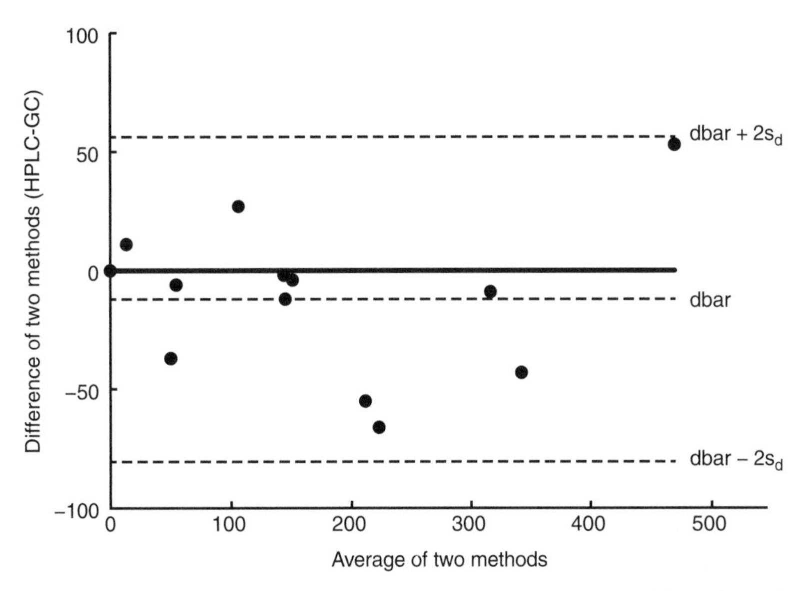

FIGURE 5.7 Bland–Altman plot for assessing agreement between two biomarkers of exposure to benzene: high-pressure liquid chromatography (HPLC) based assay and gas chromatography (GC) based assay for urinary muconic acid. Reprinted from Looney and Hagan (2008), with permission from Elsevier.

0.728 (see Section 3.8); thus, there is no evidence against the assumption that d and m are independent. The "limits of agreement" are $\bar{d} - 2s_d = -11.9 - 2(34.2) = -80.3$ to $\bar{d} + 2s_d = -11.9 + 2(34.2) = 56.5$; these are represented (along with $\bar{d}$) by dotted lines in Figure 5.7. (Note that all of the differences fall within the limits $\bar{d} - 2s_d$ to $\bar{d} + 2s_d$.) If differences as large as 80.3 in absolute value are not clinically relevant, then the two methods can be used interchangeably. However, given the order of magnitude of the measurements in Table 5.30, a difference of 80 ng/mL is likely to be clinically important, so a reasonable conclusion would be that there is inadequate agreement between the two methods. This was not obvious from the standard scatterplot of the data given in Figure 5.6, nor from the results of the traditional measures of agreement summarized in Table 5.31.

Deming Regression Strike (1996, pp. 155–164) describes a methodology that can be used to determine the type of disagreement that may be present in a method comparison study. In the context of the analysis of biomarker data, his approach is most likely to be applicable when one of the methods (say, Method X) is a *reference* method (perhaps a biomarker that is already in routine use) and the other method (say, Method Y) is a *test* method (most commonly, a new biomarker that is being evaluated). Any systematic difference (or *bias*) between the two determinations is relative in nature, since neither Method X nor Method Y is assumed to represent the true value of the analyte (i.e., neither is the gold standard).

As in the Bland–Altman method, the first step is to construct a scatterplot of Y versus X and superimpose the line of perfect agreement $Y = X$. Any systematic discrepancy between Methods X and Y will be indicated on this plot by a general shift in the location of the plotted points away from the line $Y = X$. Strike makes the assumption that systematic differences between Methods X and Y can be attributed to either *constant bias*, *proportional bias*, or both, and assumes the following underlying model:

$$X_i = \xi_i + \delta_i, \quad 1 \le i \le n \tag{5.47}$$

$$Y_i = \eta_i + \varepsilon_i, \quad 1 \le i \le n,$$

where

X_i = observed value for Method X,
ξ_i = true value for Method X,
δ_i = random error for Method X,
Y_i = observed value for Method Y,
η_i = true value for Method Y,
ε_i = random error for Method Y.

Strike makes the additional assumption that the errors δ_i and ε_i are stochastically independent of each other and normally distributed with constant variance (σ_δ^2 and σ_ε^2, respectively). Strike points out that constant variance assumptions such as these are usually unrealistic in practice and recommends a computationally intensive method, called *weighted Deming regression*, which can account for this heterogeneity (Linnet, 1990, 1993). This method, along with (unweighted) Deming regression, is available in the CBstat software package. It is freely available and can be downloaded from http://cbstat5.software.informer.com/. SAS code for performing unweighted Deming regression was provided by Deal et al. (2009) and is included on the companion website.

Strike further assumes that any systematic discrepancy between Methods X and Y can be represented by the following linear model:

$$\eta_i = \beta_0 + \beta_1 \xi_i. \tag{5.48}$$

In this model, *constant bias* is indicated by deviations of β_0 from 0 and *proportional bias* by deviations of β_1 from 1. (This is the same terminology used by Westgard and Hunt (1973)). If we now incorporate Equation (5.48) into the equation for Y_i in Equation (5.47), we have

$$Y_i = \beta_0 + \beta_1 X_i + (\epsilon_i - \beta_1 \delta_i). \tag{5.49}$$

The model represented in (5.49) is sometimes called a *functional errors-in-variables model* and assessing agreement between Methods X and Y requires estimation of β_0 and β_1. Strike recommends a method that requires an estimate of the ratio of the error variances $\lambda = \sigma_\epsilon^2/\sigma_\delta^2$. The method that Strike describes is generally referred to in the clinical laboratory literature as "Deming regression"; however, this is somewhat of a misnomer since Deming was concerned with generalizing the errors-in-variables model to nonlinear relationships, not the present modeling situation. Strike points out that the method he advocates for estimating β_0 and β_1 is actually due to Kummel (1879).

The estimates of β_0 and β_1 recommended by Strike are

$$\hat{\beta}_1 = \frac{(S_{yy} - \hat{\lambda} S_{xx}) + \sqrt{(S_{yy} - \hat{\lambda} S_{xx})^2 + 4\hat{\lambda} S_{xy}^2}}{2S_{xy}}, \tag{5.50}$$

$$\hat{\beta}_0 = \bar{Y} - \hat{\beta}_1 \bar{X},$$

where

$$\hat{\lambda} = \hat{\sigma}_\epsilon^2 / \hat{\sigma}_\delta^2,$$

$$S_{yy} = \sum_{i=1}^{n} (y_i - \bar{y})^2, \ S_{xx} = \sum_{i=1}^{n} (x_i - \bar{x})^2, \ S_{xy} = \sum_{i=1}^{n} (x_i - \bar{x})(y_i - \bar{y}).$$

The estimate $\hat{\lambda}$ can be obtained either from the error variance estimates for methods X and Y provided by the laboratory or by estimating the error variance for each method using

$$\hat{\sigma}^2 = \sum_{i=1}^{n} d_i^2/(2n),$$

where d_i is the difference between two determinations (calculated from replicate samples) for a given method for specimen i. (The error variance can also be estimated from the assessment of reliability recommended by Taioli et al. (1994) that we described in Section 5.3.4.) It is important to note that the "Deming regression" approach described by Strike *cannot* be applied without an estimate of the ratio of error variances of the two methods. If no data are available, $\hat{\sigma}^2$ can be set equal to 1, but this yields only approximate, and possibly inaccurate, results.

Significance tests for β_0 and β_1 require formulas for the ASEs of $\hat{\beta}_0$ and $\hat{\beta}_1$; the approximations that Strike recommends for routine use are given by

$$\text{ASE}(\hat{\beta}_1) = \left\{ \frac{\hat{\beta}_1^2[(1-r^2)/r^2]}{n-2} \right\}^{1/2}, \tag{5.51}$$

$$\text{ASE}(\hat{\beta}_0) = \left\{ \frac{[\text{ASE}(\hat{\beta}_1)]^2 \sum_{i=1}^{n} x_i^2}{n} \right\}^{1/2},$$

where

$$r^2 = [S_{xy}^2/(S_{xx}S_{yy})]$$

is the usual "R^2" value for the regression of Y on X. Tests of $H_0 : \beta_1 = 1$ and $H_0 : \beta_0 = 0$ can be performed by comparing $t_{01} = (\hat{\beta}_1 - 1)/\text{ASE}(\hat{\beta}_1)$ and $t_{00} = \hat{\beta}_0/\text{ASE}(\hat{\beta}_0)$, respectively, with the t distribution with $n - 2$ degrees of freedom.

Example 5.33 Use of Deming Regression to Examine Consistency Between Biomarkers

Consider once again the data in Table 5.10 that were discussed in Section 5.2.2. The scatterplot of Y versus X in Figure 5.1 indicated substantial lack of agreement between X and Y and this was confirmed by the ICCs ($r_I = 0.095$, $r_I^* = 0.307$) and Lin's coefficient (LCC = 0.088), all of which indicated substantial disagreement. We apply the methodology recommended by Strike in order to gain a better understanding of the nature and extent of this disagreement.

Using Equations (5.50) and (5.51), we obtain $\hat{\beta}_1 = 0.158$, $\text{ASE}(\hat{\beta}_1) = 0.008$, $\hat{\beta}_0 = -1.318$, $\text{ASE}(\hat{\beta}_0) = 0.691$. For the test of $H_0 : \beta_1 = 1$, this yields

$$t_{01} = \frac{\hat{\beta}_1 - 1}{SE(\hat{\beta}_1)} = \frac{0.158 - 1}{0.008} = -152.88,$$

and using a t-distribution with $df = n - 2 = 9$, we find $p < 0.0001$. Therefore, there is significant proportional bias (which in this case is negative since $\hat{\beta}_1 < 1.0$). For the test of $H_0 : \beta_0 = 0$, we have

$$t_{00} = \frac{\hat{\beta}_0}{SE(\hat{\beta}_0)} = \frac{-1.318}{0.691} = -1.91,$$

and again using a t-distribution with $df = 9$, we have $p = 0.089$. Thus, the constant bias is not statistically significant.

SAS code for performing these analyses is provided on the companion website.

Spearman's Correlation Another method that can be used to measure consistency between measurements in a method comparison study is SCC, denoted by r_s. (See Section 4.5.1.1 for a general description.) This method is useful, and to be preferred over PCC, when examining the agreement between two biomarkers whose determinations are in different units, or between a biomarker and some other measure of exposure such as environmental monitoring. For example, Coultas et al. (1990) used the SCC to measure the consistency between various measures of exposure to environmental tobacco smoke at work (e.g., nicotine exposure measured with a personal monitoring pump vs. post-shift urinary cotinine).

Suppose that one wishes to use the SCC to measure the agreement between two biomarkers that are measured in different units. If the value of the SCC is close to one, the implication is that a subject with high levels of exposure according to Biomarker A will also tend to have high levels of exposure according to Biomarker B. Therefore, regardless of which biomarker is used, there is support for the assumption that subjects will be assigned to a high (or low) exposure group in a consistent manner. However, the PCC is not recommended for measuring consistency between biomarker determinations; one of the main reasons is that r may be low even though high levels of exposure according to Biomarker A are associated with high levels of exposure according to Biomarker B. This can occur, for example, if the relationship between the two biomarkers is nonlinear. SCC will have a large value if the two biomarker determinations are strongly related according to *any* monotonic relationship.

Example 5.34 Use of Spearman Correlation to Measure Consistency Between Biomarkers

Consider the data in Table 5.32 on concentrations of o-cresol and hippuric acid in urine samples of workers exposed to toluene (Amorim and Alvarez-Leite, 1997),

TABLE 5.32 Data on Concentrations of *o*-Cresol and Hippuric Acid Concentrations in Urine Samples

Specimen Number	*o*-Cresol (μg/mL)	Rank of *o*-Cresol	Hippuric Acid (mg/mL)	Rank of Hippuric Acid
1	0.21	1.5	0.30	2.0
2	0.21	1.5	0.80	5.0
3	0.25	3.0	0.40	3.0
4	0.28	4.0	0.50	4.0
5	0.32	5.0	1.10	7.5
6	0.34	6.0	1.19	9.0
7	0.41	7.0	1.30	12.0
8	0.44	8.5	1.08	6.0
9	0.44	8.5	1.10	7.5
10	0.51	10.0	1.20	10.5
11	0.59	11.0	1.20	10.5
12	0.76	12.0	1.33	13.0
13	1.25	13.0	0.20	1.0
14	1.36	14.0	2.10	14.0
15	2.80	15.0	3.02	15.0

Source: Adapted, with permission, from Tables 1–3 of Amorim and Alvarez-Leite (1997), reprinted by permission of Taylor & Francis Ltd.

which have been ranked according to the magnitude of the *o*-cresol value. Applying the formula in Equation (4.55), we obtain $r_s = 0.632$, which indicates a moderate degree of consistency between the two measurements using the Morton et al. criteria for interpreting correlation coefficients (see Section 4.5.3). However, even though this correlation is statistically significant ($p = 0.019$), the 95% CI (obtained using Equation (4.65)) is extremely wide due to the small sample size ($n = 15$): (0.124, 0.877). The consistency between *o*-cresol and hippuric acid as biomarkers for toluene exposure using the Amorim and Alvarez-Leite data is examined in greater detail in Example 4.31.

5.4.4 Assessing Criterion Validity in Method Comparison Studies

There are two types of validity that should be examined when validating a biomarker in the absence of a gold standard. *Criterion validity* is assessed by correlating the biomarker with measures of other phenomena that are expected to be correlated with the exposure or outcome that the biomarker represents. There are two types of criterion validity, *concurrent* and *predictive*. *Concurrent* refers to other phenomena that are contemporaneous with the biomarker, whereas *predictive* refers to phenomena that occur at some future time point.

For example, one could assess the concurrent validity of urinary *o*-cresol as a biomarker of exposure to toluene for the study described in Example 5.34 by correlating the concentration of *o*-cresol in the urine of workers exposed to toluene with urinary hippuric acid, which is the most frequently used biomarker for occupational exposure to toluene (Amorim and Alvarez-Leite 1997). As an example of predictive validity, in a study of the usefulness of plasma cotinine as a biomarker for environmental tobacco smoke, the authors examined the correlation between plasma cotinine and the metabolic clearance of theophylline, a drug whose metabolism is known to be increased in nonsmokers by the presence of cigarette smoke (Matsunga et al. 1989). The PCC is typically used to measure criterion validity; however, we recommend that the SCC be used instead since the PCC only measures the degree of linear relationship, whereas the SCC is sensitive to any monotonic relationship between the biomarker and the criterion.

5.4.5 Assessing Construct Validity in Method Comparison Studies

The other type of validity that should be assessed in the absence of a gold standard is *construct validity*, which is assessed by testing hypotheses formulated by the investigator about the characteristics of those who should have high levels of the exposure represented by the biomarker vs. those who should have low levels. For example, Hüttner et al. (1999) evaluated chromosomal aberrations in human peripheral blood lymphocytes as a biomarker of chronic exposure to heavy metals and dioxins/furans over a long period of time. As part of their examination of construct validity, they compared 52 exposed individuals from a polluted area with 51 matched controls from a distant non-industrialized area and found a statistically significant increase in the frequency of chromosomal aberrations in human peripheral blood lymphocytes in the exposed group (*t*-test; $p < 0.001$). Construct validity is generally assessed by performing the appropriate statistical test to carry out the comparison of interest. For example, Hüttner, Götze, and Nikolova used Fisher's exact test to compare the exposed and unexposed individuals in terms of the dichotomous outcome: chromosomal aberration vs. no chromosomal aberration. For continuous outcomes, the appropriate normal-theory test should be used if the outcome appears to follow a normal distribution (*t*-test for the comparison of two groups, one-way ANOVA for more than two groups). If the outcome data are highly skewed or otherwise non-normal, the M-W-W test should be used to compare two groups, and the Kruskal–Wallis test should be used for more than two groups. See Section 4.2.3.3 for a description of how to perform these tests.

PROBLEMS

5.1. A hypothetical 2×2 table for the comparison of the biomarker proposed by Qiao et al. (1997) with their results for sputum cytology is given below. This table was derived using the assumption that their biomarker agreed with the sputum cytology result on the 12 cases diagnosed as positive using sputum cytology. Use the results in the table to assess the agreement between immunocytochemistry and sputum cytology.

Hypothetical 2 × 2 Table for Comparison of Two Biomarkers for Lung Cancer

	Immunocytochemistry		
Sputum Cytology	Positive	Negative	Total
Positive	12	0	12
Negative	53	68	121
Total	65	68	133

5.2. Suppose a study of biomarkers for Alzheimer's disease yielded the results in the table below. Evaluate the agreement between these three biomarkers.

Results of Three Biomarker Tests for Patients Screened for Alzheimer's Disease

Patient	Serum Amyloid-β	Apolipoprotein E Genotype	Magnetic Resonance Imaging of the Brain
1	Normal	Normal	Normal
2	Normal	Normal	Normal
3	Normal	Normal	Abnormal
4	Abnormal	Abnormal	Abnormal
5	Abnormal	Abnormal	Abnormal
6	Normal	Normal	Normal
7	Normal	Normal	Abnormal
8	Normal	Normal	Normal
9	Normal	Normal	Normal
10	Abnormal	Normal	Normal
11	Normal	Normal	Normal
12	Normal	Normal	Normal
13	Normal	Normal	Normal
14	Normal	Normal	Abnormal
15	Normal	Normal	Normal
16	Normal	Normal	Normal
17	Abnormal	Abnormal	Abnormal
18	Normal	Normal	Normal
19	Abnormal	Abnormal	Abnormal
20	Abnormal	Abnormal	Abnormal
21	Normal	Normal	Normal
22	Abnormal	Normal	Abnormal
23	Normal	Normal	Normal

5.3. Right Heart Catheterization (RHC) is the gold standard for diagnosis of pulmonary artery hypertension (PAH). A study of patients referred for RHC was undertaken to assess the utility of screening for PAH with a less invasive radionucleotide technique that measures the right atrial emptying rate (RAER). Use the data in the following table to assess the performance of the radionucleotide technique for diagnosing PAH by computing the following:

A) Sensitivity of RAER

B) Specificity of RAER

C) Positive predictive value of RAER

D) Negative predictive value of RAER

E) Accuracy of RAER

Results From a Radionucleotide Technique to Screen 66 Patients for PAH, Where RHC Results are Considered to Represent the True Disease State

		RHC	
		+	−
Radionucleotide technique	+	19	2
	−	6	39

5.4. Suppose a study was conducted to assess the potential utility of aberrant crypt foci (ACF) as a biomarker of colorectal cancer. For this study, endoscopists' magnification chromoendoscopic diagnosis of ACF yielded the results shown in the tables in parts (A) and (B) below.

A) Use the data in the following table to evaluate the inter-rater reliability of the endoscopists' ACF diagnoses.

Two Endoscopists' ACF Diagnoses on 213 Colorectal Biopsies

		Rater 2 ACF?	
		Yes	No
Rater 1 ACF?	Yes	43	38
	No	29	103

B) Use the data in the following table to evaluate the intra-rater reliability of the endoscopist's ACF diagnoses.

An Endoscopist's ACF Diagnosis on 213 Colorectal Biopsies Evaluated on Two Different Occasions

		Second Diagnosis ACF?	
		Yes	No
First Diagnosis ACF?	Yes	54	27
	No	19	113

REFERENCES

Aberson, C.L. (2010), *Applied Power Analysis for the Behavioral Sciences*, New York: Routledge.

Adams, G., Gulliford, M.C., Ukoumunne, O.C., Eldridge, S., Chinn, S., and Campbell, M.J. (2004), "Patterns of Intra-Cluster Correlation From Primary Care Research to Inform Study Design and Analysis," *Journal of Clinical Epidemiology*, 57, 785–794.

Agresti, A. (2007), *An Introduction to Categorical Data Analysis* (2nd ed.), New York: John Wiley & Sons.

Agresti, A., Mehta, C.R., and Patel, N.R. (1990), "Exact Inference for Contingency Tables with Ordered Categories," *Journal of the American Statistical Association*, 85, 453–458.

Ahlbom, A. (1993), *Biostatistics for Epidemiologists*, Boca Raton: Lewis Publishers.

Aldor-Noiman, S., Brown, L.D., Buja, A., Rolke, W., and Stine, R.A. (2013), "The Power to See: A New Graphical Test for Normality," *The American Statistician*, 67, 249–260.

Algina, J., Oshima, T.C., and Lin, W. (1994), "Type I Error Rates for Welch's Test and James's Second-Order Test Under Nonnormality and Inequality of Variance When There are Two Groups," *Journal of Educational and Behavioral Statistics*, 19, 275–291.

Altman, D.G. and Bland, J.M. (1983), "Measurement in Medicine: The Analysis of Method Comparison Studies," *The Statistician*, 32, 307–317.

Amorim, L.C.A. and Alvarez-Leite, E.M. (1997), "Determination of o-Cresol by Gas Chromatography and Comparison with Hippuric Acid Levels in Urine Samples of Individuals Exposed to Toluene," *Journal of Toxicology and Environmental Health*, 50, 401–407.

Analysis of Biomarker Data: A Practical Guide, First Edition. Stephen W. Looney and Joseph L. Hagan.

Ansari, A.A., Ali, S.K., and Donnon, T. (2013), "The Construct and Criterion Validity of the Mini-CES: A Meta-Analysis of the Published Research," *Academic Medicine*, 88, 413–420.

Armitage, P. (1955), "Test for Linear Trend in Proportions and Frequencies," *Biometrics*, 11, 375–386.

Atawodi, S.E., Lea, S., Nyberg, F., Mukeria, A., Constantinescu, V., Ahrens, W., Brueske-Hohlfeld, I., Fortes, C., Boffetta, P., and Friesen, M.D. (1998), "4-Hydroxyl-1-(3-Pyridyl)-1-Butanone-Hemoglobin Adducts as Biomarkers of Exposure to Tobacco Smoke: Validation of a Method to be Used in Multicenter Studies," *Cancer Epidemiology, Biomarkers and Prevention*, 7, 817–821.

Atkinson, A.C. (1973), "Testing Transformations to Normality," *Journal of the Royal Statistical Society B* 35, 473–479.

Atkinson, G. (1995), "A Comparison of Statistical Methods for Assessing Measurement Repeatability in Ergonomics Research," in *Sport, Leisure and Ergonomics*, eds. G. Atkinson and T. Reilly, London: E. & F. N. Spon, pp. 218–222.

Atkinson, G. and Nevill, A. (1997), "Comment on the Use of Concordance Correlation to Assess the Agreement Between Two Variables," *Biometrics*, 53, 775–777 (Letter to the Editor).

Ayadi, L., Chaabouni, S., Khabir, A., Amouri, H., Makni, S., Guermazi, M., Frikha, M., and Boudawara, T. (2010), "Correlation Between Immunohistochemical Biomarkers Expression and Prognosis of Ovarian Carcinomas in Tunisian Patients," *World Journal of Oncology*, 1, 118–128.

Barnett, V. and Lewis, T. (1995), *Outliers in Statistical Data* (3rd ed.), Chichester: John Wiley & Sons.

Bartczak, A., Kline, S.A., Yu, R., Weisel, C.P., Goldstein, B.D., Witz, G., and Bechtold, W.E. (1994), "Evaluation of Assays for the Identification and Quantitation of Muconic Acid, a Benzene Metabolite in Human Urine," *Journal of Toxicology and Environmental Health*, 42, 245–258.

Bartko, J.J. (1994), "General Methodology II. Measures of Agreement: A Single Procedure," *Statistics in Medicine*, 13, 737–745.

BDWG (Biomarkers Definitions Working Group) (2001), "Biomarkers and Surrogate Endpoints: Preferred Definitions and Conceptual Framework," *Clinical Pharmacology and Therapeutics*, 69, 89–95.

Berenson, M.L., Levine, D.M., and Goldstein, M. (1983), *Intermediate Statistical Methods: A Computer Package Approach*, Englewood Cliffs, NJ: Prentice-Hall, pp. 319–320.

Bernstein, C., Bernstein, H., Garewal, P., Dinning, R., Jabi, R.E., Sampliner, M.K., McCluskey, M., Panda, D.J., Roe, L.L., L'Heureux, L., and Payne, C. (1999), "A Bile Acid-Induced Apoptosis Assay for Colon Cancer Risk and Associated Quality Control Studies," *Cancer Research*, 59, 2353–2357.

Bland, J.M. and Altman, D.G. (1986), "Statistical Methods for Assessing Agreement Between Two Methods of Clinical Measurement," *The Lancet*, 8, 307–310.

Bland, J.M. and Altman, D.G. (1990), "A Note on the Use of the Intraclass Correlation Coefficient in the Evaluation of Agreement Between Two Methods of Measurement," *Computers in Biology and Medicine*, 20, 337–340.

Blankenberg, S., Zeller, T., Saarela, O., Havulinna, A.S., Kee, F., Tunstall-Pedoe, H., Kuulasmaa, K., Yarnell, J., Schnabel, R.B., Wild, P.S., Münzel, T.F., Lackner, K.J.,

Tiret, L., Evans, A., and Salomaa, V. (2010), "Contribution of 30 Biomarkers to 10-Year Cardiovascular Risk Estimation in 2 Population Cohorts," *Circulation*, 121, 2388–2397.

Bonett D.G. and Wright T.A. (2000), "Sample Size Requirements for Estimating Pearson, Kendall, and Spearman Correlations," *Psychometrika*, 65, 23–28.

Box, G.E.P. and Cox D.R. (1964), "An Analysis of Transformations," *Journal of the Royal Statistical Society B*, 26, 211–252.

Box, G.E. and Draper, N.R. (1987), *Empirical Model-Building and Response Surfaces*, New York: John Wiley & Sons.

Bradley, J.V. (1978), "Robustness?" *British Journal of Mathematical and Statistical Psychology*, 31, 144–152.

Brown, B.W. (1980), "Prediction Analyses for Binary Data," in *Biostatistics Casebook*, eds. R.G. Miller, B. Efron, B.W. Brown, and L.E. Moses, New York: John Wiley & Sons, pp. 3–18.

Brown, M.B. and Forsythe, A.B. (1974), "Robust Tests for the Equality of Variances," *Journal of the American Statistical Association*, 69, 364–367.

Buckley, T.J., Waldman, J.M., Dhara, R., Greenberg, A., Ouyang, Z., and Lioy, P.J. (1995), "An Assessment of Urinary Biomarker for Total Human Environmental Exposure to Benzo[α]pyrene," *International Archives of Occupational and Environmental Health*, 67, 257–266.

Burzykowski, T., Molenberghs, G., and Buyse, M. (eds.) (2005), *The Evaluation of Surrogate Endpoints*, New York: Springer.

Buss, I.H., Senthilmohan, R., Darlow, B.A., Mogridge, N., Kettle, A.J., and Winterbourn, C.C. (2003), "3-Chlorotyrosine as a Marker of Protein Damage by Myeloperoxidase in Tracheal Aspirates from Preterm Infants: Association With Adverse Respiratory Outcome," *Pediatric Research*, 53, 455–462.

Buyse, M. and Molenberghs, G. (1998), "Criteria for the Validation of Surrogate Endpoints in Randomized Experiments," *Biometrics*, 54, 1014–1029.

Buyse, M., Molenberghs, G., Burzykowski, T., Renard, D., and Geys, H. (2000), "The Validation of Surrogate Endpoints in Meta-Analyses of Randomized Experiments," *Biostatistics*, 1(1), 49–67.

Byrt, T., Bishop, J., and Carlin, J.B. (1993), "Bias, Prevalence, and Kappa," *Journal of Clinical Epidemiology*, 46, 423–429.

Carroll, R.J. and Ruppert, D. (1988), *Transformations and Weighting in Regression*, New York: Chapman & Hall.

Casella, G. and Berger, R.L. (2002), *Statistical Inference* (2nd ed.), Pacific Grove, CA: Duxbury.

Chauvenet, W. (1863), "Method of Least Squares," Appendix to *Manual of Spherical and Practical Astronomy*, Vol. 2, Philadelphia: Lippincott, pp. 469–566. Reprinted (1960), (5th ed.), New York: Dover.

Cheng, N.F. and Gansky, S.A. (2006), "A SAS Macro to Compute Lin's Concordance Correlation with Confidence Intervals." Supported by NIH grant number U54DE014251. UCSF CAN-DO website. Available at http://www.cando.ucsf.edu/#!publications/csll. Accessed December 29, 2006.

Chiaradia, M., Gulson, B.L., and MacDonald, K. (1997), "Contamination of Houses by Workers Occupationally Exposed in a Lead-Zinc-Copper Mine and Impact on Blood Lead

Concentrations in the Families," *Occupational and Environmental Medicine*, 54, 117–124.

Chow, S-C. and Liu, J-P. (2013), *Design and Analysis of Clinical Trials: Concepts and Methodologies* (3rd ed.), Hoboken, NJ: John Wiley & Sons.

Cicchetti, D.V. and Feinstein, A.R. (1990), "High Agreement but Low Kappa: II. Resolving the Paradoxes," *Journal of Clinical Epidemiology*, 43, 551–558.

Cochran, W.G. (1950), "The Comparison of Percentages in Matched Samples," *Biometrika*, 37, 256–266.

Cochran, W.G. (1954), "Some Methods for Strengthening the Common χ^2 Tests," *Biometrics*, 10, 417–454.

Cohen, J. (1960), "A Coefficient of Agreement for Nominal Scales," *Educational and Psychological Measurement*, 20, 37–46.

Cohen, J. (1988), *Statistical Power Analysis for the Behavioral Sciences* (2nd ed.), Hillsdale, NJ: Lawrence Erlbaum Associates.

Coleman, C.D. (2004), "A Fast, High-Precision Implementation of the Univariate One-Parameter Box-Cox Transformation Using the Golden Section Search in SAS/IML®," *Proceedings of the 17th Northeast SAS Users Group (NESUG) Conference*. Available at http://www.nesug.org/proceedings/nesug04/an/an12.pdf. Accessed September 23, 2013.

Connor, R.J. (1987), "Sample Size for Testing Differences in Proportions for the Paired-Sample Design," *Biometrics*, 43, 207–211.

Conover, W.J. (1999), *Practical Nonparametric Statistics* (3rd ed.), New York: John Wiley & Sons.

Conover, W.J. and Iman, R.L. (1981), "Rank Transformations as a Bridge Between Parametric and Nonparametric Statistics," *The American Statistician*, 35, 124–129.

Conover, W.J., Johnson, M.E., and Johnson M.M. (1981), "A Comparative Study of Tests for Homogeneity of Variances, with Applications to the Outer Continental Shelf Bidding Data," *Technometrics*, 23, 351–361.

Cook, D.G., Whincup, P.H., Papacosta, O., Strachan, D.P., Jarvis, M.J., and Bryant, A. (1993), "Relation of Passive Smoking as Assessed by Salivary Cotinine Concentration and Questionnaire to Spirometric Indices in Children," *Thorax*, 48, 14–20.

Coultas, D.B., Samet, J.M., McCarthy, J.F., and Spengler, J.D. (1990), "A Personal Monitoring Study to Assess Workplace Exposure to Environmental Tobacco Smoke," *American Journal of Public Health*, 80, 988–990.

Cox, D.R. and Hinkley, D.V. (1974), *Theoretical Statistics*, London: Chapman & Hall.

Cummings, S.R., Duong, T., Kenyon, E., Cauley, J.A., Whitehead, M., and Krueger, K.A. (2002), "Serum Estradiol Level and Risk of Breast Cancer During Treatment With Raloxifene," *Journal of the American Medical Association*, 287, 216–220.

D'Agostino, R.B. (1986), "Graphical Analysis," in *Goodness-of-Fit Techniques*, eds. R.B. D'Agostino and M.A. Stephens, New York: Marcel Dekker, pp. 7–62.

D'Agostino, R.B., Belanger, A., and D'Agostino, R.B., Jr. (1990), "A Suggestion for Using Powerful and Informative Tests for Normality," *The American Statistician*, 44(4), 316–321.

D'Agostino, R.B. and Stephens, M.A. (eds.) (1986), *Goodness-of-Fit Techniques*, New York: Marcel Dekker.

Daniels, M.J. and Hughes, M.D. (1997), "Meta-Analysis for the Evaluation of Potential Surrogate Markers," *Statistics in Medicine*, 16, 1965–1982.

Davis, L.J. (1986), "Exact Tests for 2 × 2 Contingency Tables," *The American Statistician*, 40(2), 139–141.

Deal, A.M., Pate, V.W., and El Rouby, S. (2009), "A SAS® Macro for Deming Regression," Paper CC-014 presented at the 17th annual SouthEast SAS Users Group (SESUG) Conference, Birmingham, AL. Available at http://analytics.ncsu.edu/sesug/2009/CC014.Deal.pdf. Accessed February 3, 2011.

DeCaprio, A.P. (2006), "Introduction to Toxicologic Biomarkers," in *Toxicologic Biomarkers*, ed. A.P. DeCaprio, New York: Marcel Dekker, pp. 1–15.

Delfino, R.J., Staimer, N., Tjoa, T., Gillen, D.L., Polidori, A., Arhami, M, Kleinman, M.T., Vazir, N.D., Longhurst, J., and Sioutas, C. (2009), "Air Pollution Exposures and Circulating Biomarkers of Effect in a Susceptible Population: Clues to Potential Causal Component Mixtures and Mechanisms," *Environmental Health Perspectives*, 117, 1232–1238.

DeLong, E.R., DeLong, D.M., and Clarke-Pearson, D.L. (1988), "Comparing the Areas Under Two or More Correlated Receiver Operating Characteristic Curves: A Nonparametric Approach," *Biometrika*, 44, 837–845.

DeMattos, R.B., Bales, K.R., Cummins, D.J., Paul, S.M., and Holtzman, D.M. (2002), "Brain to Plasma Amyloid-β Efflux: A Measure of Brain Amyloid Burden in a Mouse Model of Alzheimer's Disease," *Science*, 295, 2264–2267.

Dimakos, I.C. (1997), "Power Transformations Using SAS/IML Software," *Proceedings of the Twenty-Second Annual SAS® Users Group International Conference*, San Diego, CA, March 16–19, 1997. Available at http://www2.sas.com/proceedings/sugi22/CODERS/PAPER95.PDF. Accessed September 19, 2013.

Dodge, Y. (ed.) (2003), *The Oxford Dictionary of Statistical Terms*, Oxford, UK: Oxford University Press.

Donner, A., and Klar, N. (2010), *Design and Analysis of Cluster Randomization Trials in Health Research*, Hoboken, NJ: John Wiley & Sons.

Duncan, R., Dey, R., Tomioka, K., Hairston, H., Selvapandiyan, A., and Nakhasi, H.L. (2009), "Biomarkers of Attenuation in the Leishmania donovani Centrin Gene Deleted Cell Line - Requirements for Safety in a Live Vaccine Candidate," *The Open Parasitology Journal*, 3, 14–23.

Dunnett, C.W. (1980a), "Pairwise Multiple Comparisons in the Homogeneous Variance, Unequal Sample Size Case," *Journal of the American Statistical Association*, 75, 789–795.

Dunnett, C.W. (1980b), "Pairwise Multiple Comparisons in the Unequal Variance Case," *Journal of the American Statistical Association*, 75, 796–800.

England, L.J., Levine, R.J., Qian, C., Soule, L.M., Schisterman, E.F., Yu, K.F., and Catalano, P.M. (2004), "Glucose Tolerance and Risk of Gestational Diabetes Mellitus in Nulliparous Women who Smoke During Pregnancy," *American Journal of Epidemiology*, 160, 1205–1213.

Faupel-Badger, J.M., Prindiville, S.A., Venzon, D., Vonderhaar, B.K., Zujewski, J.A., and Eng-Wong, J. (2006), "Effects of Raloxifene on Circulating Prolactin and Estradiol Levels in Premenopausal Women at High Risk for Developing Breast Cancer," *Cancer Epidemiology, Biomarkers and Prevention*, 15, 1153–1158.

Feinstein, A.R. and Cicchetti, D.V. (1990), "High Agreement but Low Kappa: I. The Problems of Two Paradoxes," *Journal of Clinical Epidemiology*, 43, 543–549.

Fieller E.C., Hartley, H.O., and Pearson, E.S. (1957), "Tests for Rank Correlation Coefficients," *Biometrika*, 44, 470–481.

Fleiss, J.L. (1971), "Measuring Nominal Scale Agreement Among Many Raters," *Psychological Bulletin*, 76, 378–382.

Fleiss, J.L. and Cohen, J. (1973), "The Equivalence of Weighted Kappa and the Intraclass Correlation Coefficient as Measures of Reliability," *Educational and Psychological Measurement*, 33, 613–619.

Fleiss, J.L. and Cuzick, J. (1979), "The Reliability of Dichotomous Judgments: Unequal Numbers of Judges per Subject," *Applied Psychological Measurement*, 3, 537–542.

Fleiss, J.L., Levin, B., and Paik, M.C. (2003), *Statistical Methods for Rates and Proportions* (3rd ed.), Hoboken, NJ: John Wiley & Sons.

Freedman, L.S. (2008), "An Analysis of the Controversy Over Classical One-Sided Tests," *Clinical Trials*, 5, 635–640. Corrigendum (2009), 6, 198.

Freedman, L.S., Graubard, B.I., and Schatzkin, A. (1992), "Statistical Validation of Intermediate Endpoints for Chronic Diseases," *Statistics in Medicine*, 11, 167–178.

Freeman, G.H., and Halton, J.H. (1951), "Note on Exact Treatment of Contingency, Goodness of Fit, and Other Problems of Significance," *Biometrika*, 38, 141–149.

Freund, R.J. and Littell, R.C. (2000), *SAS® System for Regression* (3rd ed.), Cary, NC: SAS Institute Inc.

Fritsma, G.A. and McGlasson, D.L. (2012), *Quick Guide to Laboratory Statistics and Quality Control*, Washington, DC: American Association for Clinical Chemistry.

Gail, M.H., Pfeiffer, R., Van Houwelingen, H.C., and Carroll, R.J. (2000), "On Meta-Analytic Assessment of Surrogate Outcomes," *Biostatistics* 1, 231–246.

Gerson, M. (1975), "The Techniques and Uses of Probability Plots," *The Statistician*, 24, 235–257.

Gibbons, J.D. and Chakraborti, S. (2003), *Nonparametric Statistical Inference* (4th ed.), New York: Marcel Dekker.

Goldberg, J.F., Shah, M.D., Chiou, K., Hanna, J., Hagan, J.L., Cabrera, A.G., Jeewa, A., and Price, J.F. (2014), "Anemia Is Associated With Adverse Clinical Outcomes in Children Hospitalized With Acute Heart Failure," Presented at the 18th Annual Scientific Meeting of the Heart Failure Society of America, Las Vegas, NV, September 14–17, 2014.

Goldsmith, L.J. (2001), "Power and Sample Size Considerations in Molecular Biology," in *Methods in Molecular Biology, Vol. 184: Biostatistical Methods*, ed. S.W. Looney, Totowa, NJ: Humana Press, pp. 111–130.

Gönen, M. (2007), *Analyzing Receiver Operating Characteristic Curves with SAS*, Cary, NC: SAS Institute Inc.

Gordis, L. (2004), *Epidemiology* (3rd ed.), Bridgewater, NJ: Elsevier.

Graham, P. and Bull, B. (1998), "Approximate Standard Errors and Confidence Intervals for Indices of Positive and Negative Agreement," *Journal of Clinical Epidemiology*, 51, 763–771.

Granella M., Priante E., Nardini B., Bono R., and Clonfero E. (1996), "Excretion of Mutagens, Nicotine and Its Metabolites in Urine of Cigarette Smokers," *Mutagenesis*, 11, 207–211.

Grosskurth, H., Mosha, F., Todd, J., Mwijarubi, E., Klokke, A., Senkoro, K., Mayaud, P., Changalucha, J., Nicol, A., ka-Gina, G., Newell, J., Mugeye, K., Mabey, D., and Hayes, R. (1995), "Impact of Improved Treatment of Sexually Transmitted Diseases on HIV Infection in Rural Tanzania: Randomised Controlled Trial," *The Lancet*, 346, 530–536.

Grubbs, F.E. (1950), "Sample Criteria for Testing Outlying Observations," *Annals of Mathematical Statistics*, 21, 27–58.

Grubbs, F.E. and Beck, G. (1972), "Extension of Sample Sizes and Percentage Points for Significance Tests of Outlying Observations," *Technometrics*, 14, 847–854.

Hagan, J.L. and Looney, S.W. (2004), "Frequency of Use of Statistical Techniques for Assessing Agreement Between Continuous Measurements," *Proceedings of the ASA Biometrics Section, 2004 Joint Statistical Meetings*, Alexandria, VA: American Statistical Association, pp. 344–350.

Hanley, J.A. and McNeil, B.J. (1982), "The Meaning and Use of the Area under a Receiver Operating Characteristic (ROC) Curve," *Radiology*, 143, 29–36.

Hartung, D.M., Touchette, D.T., Bultemeier, N.C., and Haxby, D.G. (2005), "Risk of Hospitalization for Heart Failure Associated with Thiazolidinedione Therapy: A Medicaid Claims–Based Case-Control Study," *Pharmacotherapy: The Journal of Human Pharmacology and Drug Therapy*, 25, 1329–1336.

Hauck, W.W., Gilliss, C.L., Donner, A., and Gortiner, S. (1991), "Randomization by Cluster," *Nursing Research*, 40, 356–358.

Hazelton, M.L. (2003), "A Graphical Tool for Assessing Normality," *American Statistician*, 57, 285–288.

Healy, M.J.R. (1968), "Multivariate Normal Plotting," *Applied Statistics*, 17, 157–161.

Hedeker, D. and Gibbons, R.D. (2006), *Longitudinal Data Analysis*, Hoboken, NJ: John Wiley & Sons.

Heist, R.S., Duda, G. D., Sahani, D., Pennell, N.A., Neal, J.W., Ancukiewicz, M., Engelman, J.A., Lynch, T.J., and Jain, R.K. (2010), "In Vivo Assessment of the Effects of Bevacizumab in Advanced Non-Small Cell Lung Cancer (NSCLC)," *Journal of Clinical Oncology*, 28, 7612 (Abstract).

Helsel, D. (2012), *Statistics for Censored Environmental Data Using Minitab and R* (2nd ed.), Hoboken, NJ: John Wiley & Sons.

Henderson, A.R. (2006), "Testing Experimental Data for Univariate Normality," *Clinica Chimica Acta*, 366, 112–129.

Henderson, F.W., Reid, H.F., Morris, R., Wang, O.L., Hu, P.C., Helms, R.W., Forehand, L., Mumford, J., Lewtas, J., Haley, N.J. et al. (1989), "Home Air Nicotine Levels and Urinary Cotinine Excretion in Preschool Children," *American Journal of Respiratory Disorders and Critical Care Medicine*, 140, 197–201.

Hettmansperger, T.P. and McKean, J.W. (1998), *Robust Nonparametric Statistical Methods*, London: Arnold.

Hirji, K.F., Tan, S.J., and Elashoff, R.M. (1991), "A Quasi-Exact Test for Comparing Two Binomial Proportions," *Statistics in Medicine*, 10, 1137–1153.

Hobbs, C.A., Cleves, M.A., Melnyk, S., Zhao, W., and James, S.J. (2005), "Congenital Heart Defects and Abnormal Maternal Biomarkers of Methionine and Homocysteine Metabolism," *The American Journal of Clinical Nutrition*, 81, 147–153.

Hosmer, D.W. and Lemeshow, S. (2000), *Applied Logistic Regression* (2nd ed.), Hoboken, NJ: John Wiley & Sons.

Huber, P.J. (1996), *Robust Statistical Procedures* (2nd ed.), Philadelphia, PA: Society for Industrial and Applied Mathematics.

Huber-Carol, C., Balakrishnan, N., Nikulin, M.S., and Mesbah, M. (eds.) (2002), *Goodness-of-Fit Tests and Model Validity*, New York: Springer.

Hulley, S.B., Cummings, S.R., Browner, W.S., Grady, D.G., and Newman, T.B. (2013), *Designing Clinical Research* (4th ed.), Philadelphia: Lippincott Williams and Wilkins.

Hunter, A., Kalathingal, S., Shrout, M., Plummer, K., and Looney, S. (2014), "The Effectiveness of a Pre-Procedural Mouth Rinse in Reducing Bacteria on Radiographic Phosphor Plates," *Imaging Science in Dentistry*, 44(2), 149–154.

Hüttner, E., Götze, A., and Nikolova, T. (1999), "Chromosomal Aberrations in Humans as Genetic Endpoints to Assess the Impact of Pollution," *Mutation Research*, 445, 251–257.

Hwang, J., Na, S., Lee, H., and Lee, D. (2009), "Correlation Between Preoperative Serum Levels of Five Biomarkers and Relationships Between These Biomarkers and Cancer Stage in Epithelial Ovarian Cancer," *Journal of Gynecologic Oncology*, 20, 169–175.

Iman, R.L. (1976), "An Approximation to the Exact Distribution of the Wilcoxon-Mann-Whitney Rank Sum Statistic," *Communications in Statistics - Theory and Methods*, A5, 587–598.

Iman, R.L. and Davenport, J.M. (1976), "New Approximations to the Exact Distribution of the Kruskal-Wallis Test Statistic," *Communications in Statistics - Theory and Methods*, A5, 1335–1348.

Iyer, R.R., Eisen, M.B., Ross, D.T., Schuler, G., Moore, T., Lee, J.C.F., Trent, J.M., Staudt, L.M., Hudson, J., Boguski, M.S., Lashkari, D., Shalon, D., Botstein, D., and Brown, P.O. (1999), "The Transcriptional Program in the Response of Human Fibroblasts to Serum," *Science*, 283, 83–87.

Jayakumar, C., Ranganathan, P., Devarajan, P., Krawczeski, C.D., Looney, S., and Ramesh, G. (2013), "Semaphorin 3A Is a New Early Diagnostic Biomarker of Experimental and Pediatric Acute Kidney Injury," *PLoS ONE*, 8, e58446, doi:l0.1371/journal.pone.0058446.

Johnson, N.L. (1949), "Systems of Frequency Curves Generated by Methods of Translation," *Biometrika*, 36, 149–176.

Jones, L., Parker, J.D., and Mendola, P. (2010), "Blood Lead and Mercury Levels in Pregnant Women in the United States, 2003-2008," NCHS Data Brief, Number 52. Available at http://www.cdc.gov/nchs/data/databriefs/db52.pdf. Accessed March 8, 2014.

Jones, M.C. and Daly, F. (1995), "Density Probability Plots," *Communications in Statistics – Simulation and Computation*, 24, 911–927.

Jones, R. and Payne, B. (1997), *Clinical Investigation and Statistics in Laboratory Medicine*, Washington, DC: American Association for Clinical Chemistry.

Joseph, A.M., Hecht S.S., Murphy, S.E., Carmella, S.G., Le, C.T., Zhang, Y., Shaomei, H., and Hatsukami, D.K. (2005), "Relationships Between Cigarette Consumption and Biomarkers of Tobacco Toxin Exposure," *Cancer Epidemiology, Biomarkers and Prevention*, 14, 2963–2968.

Juneau, P. (2004), "Simultaneous Nonparametric Inference in a One-Way Layout Using the SAS® System," Paper SP04, presented at the June 2004 meeting of the Michigan SAS User's Group. Available at http://www.misug.org/presentations.html. Accessed February 11, 2014. SAS code available at http://www.misug.org/uploads/8/1/9/1/8191072/pjuneau_nonparam_comp.zip.

Kim, B., Lee, H.J., Choi, H.Y., Shin, Y., Nam, S., Seo, G., Son, D.S., Jo, J., Kim, J., Lee, J., Kim, J., Kim, K., and Lee, S. (2007), "Clinical Validity of the Lung Cancer Biomarkers Identified by Bioinformatics Analysis of Public Expression Data," *Cancer Research*, 67, 7431–7438.

Kleinbaum, D.G., Kupper, L.L., and Morgenstern, H. (1982), *Epidemiological Research*, New York: Van Nostrand Reinhold.

Knapp, R.G. and Miller, M.C. (1992), *Clinical Epidemiology and Biostatistics*, Philadelphia, PA: Harwal Publishing Company.

Kraemer, H.C. (1980), "Extension of the kappa Coefficient," *Biometrics*, 36, 207–216.

Krishnamoorthy, K. (2006), *The Handbook of Statistical Distributions with Applications*, Boca Raton, FL: CRC Press.

Kummel, C.H. (1879), "Reduction of Observation Equations Which Contain More Than One Observed Quantity," *The Analyst*, 6, 97–105.

Kutner, M., Nachtsheim, C., Neter, J., and Li, W. (2004), *Applied Linear Statistical Models* (5th ed.), Chicago, IL: McGraw-Hill/Irwin.

Lachin, J.M. (1992), "Power and Sample Size Evaluation for the McNemar Test With Application to Matched Case-Control Studies," *Statistics in Medicine*, 11, 1239–1251.

Lagorio, S., Crebelli, R., Ricciarello, R., Conti, L., Iavarone, I., Zona, A., Ghittori, S., and Carere, A. (1998), "Methodological Issues in Biomonitoring of Low Level Exposure to Benzene," *Occupational Medicine*, 8, 497–504.

Landis, J.R. and Koch, G.G. (1977), "The Measurement of Observer Agreement for Categorical Data," *Biometrics*, 33, 159–174.

Lang, T.A. and Secic, M. (eds.) (2006), *How to Report Statistics in Medicine* (2nd ed.), Philadelphia: American College of Physicians.

Lata, S., Cuchacovich, R., Hagan, J.L., Patel, N., and Espinoza, R. (2010a), "Do Adipocytokines Play a Role in Bone Turnover in Spondyloarthropathies?" *Journal of Investigative Medicine*, 58, 443 (Abstract).

Lata, S., Cuchacovich, R., Hagan, J.L., Patel, N., and Espinoza, R. (2010b), "Genes and Cytokine Expression Profile in Idiopathic Juvenile Osteoporosis," *Journal of Investigative Medicine*, 58, 470–471 (Abstract).

Lee, J., Koh, D., and Ong, C.N. (1989), "Statistical Evaluation of Agreement Between Two Methods for Measuring a Quantitative Variable," *Computers in Biology and Medicine*, 19, 61–70.

Lehmann, E.L. (1975), *Nonparametrics: Statistical Methods Based on Ranks*, San Francisco: Holden-Day.

Lemoine, A., Hagan, J.L., and Miller, J.M., Jr. (2013), "Umbilical Cord Coiling and Maternal Diabetes," Presented at Louisiana State University Health Sciences Center, Department of Obstetrics and Gynecology Resident Research Day, May 2013.

Li, L., Wang, W., and Chan, I. (2005), "Correlation Coefficient Inference on Censored Bioassay Data," *Journal of Biopharmaceutical Statistics*, 15, 501–512.

Lin, D.Y., Fleming T.R., and DeGruttola, V. (1997), "Estimating the Proportion of Treatment Effect Explained by a Surrogate Marker," *Statistics in Medicine*, 997, 1515–1527.

Lin, L.I. (1989), "A Concordance Correlation Coefficient to Evaluate Reproducibility," *Biometrics*, 45, 255–268.

Lin, L.I. (2000), "A Note on the Concordance Correlation Coefficient," *Biometrics*, 56, 324–325.

Lin, L.I. and Chinchilli, V. (1997), "Rejoinder to the Letter to the Editor From Atkinson and Nevill," *Biometrics*, 53, 777–778.

Linnet, K. (1990), "Estimation of the Linear Relationship Between the Measurements of Two Methods with Proportional Errors," *Statistics in Medicine*, 9, 1463–1473.

Linnet, K. (1993), "Evaluation of Regression Procedures for Methods Comparison Studies," *Clinical Chemistry*, 39, 424–432.

Littell, R.C., Milliken, G.A., Stroup, W.W., Wolfinger, R.D., and Schabenberger, O. (2006), *SAS® for Mixed Models* (2nd ed.), Cary, NC: SAS Institute Inc.

Littell, R.C., Stroup, W.W., and Freund, R.J. (2002), *SAS® System for Linear Models* (4th ed.), Cary, NC.: SAS Institute Inc.

Lombardi, C.M. and Hurlbert, S.H. (2009), "Misprescription and Misuse of One-Tailed Tests," *Austral Ecology*, 34, 447–468.

Looney, S.W. (1996), "Sample Size Determination for Correlation Coefficient Inference: Practical Problems and Practical Solutions," *Proceedings of the ASA Statistical Computing Section, 1996 Joint Statistical Meetings*, Alexandria, VA: American Statistical Association, pp. 240–0245.

Looney, S.W. (2001), "Statistical Methods for Assessing Biomarkers," in *Methods in Molecular Biology, Vol. 184: Biostatistical Methods*, ed. S.W. Looney, Totowa, NJ: Humana Press, pp. 81–109.

Looney, S.W. and Gulledge, T.R., Jr. (1984), "Regression Tests of Fit and Probability Plotting Positions," *Journal of Statistical Computation and Simulation*, 20, 115–127.

Looney, S.W. and Gulledge, T.R., Jr. (1985a), "Use of the Correlation Coefficient with Normal Probability Plots," *The American Statistician*, 39, 75–79.

Looney, S.W. and Gulledge, T.R., Jr. (1985b), "Probability Plotting Positions and Goodness of Fit for the Normal Distribution," *The Statistician*, 34, 297–303.

Looney, S. and Hagan, J. (2006a), "On Methods for Handling Biomarker Data Below the Analytic Limit of Detection," *Proceedings of the ASA Section on the Environment, 2006 Joint Statistical Meetings*, Alexandria, VA: American Statistical Association, pp. 2477–2481.

Looney, S.W. and Hagan, J.L. (2006b), "Challenges in the Statistical Analysis of Biomarker Data," in *Toxicologic Biomarkers*, ed. A.P. DeCaprio, New York: Marcel Dekker, pp. 17–38.

Looney, S.W. and Hagan, J.L. (2008), "Statistical Methods for Assessing Biomarkers and for Analyzing Biomarker Data," in *Handbook of Statistics*. eds. C.R. Rao, J.P. Miller, and D.C. Rao, *Vol. 27: Epidemiology and Medical Statistics*, Amsterdam: Elsevier, pp. 109–147.

López, V.M., Galán, J.A., Fernández-Suárez, A., López-Celada, S., Alcover, J., and Filella, X. (2003), "Usefulness of Tissue Polypeptide Antigen in the Follow-Up of Bladder Cancer," *Urology*, 62, 243–248.

Lund, B.C., Perry, P.J., Brooks, J.M., and Arndt, S. (2001), "Euglycemic Clamp Study in Clozapine-Induced Diabetic Ketoacidosis. Clozapine Use in Patients with Schizophrenia and the Risk of Diabetes, Hyperlipidemia, and Hypertension: A Claims-Based Approach," *Archives of General Psychiatry*, 58, 1172–1176.

Lyles, R.H., Williams, J.K., and Chuachoowong, R. (2001), "Correlating Two Viral Load Assays With Known Detection Limits," *Biometrics*, 57, 1238–1244.

Lynn, H. (2001), "Maximum Likelihood Inference for Left-Censored HIV RNA Data," *Statistics in Medicine*, 20, 33–45.

MacRae, A.R., Gardner, H.A., Allen, L.C., Tokmakejian, S., and Lepage, N. (2003), "Outcome Validation of the Beckman Coulter Access Analyzer in a Second-Trimester Down Syndrome Serum Screening Application," *Clinical Chemistry*, 49, 69–76.

Mak, T.K. (1988), "Analysing Intraclass Correlation for Dichotomous Variables," *Applied Statistics*, 37(3), 344–352.

Markowski, C.A. and Markowski, E.P. (1990), "Conditions for the Effectiveness of a Preliminary Test of Variance," *American Statistician*, 44, 322–326.

Matsunga, S.K., Plezia, P.M., Karol, M.D., Katz, M.D., Camilli, A.E., and Benowitz, N.L. (1989), "Effects of Passive Smoking on Theophylline Clearance," *Clinical Pharmacology and Therapeutics*, 46, 399–407.

Maxwell, S.E. and Delaney, H.D. (2004), *Designing Experiments and Analyzing Data: A Model Comparison Perspective* (2nd ed.), Mahwah, NJ: Lawrence Erlbaum.

McCracken, C.E. (2013), "Correlation Coefficient Inference for Left-Censored Biomarker Data with Known Detection Limits," unpublished Ph.D. dissertation, Department of Biostatistics, Georgia Regents University.

McNemar, Q. (1947), "Note on the Sampling Error of the Difference Between Correlated Proportions or Percentages," *Psychometrika*, 12, 153–157.

Mehrotra, D.V., Chan, I.S.F., and Berger, R.L. (2003), "A Cautionary Note on Exact Unconditional Inference for a Difference Between Two Independent Binomial Proportions," *Biometrics*, 59, 441–450.

Mehta, C. and Patel, N. (2010), *StatXact 9*, Cambridge, MA: CYTEL Software Corporation.

Mehta, C.R., Patel, N.R., and Gray, R. (1985), "On Computing an Exact Confidence Interval for the Common Odds Ratio in Several 2×2 Contingency Tables," *Journal of the American Statistical Association*, 80, 969–973.

Mercaldo, N.D., Lau, K.F., and Zhou, X.H. (2007), "Confidence Intervals for Predictive Values With an Emphasis to Case–Control Studies," *Statistics in Medicine*, 26, 2170–2183.

Micheel, C.M. and Ball, J.R. (eds) (2010), *Evaluation of Biomarkers and Surrogate Endpoints in Chronic Disease*, Washington, DC: National Academies Press.

Mildvan, D., Landay, A., De Gruttola, V., Machado, S.G., and Kagan, J. (1997), "An Approach to the Validation of Markers for use in AIDS Clinical Trials," *Clinical Infectious Diseases* 24, 764–774.

Miller, C.S., King, C.P., Langub, M.C., Kryscio, R.J., and Thomas, M.V. (2006), "JADA Continuing Education: Salivary Biomarkers of Existing Periodontal Disease: A Cross-Sectional Study," *The Journal of the American Dental Association*, 137, 322–329.

Milliken, G.A. and Johnson, D.E. (1984), *Analysis of Messy Data: Volume I: Designed Experiments*, New York: Van Nostrand Reinhold.

Molenberghs, G., Buyse, M., Geys, H., Renard, D., Burzykowski, T., and Alonso, A., (2002), "Statistical Challenges in the Evaluation of Surrogate Endpoints in Randomized Trials," *Controlled Clinical Trials*, 23, 607–625.

Montgomery, T.C., Peck, E.A., and Vining, G.G. (2012), *Introduction to Linear Regression Analysis*, Hoboken, NJ: John Wiley & Sons.

Morton, R.F., Hebel, J.R., and McCarter, R.J. (1996), *A Study Guide to Epidemiology and Biostatistics*, Gaithersburg, MD: Aspen Publishers.

Moser, B.K. and Stevens, G.R. (1992), "Homogeneity of Variance in the Two-Sample Means Test," *The American Statistician*, 46, 19–21.

Moser, B.K., Stevens, G.R., and Watts, C.L. (1989), "The Two-sample T Test Versus Satterthwaite's Approximate F Test," *Communications in Statistics Part A-Theory and Methods*, 18, 3963–3975.

Murphy, S.E., Link, C.A., Jensen, J., Le, C., Puumala, S.S., Hecht, S.S., Carmella, S.G., Losey, L., and Hatsukami, D.K. (2004), "A Comparison of Urinary Biomarkers of Tobacco and Carcinogen Exposure in Smokers," *Cancer Epidemiology, Biomarkers and Prevention*, 13, 1617–1623.

Muscat, J.E., Djordjevic, M.J., Colosimo, S., Stellman, S.D., and Ritchie, J.P. (2005), "Racial Differences in Exposure and Glucuronidation of the Tobacco-Specific Carcinogen 4-(Methylnitrosamino)-1-(3-Pyridyl)-1-Butanone (NNK)," *Cancer*, 103, 1420–1426.

Myers, R.H., Montgomery, D.C., Vining, G.G., and Robinson, T.J. (2010), *Generalized Linear Models* (2nd ed.), Hoboken, NJ: John Wiley & Sons.

Naylor, G.J., Dick, D.A.T., and Dick, E.G. (1976), "Erythrocyte Membrane Cation Carrier, Relapse Rate of Manic-Depressive Illness and Response to Lithium," *Psychological Medicine*, 6, 257–263.

Neuhäuser, M. and Hothorn, L.A. (1999), "An Exact Cochran-Armitage Test for Trend When Dose-Response Shapes are a Priori Unknown," *Computational Statistics and Data Analysis*, 30, 403–412.

Newcombe, R.G. (1998), "Improved Confidence Intervals for the Difference between Binomial Proportions Based on Paired Data," *Statistics in Medicine*, 17, 2635–2650.

Newton, E. and Rudel, R. (2007), "Estimating Correlation With Multiply Censored Data Arising From the Adjustment of Singly Censored Data," *Environmental Science and Technology*, 41, 221–228.

NRC (National Research Council) (1987), "Biological Markers in Environmental Health," *Environmental Health Perspectives*, 74, 3–9.

Ogus, E., Yazici, A.C., and Gurbuz, F. (2007), "Evaluating the Significance Test When the Correlation Coefficient is Different from Zero in the Test of Hypothesis," *Communications in Statistics - Simulation and Computation*, 36, 847–854.

Pearson, E.S., D'Agostino, R.B., and Bowman, K.O. (1977), "Tests for Departure from Normality: Comparison of Powers," *Biometrika*, 64, 231–246.

Pepe, M.S. (2003), *The Statistical Evaluation of Medical Tests for Classification and Prediction*, New York: Oxford University Press.

Pérez-Stable, E.J., Benowitz, N.L., and Marín, G. (1995), "Is Serum Cotinine a Better Measure of Cigarette Smoking Than Self-Report," *Preventive Medicine*, 24, 171–179.

Piantadosi, S. (2005), *Clinical Trials: A Methodological Perspective* (2nd ed.), New York: John Wiley & Sons.

Porta, M. (2008), *A Dictionary of Epidemiology* (5th ed.), New York: Oxford University Press.

Prentice, R.L. (1989), "Surrogate Endpoints in Clinical Trials: Definition and Operational Criteria," *Statistics in Medicine*, 8, 431–440.

Preusser, M., Janzer, R.C., Felsberg, J., Reifenberger, G., Hamou, M-F., Diserens, A-C., Stupp, R., Gorlia, T., Marosi, C., Heinzl, H., Hainfellner, J.A., and Hegi, M. (2008), "Anti-O6-Methylguanine-Methyltransferase (MGMT) Immunohistochemistry in Glioblastoma Multiforme: Observer Variability and Lack of Association with Patient Survival Impede Its Use as Clinical Biomarker," *Brain Pathology*, 18, 520–532.

Prigent, F.M., Maddahi, J., Van Train, K.F., and Berman, D.S. (1991), "Comparison of Thallium-201 SPECT and Planar Imaging Methods for Quantification of Experimental Myocardial Infarct Size," *American Heart Journal*, 122, 972–979.

Qiao, Y-L., Tockman, M.S., Li, L., Erozan, Y.S., Yao, S.X., Barrett, M.J., Zhou, W.H., Giffen, C.A., Luo, X.C., and Taylor, P.R. (1997), "A Case-Cohort Study of an Early Biomarker of Lung Cancer in a Screening Cohort of Yunnan Tin Miners in China," *Cancer Epidemiology, Biomarkers and Prevention*, 6, 893–900.

R Core Development Team. (2014), R: A Language and Environment for Statistical Computing, Vienna, Austria: R Foundation for Statistical Computing, ISBN 3-900051-07-0 Available at http://www.R-project.org. Accessed January 8, 2014.

Rabinovitch, N., Reisdorph, N., Silveira, L., and Gelfand, E.W. (2011), "Urinary Leukotriene E4 Levels Identify Children With Tobacco Smoke Exposure at Risk for Asthma Exacerbation," *Journal of Allergy and Clinical Immunology*, 128, 323–327.

Ramsey, P. (1980), "Exact Type I Error Rates for Robustness of Student's t-test with Unequal Variances," *Journal of Educational Statistics*, 5, 337–349.

Razali, N. and Wah, Y.B. (2011), "Power Comparisons of Shapiro-Wilk, Kolmogorov-Smirnov, Lilliefors and Anderson-Darling Tests," *Journal of Statistical Modeling and Analytics*, 2, 21–33.

Reid, M.D., Osunkoya, A.O., Siddiqui, M.T., and Looney, S.W. (2012), "Accuracy of Grading of Urothelial Carcinoma on Urine Cytology: An Analysis of Interobserver and Intraobserver Agreement," *International Journal of Clinical and Experimental Pathology*, 5, 882–891.

Rosner, B. (2011), *Fundamentals of Biostatistics* (7th ed.), Boston, MA: Brooks/Cole.

Ross, R.K., Yuan, J., Yu, M.C., Wogan, G.N., Qian, G., Tu, J., Groopman, J.D., Gao, Y., and Henderson, B.E. (1992), "Urinary Aflatoxin Biomarkers and Risk of Hepatocellular Carcinoma," *The Lancet*, 339 (8799), 943–945.

Royston, J.P. (1982), "An Extension of Shapiro and Wilk's W Test for Normality to Large Samples," *Journal of the Royal Statistical Society: Series C (Applied Statistics)*, 31, 115–124.

Royston, J.P. (1989), "Correcting the Shapiro-Wilk W for Ties," *Journal of Statistical Computation and Simulation*, 31, 237–249.

Royston, J.P. (1992), "Approximating the Shapiro-Wilk's W Test for Non-Normality," *Statistics and Computing*, 2, 117–119.

Salmi, M., Stolen, C., Jousilahti, P., Yegutkin, G.G., Tapanainen, P., Janatuinen, T., Knip, M., Jalkanen, S., and Salomaa, V. (2002), "Insulin-Regulated Increase of Soluble Vascular Adhesion Protein-1 in Diabetes," *The American Journal of Pathology*, 161, 2255–2262.

Satterthwaite, F.E. (1946), "An Approximate Distribution of Estimates of Variance Components," *Biometrics Bulletin*, 2, 110–114.

Scheffé, H. (1959), *The Analysis of Variance*, New York: John Wiley & Sons, pp. 331–368.

Scheuren, F. (2005), "Multiple Imputation: How It Began and Continues," *The American Statistician*, 59, 315–319.

Semmler, A., Simon, M., Moskau, S., and Linnebank, M. (2008), "Polymorphisms of Methionine Metabolism and Susceptibility to Meningioma Formation," *Journal of Neurosurgery*, 108, 999–1004.

Shapiro, S.S. and Wilk, M.B. (1965), "An Analysis of Variance Test for Normality (Complete Samples)," *Biometrika*, 52, 591–611.

Shapiro, S.S., Wilk, M.B., and Chen, H.J. (1968), "A Comparative Study of Various Tests for Normality," *Journal of the American Statistical Association*, 63, 1343–1372.

Sheskin, D.J. (2007), *Handbook of Parametric and Nonparametric Statistical Procedures* (4th ed.), Boca Raton, FL: CRC Press.

Shiffler, R.E. (1988), "Maximum Z Scores and Outliers," *The American Statistician*, 42, 79–80.

Shlipak, M.G., Fried, L.F., Crump, C., Bleyer, A.J., Manolio, T.A., Russell, P.T., Furberg, C.D., and Psaty, B.M. (2003), "Elevations of Inflammatory and Procoagulant Biomarkers in Elderly Persons with Renal Insufficiency," *Circulation*, 107, 87–92.

Shoukri, M.M. (2004), *Measures of Interobserver Agreement*, Boca Raton, FL: CRC Press.

Shoukri, M.M. (2011), *Measures of Interobserver Agreement and Reliability* (2nd ed.), Boca Raton, FL: CRC Press.

Shoukri, M.M. and Chaudhary, M.A. (2007), *Analysis of Correlated Data with SAS® and R* (3rd ed.), Boca Raton, FL: CRC Press.

Shrout, P.E. and Fleiss, J.L. (1979), "Intraclass Correlations: Uses in Assessing Rater Reliability," *Psychological Bulletin*, 86, 420–428.

Siegel, S. and Castellan, N.J. (1988), *Nonparametric Statistics for the Behavioral Sciences* (2nd ed.), New York: McGraw-Hill.

Singer, J.D. (1995), "Using SAS PROC MIXED to Fit Multilevel Models, Hierarchical Models, and Individual Growth Models," *Journal of Educational and Behavioral Statistics*, 24, 323–355.

Snedecor, G.W. and Cochran, W.G. (1980), *Statistical Methods* (7th ed.), Ames, IA: Iowa State University Press.

Södergren, A., Karp, K., Boman, K., Eriksson, C., Lundström, E., Smedby, T., Söderlund, L., Rantapää-Dahlqvist, S., and Wållberg-Jonsson, S. (2010), "Atherosclerosis in Early Rheumatoid Arthritis: Very Early Endothelial Activation and Rapid Progression of Intima Media Thickness," *Arthritis Research and Therapy*, 12, R158. Available at http://arthritis-research.com/content/12/4/R158. Accessed July 17, 2013.

Solak, M.K. (2009), "Detection of Multiple Outliers in Univariate Data Sets," Paper SP06-2009, presented at the 2009 PharmaSUG meeting, Portland, OR, May 31–June 3, 2009. Available at http://www.lexjansen.com/pharmasug/2009/sp/sp06.pdf. Accessed January 22, 2014.

Stattin, P., Björ, O., Ferrari, P., Lukanova, P., Lenner, P., Lindahl, B., Hallmans, G., and Kaaks, R. (2007), "Prospective Study of Hyperglycemia and Cancer Risk," *Diabetes Care*, 30, 561–567.

Staudte, R.G. and Sheather, S.J. (1990), *Robust Estimation and Testing*, New York: John Wiley & Sons.

Steigen, T.K., Maeng, M., Wiseth, R., Erglis, A., Kumsars, I., Narbute, I., Gunnes, P., Mannsverk, J., Meyerdierks, O., Rotevatn, S., Niemelä, M., Kervinen, K., Jensen, J.S., Galløe, A., Nikus, K., Vikman, S., Ravkilde, J., James, S., Aarøe, J., Ylitalo, A., Helqvist, S., Sjögren, I., Thayssen, P., Virtanen, K., Puhakka, M., Airaksinen, J., Lassen, J.F., and Thuesen, L. (2006), "Randomized Study on Simple Versus Complex Stenting of Coronary Artery Bifurcation Lesions: The Nordic Bifurcation Study," *Circulation*, 14, 1955–1961.

Steiger, J.H. (1980), "Tests for Comparing Elements of a Correlation Matrix," *Psychological Bulletin*, 87, 245–261.

Stengel, B., Watier, L., Chouquet, C., Cénée, S., Philippon, C., and Hémon, D. (1999), "Influence of Renal Biomarker Variability on the Design and Interpretation of Occupational or Environmental Studies," *Toxicology Letters*, 106, 69–77.

St. Laurent, R.T. (1998), "Evaluating Agreement with a Gold Standard in Method Comparison Studies," *Biometrics*, 54, 537–545.

Stokes, M.E., Davis, C.S., and Koch, G.G. (2012), *Categorical Data Analysis Using SAS®* (3rd ed.), Cary, NC: SAS Institute Inc.

Strachan, D.P., Jarvis, M.J., and Feyerabend, C. (1990), "The Relationship of Salivary Cotinine to Respiratory Symptoms, Spirometry, and Exercise-Induced Bronchospasm in Seven-Year-Old Children," *American Review of Respiratory Disease*, 142, 147–151.

Strickland, P. and Kang, D. (1999), "Urinary 1-Hydroxypyrene and Other PAH Metabolites as Biomarkers of Exposure to Environmental PAH in Air Particulate Matter," *Toxicology Letters*, 108, 191–199.

Strike, P.W. (1991), *Statistical Methods in Laboratory Medicine*, Oxford, UK: Butterworth-Heinemann.

Strike, P.W. (1996), *Measurement in Laboratory Medicine: A Primer on Control and Interpretation*, Oxford, UK: Butterworth-Heinemann, pp. 147–172.

Stuart, M. (2013), "Identification of Novel Molecular Biomarkers for Diagnosis of Salivary Dysfunction," unpublished Master's thesis, Department of Oral Biology, Georgia Regents University.

Stuart, A. and Ord, J.K. (1987), *Kendall's Advanced Theory of Statistics: Volume 1: Distribution Theory* (5th ed.), New York: Oxford University Press.

Subar, A.F., Kipnis, F., Troiano, R.P., Midthune, D., Schoeller, D.A., Bingham, S., Sharbaugh, C.O., Trabulsi, J., Runswick, S., Ballard-Barbash, R., Sunshine, J., and Schatzkin, A. (2003), "Using Intake Biomarkers to Evaluate the Extent of Dietary Misreporting in a Large Sample of Adults: The OPEN Study," *American Journal of Epidemiology*, 158, 1–13.

Suissa, S. and Shuster, J. (1991). "The 2 × 2 Matched-Pairs Trial: Exact Unconditional Design and Analysis," *Biometrics*, 47, 361–372.

Susanto, H., Nesse, W., Dijkstra, P.U., Hoedemaker, E., van Reenen, Y.H., Agustina, D., Vissink, A., and Abbas, F. (2012), "Periodontal Inflamed Surface Area and C-Reactive Protein as Predictors of HbA1c: A Study in Indonesia," *Clinical Oral Investigations*, 16, 1237–1242.

Taioli, E., Kinney, P., Zhitkovich, A., Fulton, H., Voitkun, V., Cosma, G., Frenkel, K., Toniolo, P., Garte, S., and Costa, M. (1994), "Application of Reliability Models to Studies of Biomarker Validation," *Environmental Health Perspectives*, 102, 306–309.

Taylor, D.J., Kupper, L.L., Rappaport, S.M., and Lyles, R.H. (2001), "A Mixture Model for Occupational Exposure Mean Testing With a Limit of Detection," *Biometrics*, 57, 681–688.

Thode, H.C. (2002), *Testing for Normality*, New York: Marcel Dekker.

Tian, J., Barrantes, F., Amoateng-Adjepong, Y., and Manthous, C.A. (2009), "Rapid Reversal of Acute Kidney Injury and Hospital Outcomes: A Retrospective Cohort Study," *American Journal of Kidney Diseases*, 53, 974–981.

Tockman, M.S., Gupta, P.K., Myers, J.D., Frost, J.K., Baylin, S.B., Gold, E.B., Chase, A.M., Wilkinson, P.H., and Mulshine, J.L. (1988), "Sensitive and Specific Monoclonal Antibody Recognition of Human Lung Cancer Antigen on Preserved Sputum Cells: A New Approach to Early Lung Cancer Detection," *Journal of Clinical Oncology*, 6, 1685–1693.

Triola, M.M. and Triola, M.F. (2005), *Biostatistics for the Biological and Health Sciences*, Upper Saddle River, NJ: Pearson Education.

Tsai, M., Chang, C., and Huang, T. (2010), "Changes in High-Density Lipoprotein and Homeostasis Model Assessment of Insulin Resistance in Medicated Schizophrenic Patients and Healthy Controls," *Chang Gung Medical Journal*, 33, 613–618.

Tukey, J.W. (1977), *Exploratory Data Analysis*, Reading, MA: Addison-Wesley.

Tunstall-Pedoe, H., Brown, C.A., Woodward, M., and Tavendale, R. (1995), "Passive Smoking by Self-Report and Serum Cotinine and the Prevalence of Respiratory and Coronary Heart Disease in the Scottish Heart Health Study," *Journal of Epidemiology and Community Health*, 49, 139–143.

Van Roosbroeck, S., Li, R., Hoek G., Lebret, E., Brunekreef, B., and Spiegelman, D. (2008), "Traffic-Related Outdoor Air Pollution and Respiratory Symptoms in Children: The Impact of Adjustment for Exposure Measurement Error," *Epidemiology*, 19, 409–416.

Van Winden, A., Gast, M., Beijnen, J.H., Rutgers, E., Grobbee, D.E., Peeters, P., and van Gils, C.H. (2009), "Validation of Previously Identified Serum Biomarkers for Breast Cancer With SELDI-TOF MS: A Case Control Study," *BMC Medical Genomics*, 2:4, doi:10.1186/1755-8794-2-4.

Wang, H. (2006), "Correlation Analysis for Left-Censored Biomarker Data With Known Detection Limits," unpublished Master's thesis, Biostatistics Program, School of Public Health, Louisiana State University Health Sciences Center.

Wang, H.L., Chen, X.T., Yang, B., Ma, F.L., Wang, S., Tang, M.L., Hao, M.G., and Ruan, D.Y. (2008), "Case–Control Study of Blood Lead Levels and Attention Deficit Hyperactivity Disorder in Chinese Children," *Environmental Health Perspectives*, 116, 1401–1406.

Weiss, H.L., Niwas, S., Grizzle, W.E., and Piyathilake, C. (2003–2004), "Receiver Operating Characteristic (ROC) to Determine Cut-Off Points of Biomarkers in Lung Cancer Patients," *Disease Markers*, 19, 273–278.

Welch, B.L. (1937), "The Significance of the Difference Between Two Means When the Population Variances are Unequal," *Biometrika*, 29, 350–362.

Welch, B.L. (1951), "On the Comparison of Several Mean Values: An Alternative Approach," *Biometrika*, 38, 330–336.

Westgard, J.O. and Hunt, M.R. (1973), "Use and Interpretation of Common Statistical Tests in Method-Comparison Studies," *Clinical Chemistry*, 19, 49–57.

Westlund, K.B. and Kurland, L.T. (1953), "Studies on Multiple Sclerosis in Winnipeg, Manitoba and New Orleans, Louisiana," *American Journal of Hygiene*, 57, 380–396.

Wilcox, R. (2012), *Introduction to Robust Estimation and Hypothesis Testing* (3rd ed.), Waltham, MA: Elsevier.

Wilcox, R.R. (1987), *New Statistical Procedures for the Social Sciences*, Hillsdale, NJ: Lawrence Erlbaum Associates.

Wilk, M.B. and Gnanadesikan, R. (1968), "Probability Plotting Methods for the Analysis of Data," *Biometrika*, 55, 1–19.

Wilk, M.B. and Shapiro, S.S. (1968), "The Joint Assessment of Normality of Several Independent Samples," *Technometrics*, 10, 825–839.

Zady, M.F. (2009), "Mean, Standard Deviation and Coefficient of Variation," Westgard QC website. Available at http://www.westgard.com/lesson34.htm#6. Accessed December 14, 2011.

Zar, J.H. (2010), *Biostatistical Analysis* (5th ed.), Upper Saddle River, NJ: Pearson Prentice Hall.

Zhou, X., Obuchowski, N.A., and McClish, D.K. (2011), *Statistical Methods in Diagnostic Medicine* (2nd ed.), Hoboken, NJ: John Wiley & Sons.

SOLUTIONS TO PROBLEMS

Chapter 2

2.1

Configuration		Analysis Strategy
>2 nominal rows, >2 nominal columns*	____**G**_____	**A**. Test for linear association
>2 ordinal rows, >2 ordinal columns	____**A, D**____	**B**. Mann–Whitney–Wilcoxon
2 rows, >2 nominal columns*	_____**G**_____	**C**. Pearson's correlation
2 rows, >2 ordinal columns	_____**B**_____	**D**. Spearman's rho
>2 nominal rows, 2 columns*	_____**G**_____	**E**. Fisher's exact test
>2 ordinal rows, 2 columns	___**A, H, I**__	**F**. t-test
2 rows, 2 columns*	_____**E**_____	**G**. Fisher–Freeman–Halton test
		H. Cochran–Armitage test
		I. Permutation test for trend
		J. Shapiro–Wilk test

Note: If n is "sufficiently large," Pearson's χ^2 would give acceptable results for the configurations marked with *. However, it is generally preferable to use the indicated method with a mid-P adjustment (when available).

Analysis of Biomarker Data: A Practical Guide, First Edition. Stephen W. Looney and Joseph L. Hagan.

Chapter 3

3.1. Part A)

Variable	Median	Mode	Mean	Variance	Std Dev	Coeff of Varia-tion	25th Pctl	75th Pctl	Std Error	Lower 95% CL for Mean	Upper 95% CL for Mean
SPAP	36.30	–	40.90	330.59	18.18	44.45	27.20	58.90	3.57	33.56	48.25
RAER	59.65	–	51.67	462.07	21.50	41.60	34.10	68.30	4.22	42.99	60.35

Part B)

$$\text{PCC} = -0.749$$

Yes, there is a statistically significant negative linear association between right atrial emptying rate and systolic pulmonary artery pressure ($p < 0.001$).

$$R^2 = (-0.749)^2 = 0.561,$$

so 56.1% of the variation in systolic pulmonary artery pressure is explained by right atrial emptying rate.

Part C)

$$\hat{\beta} = -0.63$$

For every count per second increase in right atrial emptying rate there is a predicted 0.63 mm Hg decrease in systolic pulmonary artery pressure.

Part D)

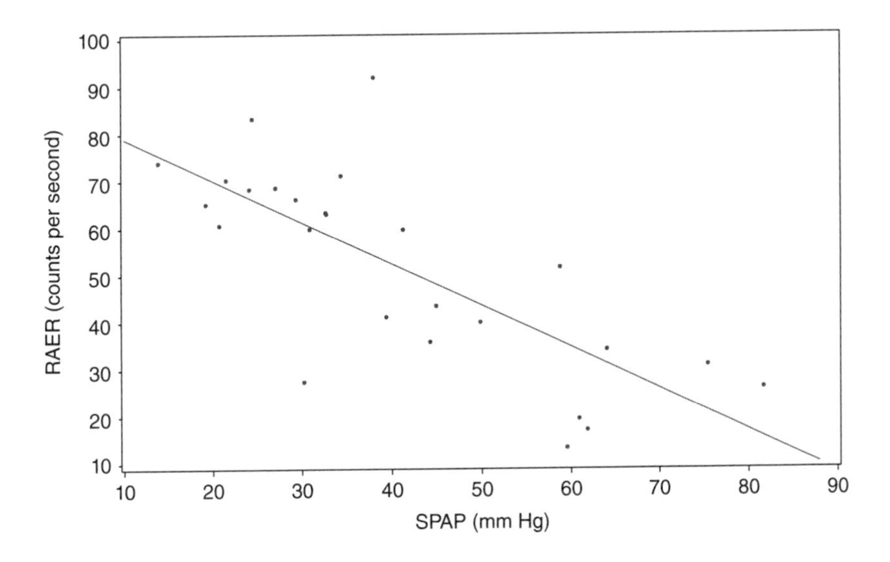

SAS code

```
data heart;
input subject SPAP RAER;
cards;
1   64.1  34.1
2   61.9  17.0
3   81.8  26.0
4   44.3  35.8
5   34.5  71.1
6   32.9  63.0
7   20.8  60.6
8   41.4  59.6
9   45.0  43.3
10  75.5  30.8
11  61.0  19.3
12  59.6  13.2
13  49.9  39.8
14  58.9  51.4
15  32.8  63.2
16  31.0  59.7
17  24.2  68.3
18  29.5  66.1
19  19.3  65.1
20  21.6  70.2
21  27.2  68.5
22  24.5  83.2
23  13.9  73.8
24  30.3  27.3
25  38.1  92.0
26  39.5  41.0
;
run;

/* 3.1 A*/
proc means data=heart median mode mean var std cv p25 p75
stderr clm maxdec=2;
var   SPAP RAER;
title 'Descriptive Statistics on SPAP RAER';
run;

/* 3.1 B*/
proc corr data=heart;
var SPAP RAER;
run;
```

```
/* 3.1 C*/
proc reg data=heart;
model SPAP= RAER;
run; quit;

/* 3.1 D*/

data heart;
set heart;
label SPAP = 'SPAP (mm Hg)'
RAER = 'RAER(counts per second)';
run;

symbol1 color=red interpol=rl
        value=dot
        height=.5;

axis1 label=(angle=90);

proc gplot data=heart;
     plot RAER*SPAP / hminor=0 hminor=0
                     vminor=0
                     caxis=black;
run;
quit;
```

3.2. The information provided in the problem yields the following 2×2 table.

Urinary Aflatoxin Detected?	Number of Subjects with Hepatocellular Carcinoma	Disease-Free Subjects
Yes	13	53
No	9	87

Since the data are obtained from a case–control study (i.e., the subjects are not selected via a simple random sample), the odds ratio should be used as the measure of association instead of the relative risk. The odds ratio for the association between presence of urinary aflatoxin and hepatocellular carcinoma is 2.4 (95% CI: 0.9–5.9) which is not a statistically significant association, since the 95% CI includes 1.

SAS code

```
data hepatic;
input Aflatoxin $ Cancer $ Count;
cards;
+ + 13
+ - 53
```

```
- + 9
- - 87
;
run;

proc freq data=hepatic;
tables Aflatoxin*Cancer /relrisk;
weight count;
exact chisq;
run;
```

3.3. The relative risk for schizophrenic patients taking Clozapine versus other antipsychotic drugs is 1.3 (0.8–2.0). There is no significant association between type of antipsychotic drug and risk of hyperlipidemia ($X^2 = 1.3$, $df = 1$, exact $p = 0.271$).

The estimated proportion (95% CI) of schizophrenic patients taking Clozapine with hyperlipidemia is 0.050 (95% CI: 0.033–0.073).

The estimated proportion (95% CI) of schizophrenic patients taking other antipsychotic drugs with hyperlipidemia is 0.039 (95% CI: 0.032–0.047).

SAS code

```
data Schizophrenia;
input Clozapine $  Hyperlipid $ Count;
cards;
+ + 26
+ - 492
- + 93
- - 2280
;
run;

proc freq data=Schizophrenia;
tables Clozapine*Hyperlipid  /relrisk;
weight count;
exact chisq;
run;

proc sort data=Schizophrenia;
by Clozapine;
run;

proc freq data=Schizophrenia;
tables Hyperlipid  /binomial;
by Clozapine;
weight count;
```

```
title 'schizophrenic patients taking
Clozapine and other antipsychotics';
run;
```

3.4. Part A)

Benign tissue: $n = 23$, $\bar{x} = 1.01$, $s = 0.30$, 95% CI: 0.93–1.19
Hyperplastic tissue: $n = 16$, $\bar{x} = 1.41$, $s = 0.56$, 95% CI: 1.11–1.71
Malignant tissue: $n = 13$, $\bar{x} = 3.95$, $s = 1.69$, 95% CI: 2.93–4.97

Part B)

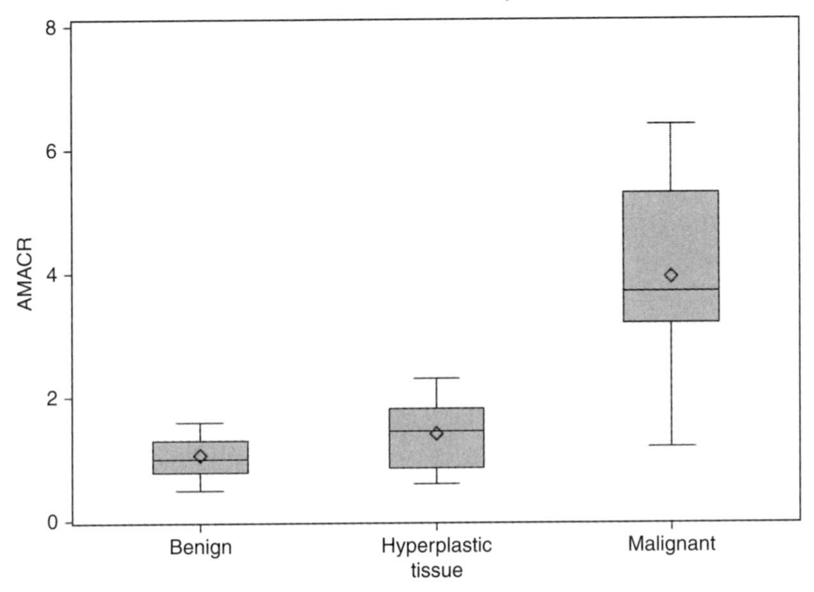

Part C)

ANOVA indicates a significant difference among the three tissue types' mean AMACR expression level ($F = 44.7$, $df = 2$ and 49, $p < 0.001$). The TK method reveals that the mean AMACR expression level in malignant tissue is significantly higher than in hyperplastic tissue ($p < 0.001$) and benign tissue ($p < 0.001$), but there is not a significant difference in the mean AMACR expression level in hyperplastic versus benign tissue ($p = 0.481$).

SAS code

```
data Benign;
input AMACR;
Tissue = 'Benign';
cards;
```

```
1.4
1.0
1.0
0.7
1.4
1.3
1.3
1.3
1.6
1.0
0.7
1.0
1.1
0.6
0.8
0.5
1.2
0.9
1.4
0.9
1.1
0.8
1.4
;
run;

data Hyperplastic;
input AMACR;
Tissue = 'Hyperplastic';
cards;
0.9
1.8
0.6
2.1
2.1
0.6
1.4
1.7
1.8
2.3
1.5
1.1
1.8
0.8
1.2
0.8
```

```
;
run;

data Malignant;
input AMACR;
Tissue = 'Malignant';
cards;
3.7
5.3
1.2
5.1
5.4
2.2
3.4
3.5
6.2
3.2
6.4
4.2
1.5
;
run;

data prostate;
set Benign Hyperplastic Malignant;
run;

/* Problem 3.4, part A */
proc means data=prostate n mean std clm;
class Tissue;
var AMACR;
run;

/* Problem 3.4, part B */
proc boxplot data=prostate ;
plot AMACR*Tissue;
run;

/* Problem 3.4, part C */

proc glm data=prostate;
class tissue;
model AMACR=Tissue;
lsmeans Tissue / adjust=Tukey;
run; quit;
```

3.5. The information provided in the problem yields the following 2 × 2 table.

Thiazolidinedione Therapy?	Number of Subjects with Heart Failure	Number of Disease-Free Subjects
Yes	59	216
No	229	1436

Subjects on Thiazolidinedione therapy have significantly higher odds of heart failure (odds ratio = 1.71, 95% CI: 1.24–2.36).

SAS code

```
data Hartung;
input hrt_fail $ Thiazo $ count;
cards;
+ + 59
+ - 229
- + 216
- - 1436
;

proc freq data=Hartung;
tables  hrt_fail*Thiazo  / cmh;
weight count;
title 'Thiazolidinedione exposure and heart failure status';
run;
```

Chapter 4

4.1. Part A)

Diabetics: $n = 21$, $\bar{x} = 8.1$, and $s = 1.8$
Non-diabetics: $n = 28$, $\bar{x} = 6.2$, and $s = 0.8$

SAS code

```
data nondiabetic;
input hgba1c @@;
cards;
5.9  5.6  6.3  5.9  6.9  6.5
7.6  6.2  5.8  6.0  6.9  5.9
6.4  5.5  7.1  5.3  6.9  5.6
5.7  6.9  4.5  7.7  5.3
6.9  7.4  5.6  5.8  6.1
;
run;

data nondiabetic;
set nondiabetic;
```

```
group = 'nondiabetic';
run;

data diabetic;
input hgba1c @@;
cards;
7.4  6.7  8.2  7.2  9.5
11.1 8.0 7.2 7.6
8.5  6.5  10.1 5.9
6.9  9.5  4.3  11.4
9.6  10.5 6.7 7.1
;
run;

data diabetic;
set diabetic;
group = 'diabetic   ';
run;

data both;
set diabetic nondiabetic;
run;

proc means data=both n mean std;
class group;
var hgba1c ;
run;
```

Part B)

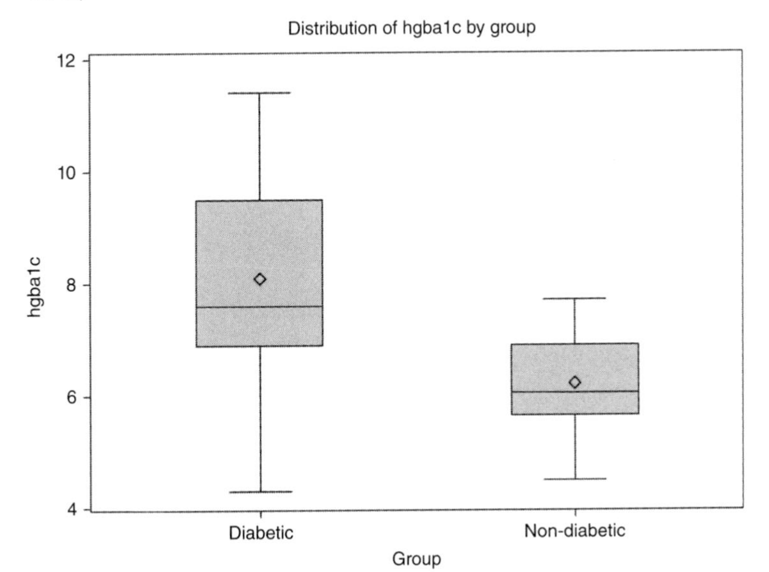

SAS code

```
proc boxplot data=both;
plot hgba1c*group;
run;
```

Part C)

Diabetics: 95% CI: 7.3–8.9
Non-Diabetics: 95% CI: 5.9–6.5

SAS code

```
proc means data=both clm;
class group;
var hgba1c ;
run;
```

Part D)

Since the hemoglobin A1c levels of both groups are normally distributed (for diabetics: $W = 1.0$, $p = 0.577$; for non-diabetics: $W = 1.0$, $p = 0.441$) a two-sample t-test is appropriate to compare the mean hemoglobin A1c levels of diabetics versus non-diabetics. Since the assumption that the variances of the two groups' hemoglobin A1c levels are equal is violated ($F = 5.6$; $df = 20, 27$; $p < 0.001$), the unequal-variance t-test should be used to compare the two groups' hemoglobin A1c levels. The unequal-variance t-test indicates that the mean preoperative hemoglobin A1c level of diabetics is significantly higher compared to non-diabetics ($t = 4.4$, $df = 25.4$, $p < 0.001$).

SAS code

```
/* assess normaility of groups'hgba1c */
proc univariate data=both normal;
by group;
var hgba1c ;
run;

/* compare mean hgba1c */
proc ttest data=both;
class group;
var hgba1c ;
run;
```

4.2. Since the fasting blood glucose levels are not normally distributed ($W = 0.4$, $p < 0.001$), Spearman's correlation should be used instead of Pearson's correlation. Using the data in the table, the null hypothesis of no correlation between age and fasting blood glucose level is not rejected ($r_s = 0.200$, $p = 0.443$).

SAS code

```
/* assess normality of age and glucose */
proc univariate data=NHANES normal;
var age glucose;
run;

/* compute Spearman's correlation coefficient */
proc corr data=NHANES spearman;
var age glucose;
run;
```

4.3. The Shapiro–Wilk test indicates that the HDL levels of both Black and Hispanic subjects are not normally distributed (for Black subjects, $W = 0.7$, $p < 0.001$; for Hispanic subjects, $W = 0.9$, $p = 0.004$). Thus, ANOVA is not appropriate for comparing ethnicities' mean HDL levels. Next the k-sample Conover test is applied and found to not indicate significant differences in the HDL variances across ethnic groups ($X^2 = 5.7$, $df = 2$, $p = 0.058$). Thus, the Kruskal–Wallis test is an appropriate method to compare the ethnic groups' HDL levels. The Kruskal–Wallis test indicates a significant difference in the ethnic groups' HDL levels ($X^2 = 8.3$, $df = 2$, $p = 0.016$). Next, Dunn's method is applied to each of the three pairs of ethnic groups. The SAS output from the macro to perform Dunn's method indicates that Blacks have significantly higher HDL levels than Hispanics.

```
  Large Sample Approximation Multiple Comparison Procedure
                          Designed for Unbalanced Data
3 Groups: black hispanic white (Respective Sample Sizes:
21 24 29)
                               Alpha = 0.05
                         Method Suggested by Dunn (1964)
                               Difference
                                  in      Cutoff
Comparison    Group           Average     at        Significance
Number     Comparisons        Ranks    Alpha=0.05 Difference = **
   1    black - hispanic   17.1815     15.3839         **
   2    black - white      14.5788     14.7521
   3    hispanic - white   2.6027      14.2072
```

SAS code

```
data white;
input hdl @@;
```

```
ethnicity='white   ';
cards;
76  40  48  43  48
35  45  65  28  50
28  59  55  15  34
24  48  39  32  60
44  74  39  90  48
25  35  45  36
;
run;

data black;
input hdl @@;
ethnicity='black   ';
cards;
32  70  44  50
49  57  53  56
49  98  40  71
49  77  29
179  43  39
75  83  45
;
run;

data hispanic;
input hdl @@;
ethnicity='hispanic';
cards;
39  62  32  69
47  37  28  38
59  31  31  32
33  48  74  40
79  31  48  35
42  43  43  42
;
run;

data all;
set white black hispanic;
run;

proc sort data=all;
by ethnicity;
run;
```

```
/* test for normality in each ethnic group */
proc univariate data = all normal;
by ethnicity;
var hdl;
run;

/* Use k-sample Conover test to test for homogeneity of
 variances  */

proc npar1way data=all conover;
class ethnicity;
var hdl ;
run; quit;

/* use Kruskal-Wallis test to compare groups' HDL levels */
proc npar1way data=all;
class ethnicity;
var hdl ;
run;

/* Use Dunn's method for post-hoc analysis   */

options nomacrogen nosymbolgen;

%macro DUNN(DSN,GROUP,VAR,ALPHA);
%*********************************************************;
%* The Dunn Macro                                        *;
%* - - - - - - - - - - - - - - - - - - - - - - - - - - - *;
%*                                                       *;
%* This macro is designed to perform all two-sided
    pairwise *;
%* comparisons of the location parameters for n groups
   (n gt 2)*;
%* in a one-way layout. The method for the procedure
   involves a*;
%* large sample approximation. The method of comparison
   employs*;
%* ranking all non-missing observations and averaging
   the ranks*;
%* for each level of the class variable (&GROUP).       *;
%*                                                      *;
%* The required inputs for the macro are a SAS data set
   (&DSN) *;
%* containing a character class variable (&GROUP),
   a response  *;
```

```
%* variable (&VAR), and a family-wise error rate (&ALPHA). *;
%*                                                          *;
%* For more details on this nonparametric multiple
   comparison  *;
%* procedure, see Hollander and Wolfe s Nonparamet-
ric      *;
%* Statistical Methods, 1/e p. 125.                        *;
%*                                                          *;
%* Overall Macro Scheme:                                    *;
%* - - - - - - - - - - - - - - - - -*;
%* The macro consists of a body of code containing one
   embedded*;
%* macro (%GROUPS). The embedded macro determines the
   number of*;
%* groups present (&NGRPS). If a group in the SAS data set
   does*;
%* not contain at least one response value, it will not be *;
%* included in the analysis. The embedded macro also
   creates       *;
%* one global macro variable that contains the group
   labels*;
%* (&GRPVEC) for the levels of the class variable.         *;
%*                                                          *;
%* The main body of the SAS macro code determines
   summary  *;
%* statistics (e.g., average ranks, sample sizes, etc.)
   This    *;
%* information is then employed to calculate the
   pair-wise *;
%* test statistics. The cutoff for the test statistic is   *;
%* calculated with PROBIT function. The results are then   *;
%* printed out with a PROC PRINT procedure.                *;
%*                                                          *;
%*If you have questions about this code or its
  application,*;
%*please do not hesitate to contact me.                    *;
%*                                                          *;
%*Paul Juneau                                              *;
%*Associate Director                                       *;
%*Midwest Nonclinical Statistics - Michigan Laboratories   *;
%*Pfizer Global Research & Development                     *;
%*734-622-1791                                             *;
%*paul.juneau@pfizer.com                                   *;
%*                                                          *;
```

```
%*2004                                                          *;
%************************************************************ ;

%*First, take the input data set &DSN and eliminate missing
   values;
data &DSN.2;
  set &DSN;
  if &VAR ne .;
run;

%macro GROUPS;
%*This macro creates two outputs:                               *;
%*(1) The total number of groups present (&NGRPS)               *;
%*(2) A macro variable that contains all of the individual*;
%*    class variable labels (&GRPVEC)                           *;

%global GRPVEC;

proc sort data=&DSN.2; by &GROUP;
run;

%*Create a data set that contains just the levels of
   the class variable (&GROUP);
data &GROUP; set &DSN.2; by &GROUP;
if first.&GROUP;
run;

proc transpose data=&GROUP out=GRPVEC; var &GROUP;
run;

%*Determine the number of levels of the class variable;
data _null_;
call symput('NGRPS',left(put(count,8.)));
stop;
set &GROUP nobs=COUNT;
run;

%*Create a global macro variable containing the labels for
each level of the class variable;
data null; set GRPVEC;

GRPVEC=
%do G=1 %to %eval(&NGRPS-1);
  trim(left(COL&G))||""||
%end;
  trim(left(COL&NGRPS));
call SYMPUT('GRPVEC',GRPVEC);
run;
```

```
%mend GROUPS;

%GROUPS

proc sort data=&DSN.2;
by &GROUP;
run;

%*Rank all non-missing responses;
proc rank data=&DSN.2 out=R&VAR;
ranks R&VAR;
var &VAR;
run;

proc sort data=R&VAR;
by &GROUP;
run;

%*Calculate the average of the ranks for each group;
proc univariate noprint data=R&VAR;
var R&VAR;
by &GROUP;
output out=S&VAR sum=S&VAR n=N&VAR;
run;

%*Determine the total sample size for the entire experiment;
proc univariate noprint data=S&VAR;
var N&VAR;
output out=SN&VAR sum=SN&VAR;
run;

%*Create a macro variable with value equal to the total
  sample size for the entire experiment;

data _null_;
set SN&VAR;

call symput("N",left(put(SN&VAR,8.)));
run;

data SR&VAR; set S&VAR;
keep S&VAR;
run;

data N&VAR; set S&VAR;
keep N&VAR;
run;
```

```
proc transpose data=SR&VAR out=SRVEC; var S&VAR;
run;
%*Create a macro variable containing the summary statis-
  tics (average ranks) for each group;

data _null_;
  set SRVEC;
SRVEC=
%do S=1 %to %eval(&NGRPS-1);
  trim(left(put(COL&S,11.3)))||""||
%end;
  trim(left(put(COL&NGRPS,11.3)));
call SYMPUT('SRVEC',SRVEC);
run;

proc transpose data=N&VAR out=nVEC; var n&VAR;
run;

%*Create a macro variable containing the sample sizes for
  each level of the class variable;

data _null_;
  set NVEC;
nVEC=
%do S2=1 %to %eval(&NGRPS-1);
  trim(left(put(COL&S2,8.)))||""||
%end;
  trim(left(put(COL&NGRPS,8.)));
call SYMPUT('NVEC',NVEC);
run;

%*Perform the pair-wise large sample approximation MCP;
data NPARMCP;

%do U=1 %to &NGRPS;

%do V=%eval(&U+1) %to &NGRPS;

%let RSUM&U=%scan(&SRVEC,&U," ");
%let N&U=%scan(&NVEC,&U," ");
%let RSUM&V=%scan(&SRVEC,&V," ");
%let N&V=%scan(&NVEC,&V," ");

c+1;
DIFFLBL="%scan(&GRPVEC,&U," ") - %scan(&GRPVEC,&V," ")";
AVDIFF=abs((&&RSUM&U/&&N&U)-(&&RSUM&V/&&N&V));
CUTOFF=probit(1-(&ALPHA/((&NGRPS*(&NGRPS-1)))))
```

```
        *(((&N*(&N+1))/12)**0.5)
        *((1/&&N&U + 1/&&N&V)**0.5);
SYMBOL="  ";
if AVDIFF ge CUTOFF then do;
 SYMBOL="**";
end;
output;
%end;

%end;

label DIFFLBL="Group@Comparisons"
    AVDIFF="Difference@in@Average@Ranks"
    CUTOFF="Cutoff@at@Alpha=&ALPHA"
    SYMBOL="Significance@Difference = **"
    c="Comparison@Number"
;

title1 "Large Sample Approximation Multiple Comparison
Procedure";
title2 "Designed for Unbalanced Data";
title3 "%trim(%left(&NGRPS)) Groups: %trim(%left(&GRPVEC))
(Respective Sample Sizes: %trim(%left(&NVEC)))";
title4 "Alpha = &ALPHA";
title5 ;
title6 "Method Suggested by Dunn (1964)";
%*Print out the results of the test;

proc print label split='@' noobs;
run;

%mend DUNN;
%DUNN(all,ethnicity,hdl,0.05);
```

4.4. Part A)

The sample correlation coefficients, 95% CI for ξ, and the p-value testing H_0: $\xi = 0$ for Pearson's, Spearman's, and Kendall's correlation between the HDL and triglyceride levels are given in the table below.

Measure of Association	Estimated Coefficient	95% CI for ξ	p-value for Test of H_0: $\xi = 0$
Pearson	−0.805	(−0.924, −0.541)	<0.001
Spearman	−0.793	(−0.858, −0.704)	<0.001
Kendall	−0.586	(−0.759, −0.334)	<0.001

ξ: Population value of measure of association ($\xi = \rho$ for Pearson's, $\xi = \rho_s$ for Spearman's, and $\xi = \tau_b$ for Kendall's).

SAS code

```
data lipids;
input Subject HDL TG;
cards;
1  57  34
2  49  118
3  59  83
4  64  101
5  51  143
6  79  63
7  52  164
8  60  141
9  40  245
10  77  54
11  82  79
12  55  207
13  58  112
14  53  191
15  38  290
16  76  39
17  42  202
18  58  118
;
run;

PROC CORR PEARSON SPEARMAN KENDALL FISHER(BIASADJ=NO)
data=lipids;
   VAR HDL  TG;
   title 'Results for Spearman Using This Fisher z Not
   Recommended';
 run;
%let rs = -0.79287;
%let n = 20;
data fisher_rs;
rs_fisher=0.5*(log((1+&rs)/(1-&rs)));
low_rsz=rs_fisher-1.96*sqrt((1+&rs**2)/2)/(sqrt(&n-3));
up_rsz=rs_fisher+1.96*sqrt((1+&rs**2)/2)/(sqrt(&n-3));
low_rs=(exp(2*low_rsz)-1)/(exp(2*low_rsz)+1);
up_rs=(exp(2*up_rsz)-1)/(exp(2*up_rsz)+1);
se_rs = sqrt(((1+&rs**2)/2)/(&n-3));
z_rs = rs_fisher/se_rs;
p_val_rs = 2*(1-(probnorm(abs(z_rs))));
run;
proc print data=fisher_rs;
```

```
title 'Spearman Coefficient Using Bonett and Wright
Transformation';
run;
%let rk =  -0.58553;
%let n = 20;

data fisher_rk;
rk_fisher=0.5*(log((1+&rk)/(1-&rk)));
low_rkz=rk_fisher-1.96*sqrt(0.437)/(sqrt(&n-4));
up_rkz=rk_fisher+1.96*sqrt(0.437)/(sqrt(&n-4));
low_rk=(exp(2*low_rkz)-1)/(exp(2*low_rkz)+1);
up_rk=(exp(2*up_rkz)-1)/(exp(2*up_rkz)+1);
se_rk = sqrt((0.437)/(&n-4));
z_rk = rk_fisher/se_rk;
p_val_rk = 2*(1-abs(probnorm(abs(z_rk))));
run;

proc print data=fisher_rk;
title 'Kendall Coefficient Using Fieller et al. (1957)
Transformation';
run;
```

Part B)

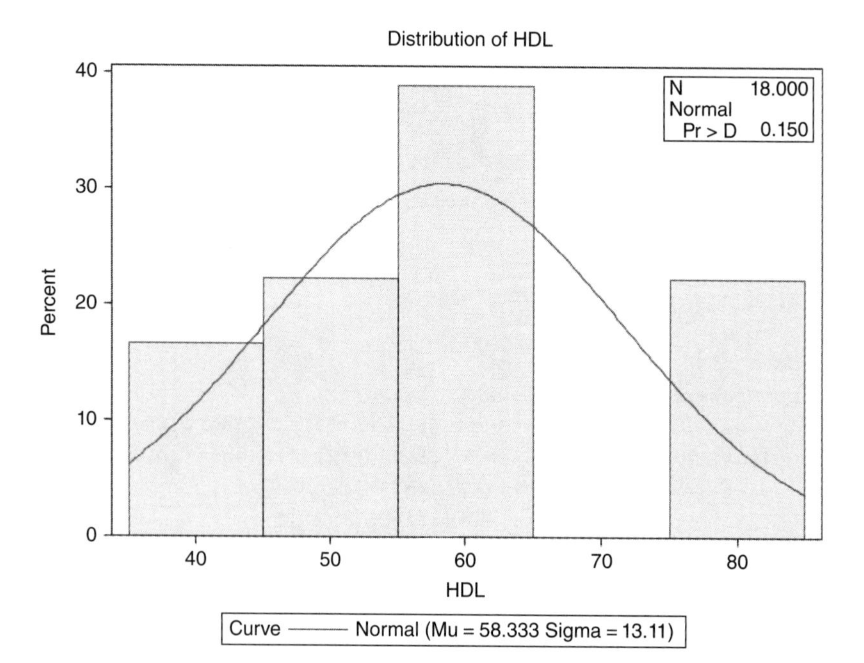

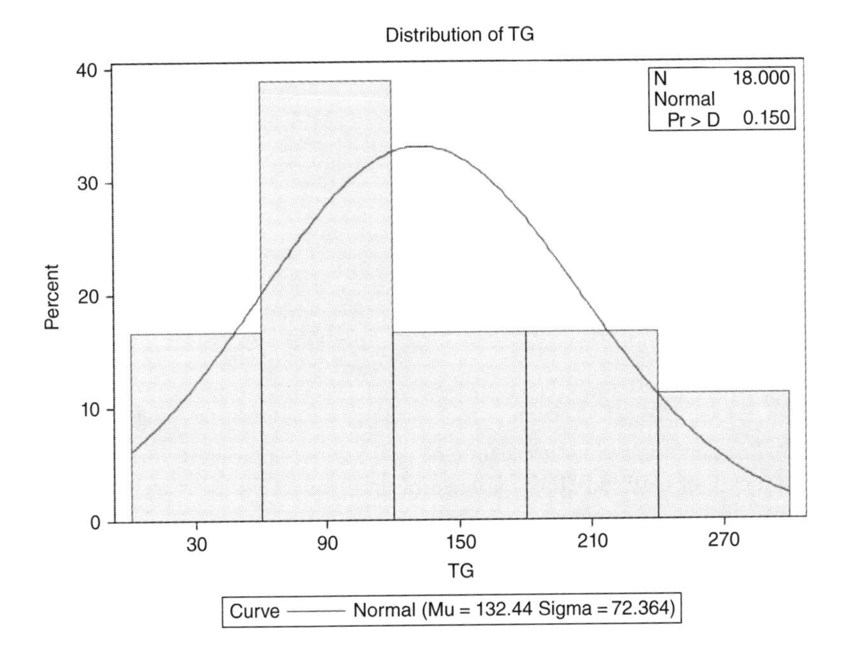

SAS code

```
proc univariate data=lipids;
 histogram hdl / normal(percents=20 40 60 80 midpercents)
                   name='MyPlot';
 inset n normal(ksdpval) / pos = ne format = 6.3;
run;

proc univariate data=lipids;
 histogram TG / normal(percents=20 40 60 80 midpercents)
                   name='MyPlot';
 inset n normal(ksdpval) / pos = ne format = 6.3;
run;
```

Part C)

HDL cholesterol: skewness = 0.40, kurtosis = −0.54
Triglycerides: skewness = 0.60, kurtosis = −0.28

SAS code

```
proc univariate data=lipids;
var HDL TG;
run;
```

Part D)

The Shapiro–Wilk test does not indicate a departure from normality for either HDL cholesterol ($W = 0.94$, $p = 0.239$) or triglycerides ($W = 0.96$, $p = 0.528$).

SAS code

```
proc univariate data=lipids normal;
  var HDL TG;
run;
```

Part E)

Pearson's correlation coefficient is the most appropriate measure for the association between HDL cholesterol and triglycerides, since both variables are normally distributed.

4.5. African American women are diagnosed with a significantly more advanced cancer stage compared to Caucasian women ($Z = 2.5$, $p = 0.014$).

SAS code

```
data cancer;
input ethnicity $ stage count;
cards;
C 1 217
C 2 102
C 3 17
AA 1 44
AA 2 33
AA 3 9
;
run;

proc npar1way data=cancer wilcoxon;
class ethnicity;
var stage;
freq count;
run;
```

4.6. Part A)

The Shapiro–Wilk test indicates that the biomarker is not normally distributed in disease-free subjects ($W = 0.9$, $p = 0.004$). The Conover test indicates a significant difference in the variability of the biomarker level of obese adults with versus without diabetes (Exact $p = 0.003$, using the Chi-square approximation, $X^2 = 8.5$, $df = 1$, $p = 0.004$). Thus, the two-sample median test should be used to compare the biomarker levels of the two groups.

SAS code

```
data obese;
input pt group  biomarker;
cards;
1   1  120
2   1  88
3   1  120
4   1  120
5   1  111
6   1  117
7   1  112
8   1  124
9   1  121
10  1  113
11  1  116
12  1  122
13  1  123
14  1  121
15  1  122
16  1  101
17  1  99
18  1  119
19  1  109
20  1  112
21  1  111
22  1  107
23  1  122
24  1  106
25  1  122
26  2  265
27  2  267
28  2  277
29  2  326
30  2  300
31  2  291
32  2  249
33  2  313
34  2  318
35  2  292
36  2  293
37  2  325
```

```
38  2  290
39  2  322
40  2  296
41  2  243
42  2  303
;
run;

proc sort data=obese;
by group;
run;

/* use Shapiro-Wilk test to test normality */
proc univariate data=obese normal;
by group;
var biomarker;
run;

/* use Conover test to test equality of variances */
proc npar1way data=obese;
class group;
var biomarker;
exact conover;
run;
```

Part B)

Obese adults with diabetes have significantly higher biomarker levels than subjects without diabetes ($X^2 = 30.8$, $df = 1$, $p < 0.001$).

SAS code

```
/* continued from Problem 4.10 */
/* use median test to compare biomarker levels of
subjects with (group=2) and without diabetes (group=1) */

proc npar1way data=obese median;
class group;
var biomarker;
run;
```

4.7. Part A)

The Shapiro–Wilk test does not indicate a departure from normality for either group (Production workers: $W = 0.89$, $p = 0.107$, Office workers:

$W = 0.94$, $p = 0.364$). The Conover test indicates a significant difference in the variability of the enzyme concentrations (Exact $p < 0.001$). Thus, the unequal-variance t-test should be used to compare the mean enzyme concentrations of the two groups.

SAS code

```
data Enzyme1;
input Enzyme;
group = 'Production';
cards;
55
54
57
56
54
59
57
57
58
58
63
64
;
run;

data Enzyme2;
input Enzyme;
group = 'Office';
cards;
118
74
133
136
144
102
147
111
106
74
155
135
143
144
178
```

```
112
77
;
run;

data Enzymes;
set Enzyme1 Enzyme2;
run;

proc sort data=Enzymes;
by group;
run;

/* use Shapiro-Wilk test to test normality */

proc univariate data=Enzymes normal;
var Enzyme;
by group;
run;

/* use Conover test to test equality of variances */

proc npar1way data=Enzymes;
class group;
var Enzyme;
exact conover;
run;
```

Part B)

The unequal-variance t-test shows that workers in the production unit have significantly higher enzyme levels than workers in the office ($t = 8.9$, $df = 16.5$, $p < 0.001$).

SAS code

```
proc ttest data=Enzymes;
class group;
var Enzyme;
run;
```

4.8. Computing the difference in CEA levels for each pair of patients and applying the paired t-test, Wilcoxon signed ranks test, and sign test to the data in the table yields the following results:

Paired t-test: $t = -2.7$, $df = 9$, $p = 0.024$. Reject the null hypothesis and conclude that patients given the "new" chemotherapy regimen have significantly lower mean CEA levels.

Wilcoxon signed ranks test: $p = 0.020$. Reject the null hypothesis and conclude that patients given the "new" chemotherapy regimen have significantly lower CEA levels.

Sign test: $p = 0.109$. Fail to reject the null hypothesis that the CEA levels of the two chemotherapy regimens are the same.

The paired t-test results should be used to compare the two chemotherapy regimens' CEA levels since a departure from normality is not detected (e.g., Shapiro–Wilk $W = 0.9$, $p = 0.146$).

SAS code

```
data cea;
input new soc;
diff = new - soc;
cards;
17 22
29 31
14 22
5  16
2  9
7  14
25 21
3  8
11 7
33 38
;
run;

proc univariate data=cea normal;
var diff;
run;
```

4.9. Using Cochran's Q test, we reject the null hypothesis that the three screening tests give the same results ($Q = 22.1$, $df = 2$, $p < 0.001$).

SAS code

```
data alz;
input ApoE$ MRI$  CFT$ count;
cards;
+   +   +   56
-   -   -   119
```

```
+ + - 23
+ - - 11
+ - + 25
- + + 7
- + - 5
- - + 44
;
run;

proc freq data=Alz;
 tables ApoE*MRI*CFT / agree noprint;
 weight Count;
run;
```

4.10. 214 observations are needed.

SAS code

```
%let rp = .51;
%let w = .2;
%let b = 3;
%let c_sq = 1;

data fisher_rp_sample;
n_0_1 = 4*(&c_sq)*((1-&rp**2)**2)*((1.96/&w)**2)+&b;
if n_0_1 < 10 then n_0 = 10;
if int(n_0_1) < n_0_1 then n_0 = int(n_0_1)+1; else n_0 =
n_0_1;
rp_fisher=0.5*(log((1+&rp)/(1-&rp)));
low_rpz=rp_fisher-1.96*sqrt(&c_sq)/(sqrt(n_0-&b));
up_rpz=rp_fisher+1.96*sqrt(&c_sq)/(sqrt(n_0-&b));
low_rp=(exp(2*low_rpz)-1)/(exp(2*low_rpz)+1);
up_rp=(exp(2*up_rpz)-1)/(exp(2*up_rpz)+1);
w_0 = up_rp -low_rp;
n_1 = (n_0 - &b)*(w_0/&w)**2+&b;
if int(n_1) < n_1 then n = int(n_1)+1; else n = n_1;
run;

proc print data=fisher_rp_sample;
TITLE 'SAMPLE SIZE CALCULATION';
title2 'Pearson';
run;
```

R code

```
# Sample Size for Pearson's CC
```

```
c_sq <- 1
e <- 0.51
z <- 1.96
w <- .2
b <- 3
n0 <- 4*c_sq*((1-e**2)**2)*(z/w)**2+b
n0
```

4.11. 28 subjects are needed for the SCC and 35 subjects are needed for KCC.

SAS code

```
%let rs = .82;
%let w = .3;
%let b = 3;

data fisher_rs_sample;
c_sq = 1+(&rs**2)/2;
n_0_1 = 4*(c_sq)*((1-&rs**2)**2)*((1.96/&w)**2)+&b;
if n_0_1 < 10 then n_0 = 10;
if int(n_0_1) < n_0_1 then n_0 = int(n_0_1)+1; else n_0 =
n_0_1;
rs_fisher=0.5*(log((1+&rs)/(1-&rs)));
low_rsz=rs_fisher-1.96*sqrt(c_sq)/(sqrt(n_0-&b));
up_rsz=rs_fisher+1.96*sqrt(c_sq)/(sqrt(n_0-&b));
low_rs=(exp(2*low_rsz)-1)/(exp(2*low_rsz)+1);
up_rs=(exp(2*up_rsz)-1)/(exp(2*up_rsz)+1);
w_0 = up_rs -low_rs;
n_1 = (n_0 - &b)*(w_0/&w)**2+&b;
if int(n_1) < n_1 then n = int(n_1)+1; else n = n_1;
run;

proc print data=fisher_rs_sample;
TITLE 'SAMPLE SIZE CALCULATION';
title2 'Spearman';
run;
%let rk = .6;
%let w = .3;
%let b = 4;
%let c_sq = .437;

data fisher_rk_sample;
n_0_1 = 4*(&c_sq)*((1-&rk**2)**2)*((1.96/&w)**2)+&b;
if n_0_1 < 10 then n_0 = 10;
if int(n_0_1) < n_0_1 then n_0 = int(n_0_1)+1; else n_0 =
n_0_1;
```

```
rk_fisher=0.5*(log((1+&rk)/(1-&rk)));
low_rkz=rk_fisher-1.96*sqrt(&c_sq)/(sqrt(n_0-&b));
up_rkz=rk_fisher+1.96*sqrt(&c_sq)/(sqrt(n_0-&b));
low_rk=(exp(2*low_rkz)-1)/(exp(2*low_rkz)+1);
up_rk=(exp(2*up_rkz)-1)/(exp(2*up_rkz)+1);
w_0 = up_rk -low_rk;
n_1 = (n_0 - &b)*(w_0/&w)**2+&b;
if int(n_1) < n_1 then n = int(n_1)+1; else n = n_1;
run;

proc print data=fisher_rk_sample;
TITLE 'SAMPLE SIZE CALCULATION';
title2 'Kendall';
run;
```

R code

```
# SCC
   e <- 0.82
   c_sq <- 1+(e**2/2)
   z <- 1.96
   w <- 0.3
   b <- 3
   n0 <- 4*c_sq*((1-e**2)**2)*(z/w)**2+b
   n0
   # KCC
   c_sq <- 0.437
   e <- 0.60
   z <- 1.96
   w <- 0.3
   b <- 4
   n0 <- 4*c_sq*((1-e**2)**2)*(z/w)**2+b
   n0
```

4.12. 51 observations are needed.

SAS code

```
%let rho_1 = .51;
%let rho_0 = .2;
%LET alpha = .05;
%LET beta = .20;
%let b = 3;
%let c_sq = 1;
data fisher_rho_sample;
z_alpha = probit(1 - &alpha);
```

```
z_beta = probit(1 - &beta);
rho_1_z = 0.5*(log((1+&rho_1)/(1-&rho_1)));
rho_0_z = 0.5*(log((1+&rho_0)/(1-&rho_0)));
n = &b + sqrt(&c_sq)*((z_alpha + z_beta) / (rho_1_z -
rho_0_z))**2;
if int(n) < n then n = int(n)+1;
run;

proc print data = fisher_rho_sample;
TITLE 'SAMPLE SIZE CALCULATION';
title2 'Pearson';
title3 'Based on Hypothesis Test';
run;
```

R code

```
za <-1.64485
   zb <-0.84162
   r1 <- 0.51
   r0 <- .2
   zr1 <- 0.5*(log((1+r1)/(1-r1)))
   zr0 <- 0.5*(log((1+r0)/(1-r0)))
   n <- 3 + ((za+zb)/(zr1-zr0))**2
   n
```

4.13. 26 observations are needed for SCC and 135 observations are needed for KCC.

SAS code

```
%let rho_s_1 = .82;
%let rho_s_0 = .5;
%LET alpha = .05;
%LET beta = .20;
%let b = 3;

data fisher_Spearman_sample;
c_sq = 1 + (&rho_s_1**2)/2;
*c_sq = 1.06;
z_alpha = probit(1 - &alpha);
z_beta = probit(1 - &beta);
rho_s_1_z = 0.5*(log((1+&rho_s_1)/(1-&rho_s_1)));
rho_s_0_z = 0.5*(log((1+&rho_s_0)/(1-&rho_s_0)));
n = &b + c_sq*((z_alpha + z_beta) / (rho_s_1_z -
rho_s_0_z))**2;
if int(n) < n then n = int(n)+1;
run;
```

```
proc print data = fisher_Spearman_sample;
TITLE 'SAMPLE SIZE CALCULATION';
title2 'Spearman';
title3 'Based on Hypothesis Test';
run;

%let tau_1 = .60;
%let tau_0 = .5;
%LET alpha = .05;
%LET beta = .20;
%let b = 4;
%let c_sq = .437;

data fisher_Kendall_sample;
z_alpha = probit(1 - &alpha);
z_beta = probit(1 - &beta);
tau_1_z = 0.5*(log((1+&tau_1)/(1-&tau_1)));
tau_0_z = 0.5*(log((1+&tau_0)/(1-&tau_0)));
n = &b + &c_sq*((z_alpha + z_beta) / (tau_1_z -
tau_0_z))**2;
if int(n) < n then n = int(n)+1;
run;

proc print data = fisher_Kendall_sample;
TITLE 'SAMPLE SIZE CALCULATION';
title2 'Kendall';
title3 'Based on Hypothesis Test';
run;
```

R code

```
# SCC
   za <-1.64
   zb <-0.84162
   rs1 <- .82
   rs0 <- .5
   zr1 <- 0.5*(log((1+rs1)/(1-rs1)))
   zr0 <- 0.5*(log((1+rs0)/(1-rs0)))
   n <- 3 + (1+(rs1**2/2))*((za+zb)/(zr1-zr0))**2
   n
   # KCC
   t1 <- .6
   t0 <- .5
   za <- 1.64
```

```
zb <- 0.84162
zt1 <- 0.5*(log((1+t1)/(1-t1)))
zt0 <- 0.5*(log((1+t0)/(1-t0)))
n <- 4 + 0.437*((za+zb)/(zt1-zt0))**2
n
```

4.14. The correlation of the two enzymes is significantly higher in babies with Type B Niemann–Pick disease than in healthy babies ($z_0 = -2.0$, $p = 0.048$).

SAS code

```
%let rs_h = .15;
%let n_h = 34;

%let rs_n = .66;
%let n_n = 18;

%let c_sq = 1.06;
%let b = 3;

data fisher_rs_ind;
rsh_fisher=0.5*(log((1+&rs_h)/(1-&rs_h)));
se_rs_h = sqrt((&c_sq)/(&n_h-&b));
rsx_fisher=0.5*(log((1+&rs_n)/(1-&rs_n)));
se_rs_n = sqrt((&c_sq)/(&n_n-&b));
se_rs_ind = sqrt(((se_rs_h)**2) + ((se_rs_n)**2));
z_rs_ind = (rsh_fisher - rsx_fisher)/se_rs_ind;
p_val_rs_ind = 2*(1-probnorm(abs((z_rs_ind))));
run;

proc print data=fisher_rs_ind;
title1 'Comparison of Independent Spearman Correlations';
title2 'Using Fieller (1957) Transformation';
run;
```

4.15. Yes, the correlation between Biomarkers A and B is significantly higher than the correlation between Biomarkers A and C ($z_0 = 2.7$, $p = 0.008$).

SAS code

```
/*
  THIS PROGRAM COMPARES TWO DEPENDENT CORRELATIONS USING THE
  METHODS DESCRIBED IN STEIGER JH. TESTS FOR COMPARING
  ELEMENTS OF A CORRELATION MATRIX.  PSYCHOLOGICAL
  BULLETIN (1980), VOL. 87: 245-261.
```

```
  R1 AND R2 ARE THE DEPENDENT CORRELATIONS TO BE COMPARED.
  R12 IS THE CORRELATION BETWEEN THE VARIABLES THAT R1 & R2
  DO NOT HAVE IN COMMON.

  FOR EXAMPLE, IF R1 IS THE CORRELATION BETWEEN X1 & X2
  AND R2 is THE CORRELATION BETWEEN X1 & X3 THEN R12 IS THE
  CORRELATION IS BETWEEN X2 & X3.
*/

%let r1 = 0.78 ;
%let r2 = 0.53 ;
%let r12 = 0.31;
%let n = 64;

%let b = 3;
%let c_sq = 1.00;

data dep_related;

z1 = log ((1 + &r1) / (1 - &r1)) / 2;
z2 = log ((1 + &r2) / (1 - &r2)) / 2;

rbar = (&r1 + &r2 ) / 2;
rbart = 1 - 2 * rbar * rbar;
rbart2 = 1 - rbar * rbar;

psi = &r12 * rbart - (rbart - &r12 * &r12) * rbar * rbar / 2;
sbar = psi / (rbart2 * rbart2);

zcal = (z1 - z2) / (sqrt(2) * sqrt (1-sbar)) / (sqrt (&c_sq
/ (&n - &b))) ;
pval = 2 * (1 - probnorm(abs(zcal)));

proc print data = dep_related;
   title 'Dependent Correlations with a Variable in Common';
   run;
```

4.16. There is no significant difference in the correlations between the two enzymes before and after the BMT ($z_0 = -1.67, p = 0.095$).

SAS code

```
%let r_xy = 0.66;
%let r_uv = 0.23;
%let r_xu = 0.48;
%let r_xv = 0.16;
```

```
%let r_yu = 0.11;
%let r_yv = 0.37;

%let n = 18;

%let b = 3;
%let c_sq = 1.06;

data dep_unrelated;

z1 = log ((1 + &r_xy) / (1 - &r_xy)) / 2;
z2 = log ((1 + &r_uv) / (1 - &r_uv)) / 2;

rbar = (&r_xy + &r_uv ) / 2;
rbar_yu = rbar*&r_yu;
rbar_xu = rbar*&r_xu;
rbar_xv = rbar*&r_xv;
rbar_yv = rbar*&r_yv;

psi = (1/2)*((&r_xu-rbar_yu)*(&r_yv-rbar_yu)+
  (&r_xv-rbar_xu)*(&r_yu-rbar_xu)+
  (&r_xu-rbar_xv)*(&r_yv-rbar_xv)+
  (&r_xv-rbar_yv)*(&r_yu-rbar_yv));

rbart2 = 1 - rbar * rbar;
sbar = psi / (rbart2 * rbart2);

z2cal = (z1 - z2) / (sqrt(2) * sqrt (1-sbar)) / (sqrt (&c_sq
/ (&n - &b)));
pval2 = 2 * (1 - probnorm(abs(z2cal)));

proc print data = dep_unrelated;
 title 'Dependent Correlations with No Variable in Common';
   run;
```

4.17. 86 CML and 86 CLL patients are needed to achieve 80% power to detect a difference in the microRNA correlations.

SAS code

```
%let rho_s_1 = 0.8762 ;
%let rho_s_2 = 0.7217;

%LET alpha =    .025;
%LET beta =     .20;
```

```
%let b = 3;
%let c_sq = 1.06;

data fisher_spearman_two_sample;
z_alpha = probit(1 - &alpha);
z_beta = probit(1 - &beta);
rho_s_1_z = 0.5*(log((1+&rho_s_1)/(1-&rho_s_1)));
rho_s_2_z = 0.5*(log((1+&rho_s_2)/(1-&rho_s_2)));
n = &b + 2*&c_sq*((z_alpha + z_beta) / (rho_s_1_z -
rho_s_2_z))**2;
if int(n) < n then n = int(n)+1;
run;

proc print data = fisher_spearman_two_sample;
TITLE 'SAMPLE SIZE CALCULATION';
title2 'Comparison of Two Independent Spearman Coefficients';
run;
```

4.18. When osteonectin is differentially expressed in ovarian versus omental tissue samples from women diagnosed with high-grade ovarian cancer, it is significantly more likely to be expressed in the ovarian sample than the omental sample ($S = 10.3$, $df = 1$, $p = 0.001$).

SAS Code

```
data Osteonectin;
input Ovarian $ Omental $ count;
cards;
+ + 39
+ - 32
- + 11
- - 124
;
run;

proc freq data=Osteonectin;
tables Ovarian*Omental / agree;
weight count;
run;
```

4.19. First the Shapiro–Wilk test is used to see if the BUN data of the other eight subjects are normally distributed. The null hypothesis of normality is not rejected ($W = 0.932$, $p = 0.538$) so, Grubbs' test can be used to determine whether or not the BUN level of subject 6 comes from the same normally distributed population as the other patients. Grubbs' test does not indicate that the BUN level of subject 6 is an outlier ($G = 1.63$, $p = 0.359$).

R code

```
# load 'outlier' package
# test normality
shapiro.test(c(11.3, 10.1, 13.0, 12.3, 10.5, 12.6, 12.8, 13.7))
# test for outlier
grubbs.test(c(11.3, 10.1, 13.0, 12.3, 10.5, 14.8, 12.6, 12.8, 13.7))
```

Chapter 5

5.1. For the data in the table, the value of Cohen's kappa is only 0.188 (95% CI: 0.089–0.287), even though the two methods agree on 60% of the specimens. These results indicate only slight agreement according to the Landis and Koch (1977) criteria for interpreting kappa. These data possess two of the characteristics that can lead to a distortion in the performance of kappa as a measure of agreement (see Section 5.2.1.1): (3) The value of kappa is affected by any discrepancy in the relative frequency of "disease" and "no disease" in the sample and (4) The value of kappa is affected by any discrepancy in the relative frequency of "disease" for Method A and the relative frequency of "disease" for Method B. For these data, the estimated relative frequency of lung cancer averaged over the two biomarkers is 28.9% (and hence the estimated average relative frequency of "no lung cancer" is 71.1%). The estimated relative frequency of lung cancer according to sputum cytology is only 9.0%, whereas it is 48.9% for immunocytochemistry. Thus, there is reason to believe that kappa is not providing an adequate measure of the agreement between the two biomarkers. However, using the PABAK coefficient provides little improvement over kappa: $PABAK = 2p_0 - 1 = 2(0.602) - 1 = 0.203$ (95% CI: 0.036–0.370), results that also indicate only slight agreement between the two biomarkers. The indices of positive and negative agreement are $p_{pos} = 2(12) / (12 + 65) = 0.312$ (95% CI: 0.177–0.446) and $p_{neg} = 2(68) / (121 + 68) = 0.720$ (95% CI: 0.647–0.792), respectively. Thus, the disagreement between the two methods can be attributed primarily to those specimens that are thought to be positive.

SAS code

```
options formchar="|-|+|-+|-/\><*";

*     Calculate coefficient kappa          ;

data ci;
input a b c d;
datalines;
```

```
12 0 53 68
;

data pos_pos;
set ci;
sputum = 1;
immuno = 1;
count =  a;
run;

data pos_neg;
set ci;
sputum = 1;
immuno = 0;
count =  b;
run;

data neg_pos;
set ci;
sputum = 0;
immuno = 1;
count =  c;
run;

data neg_neg;
set ci;
sputum = 0;
immuno = 0;
count =  d;
run;

data kappa;
set pos_pos pos_neg neg_pos neg_neg;
keep sputum immuno count;
run;

proc freq data=kappa order=data; weight count;
    tables sputum*immuno / nopercent nocol norow agree;
    title1 'Coefficient kappa';
    run;

data ci;
    set ci;
n = a+b+c+d;
p11 = a/n;
```

```
p12 = b/n;
p21 = c/n;
p22 = d/n;

/*p_pos calculation*/

o1 = 2/(2*p11+p12+p21)-4*p11/((2*p11+p12+p21)**2);
o2 = -2*p11/((2*p11+p12+p21)**2);
o3 = o2;
o4 = 0;
var_ppos = (1/n)*((o1**2)*(p11)+ (o2**2)*(p12)+
(o3**2)*(p21)+(o4**2)*(p22) ) -
((o1)*(p11)+ (o2)*(p12)+ (o3)*(p21)+(o4)*(p22))**2;
se_ppos = sqrt(var_ppos);
ppos = a/(((a+ b)+(a+c))/2);
u_ci_ppos = ppos+(1.96)*(se_ppos);
l_ci_ppos = ppos-(1.96)*(se_ppos);

/*p_neg calculation*/

y1 = 0;
y2 = (-2*p22)/(2*p22+p12+p21)**2;
y3 = y2;
y4 = 2/(2*p22+p12+p21)-((4*p22)/(2*p22+p12+p21)**2);

var_pneg = (1/n)*((y1**2)*(p11)+ (y2**2)*(p12)+
(y3**2)*(p21)+(y4**2)*(p22) ) -
((y1)*(p11)+ (y2)*(p12)+ (y3)*(p21)+(y4)*(p22))**2;
se_pneg = sqrt(var_pneg);
pneg=d/(((c+ d)+(b+ d))/2);
u_ci_pneg = pneg+(1.96)*(se_pneg);
l_ci_pneg = pneg-(1.96)*(se_pneg);

run;

data ci;
set ci;
n_positive = a+d;
n_negative = b+c;
run;

data positive;
set ci;
positive = 1;
count =  n_positive;
keep positive count;
```

```
run;
data negative;
set ci;
positive = 0;
count =  n_negative;
keep positive count;
run;

data crude;
set positive negative;
run;

proc freq data=crude;
     weight count;
     tables positive / binomial(level="1" p = .75) agree;
     exact binomial;
     output out = PABAK binomial;
     run;

data PABAK;
     set PABAK;
     crude = _BIN_;
     PABAK = 2*_BIN_-1;
     SE_PABAK = 2*E_BIN;
     LCL_PABAK_A = 2*L_BIN-1;
     UCL_PABAK_A = 2*U_BIN-1;
     LCL_PABAK_E = 2*XL_BIN-1;
     UCL_PABAK_E = 2*XU_BIN-1;
     keep crude PABAK SE_PABAK LCL_PABAK_A UCL_PABAK_A
     LCL_PABAK_E  UCL_PABAK_E;

proc print data = PABAK;
     var crude PABAK SE_PABAK LCL_PABAK_A UCL_PABAK_A
     LCL_PABAK_E UCL_PABAK_E;
     title1 'PABAK';
     run;

proc print data=ci;
     var ppos se_ppos l_ci_ppos u_ci_ppos pneg se_pneg
     l_ci_pneg u_ci_pneg ;
     title1 'Positive and Negative Agreement';
     run;
```

5.2. The “kappam.fleiss” function from the “irr” package can be used to compute Fleiss’ Kappa. For these data, $\kappa = 0.658$ indicates “substantial agreement” according to the interpretations given by Landis and Koch (1977).

R code

```
# read in the data
AmyB <- c("Normal", "Normal", "Normal", "Abnormal", "Abnormal", "Normal", "Normal", "Normal", "Normal", "Abnormal", "Normal", "Normal", "Normal", "Normal", "Normal", "Normal","Abnormal", "Normal", "Abnormal", "Abnormal", "Normal", "Abnormal", "Normal")
ApoE <- c("Normal", "Normal", "Normal", "Abnormal", "Abnormal", "Normal", "Normal", "Normal", "Normal", "Normal", "Normal", "Normal", "Normal", "Normal", "Normal", "Normal", "Abnormal", "Normal", "Abnormal", "Abnormal", "Normal", "Normal", "Normal")
MRI <- c("Normal", "Normal", "Abnormal", "Abnormal", "Abnormal", "Normal", "Abnormal", "Normal", "Normal", "Normal", "Normal", "Normal", "Normal", "Abnormal", "Normal", "Normal",
"Abnormal", "Normal", "Abnormal", "Abnormal", "Normal", "Abnormal", "Normal")
alz_biomarkers <- cbind(AmyB, ApoE, MRI)
# compute Fleiss' Kappa
install.packages("irr", dependencies=TRUE)
library(irr)
kappam.fleiss(alz_biomarkers)
```

R output:

```
Fleiss' Kappa for m Raters
Subjects = 23
Raters = 3
Kappa = 0.658
```

This indicates a "substantial" degree of agreement, according to the Landis and Koch criteria (Table 5.3).

5.3.

A. Sensitivity = 19 / (6 + 19) × 100% = 76.0%

B. Specificity = 39 / (2 + 39) × 100% = 95.1%

C. Positive Predictive Value = 19 / (19 + 2) × 100% = 90.5%

D. Negative Predictive Value = 39 / (6 + 39) × 100% = 86.7%

E. Accuracy = (19 + 39) / (19 + 2 + 6 + 39) = 87.9%

5.4. Part A)

κ = 0.318 for these data which indicates "fair" agreement according to the Landis and Koch criteria (Table 5.3).

SAS code

```
data interrater;
input rater1 $ rater2 $ count;
```

```
cards;
Y Y 43
Y N 38
N Y 29
N N 103
;
run;

proc freq data=interrater;
tables rater1*rater2;
weight count;
exact kappa;
run;
```

Part B)

$\kappa = 0.533$ for these data which indicates "moderate" agreement according to the Landis and Koch criteria (Table 5.3).

SAS code

```
data intrarater;
input time1 $ time2 $ count;
cards;
Y Y 54
Y N 27
N Y 19
N N 113
;
run;

proc freq data=intrarater;
tables time1*time2;
weight count;
exact kappa;
run;
```

INDEX

Analysis of Biomarker Data: A Practical Guide, First Edition. Stephen W. Looney and Joseph L. Hagan.